Speaking for Patients and Carers

Health Consumer Groups and the Policy Process

Rob Baggott

Judith Allsop

and

Kathryn Jones

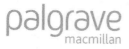

First published 2005 by
PALGRAVE MACMILLAN
Houndmills, Basingstoke, Hampshire RG21 6XS and
175 Fifth Avenue, New York, N.Y. 10010
Companies and representatives throughout the world

PALGRAVE MACMILLAN is the global academic imprint of the Palgrave Macmillan division of St. Martin's Press, LLC and of Palgrave Macmillan Ltd. Macmillan® is a registered trademark in the United States, United Kingdom and other countries. Palgrave is a registered trademark in the European Union and other countries.

ISBN 0–333–96828–X hardback
ISBN 0–333–96829–8 paperback

This book is printed on paper suitable for recycling and made from fully managed and sustained forest sources.

A catalogue record for this book is available from the British Library.

A catalog record for this book is available from the Library of Congress.

10   9   8   7   6   5   4   3   2   1
14   13 12 11 10 09 08 07 06 05

Printed in Great Britain by
Creative Print & Design (Wales), Ebbw Vale

Contents

Tables and figures

Tables

Figures

Foreword

Reading this book brought to mind many of the groups I have worked with in the health voluntary sector, locally and nationally, and their many achievements. I read it at a time when recovering from a long period of illness myself. Both hospital and community services gave me good treatment and support, but the experience was also a reminder of how patchy care can still be. It reminded me too how difficult it is, as an individual patient, to make one's voice heard. How important it is for organizations to speak for patients and carers.

In the late 1970s and 1980s, when I first worked with self-help groups, the situation for people facing serious illness was very different from that of today. I remember vividly many conversations that showed how deeply isolated people forming groups felt. Their main preoccupations were usually how best to give each other much needed mutual support, how to obtain better (or indeed any) information and how their organizations could provide some services. Deference to medical experts was the norm. Few people with serious illness then saw themselves as having the potential to challenge, or work alongside, government or powerful professionals, let alone the necessary courage, time and resources to do so. There was only slow growth in confidence that their knowledge as users of services was valid and could be useful in bringing about change. Today, in contrast, both individuals and their organizations are hugely more confident. The experience of people who use services and their carers has become central to how services are planned and delivered. As Rob Baggott, Judith Allsop and Kathryn Jones say, we have seen 'rising expectations and declining deference'.

This excellent study was undertaken with a great deal of support by the voluntary health organizations which formed the subjects of the research. It traces the historical development of advocacy by national health consumer bodies, describing the spurt in the second half of the 1990s, when doors swung open, and touching on the establishment of structures which now integrate patient involvement into the NHS. Why is it important to have done this research?

There are several key reasons, the first two spelt out by the authors. First, this study is significant because health consumer groups have become active policy advocates. Second, their activities are one way in which the democratic deficit in health care has been reduced. I'd add a third reason for the significance of this research: accountability. Substantial public and private resources have been given to the work of these organizations. Funders and donors should know what has resulted from their investment, who benefited and in what way.

One might see this book as a series of portraits in a gallery, showing different aspects of the world in which health consumer groups operate. The first portrait is a large overview, portraying many subjects. The other five are smaller, more detailed paintings, showing the variety of players, their behaviour and the minutiae of relationships between them. As one studies the portraits, one sees the interweaving of different connections and how challenging it is, for all involved, to get relationships right. While other useful studies have previously been published in this field, the De Montfort research is the most substantial and brings many fascinating perspectives to the subject.

I see three important strands running through this book: experiential knowledge, balancing acts, and collaboration. The first strand, experiential knowledge, or knowledge gained through experience of living with a condition or situation, underlies much advocacy work. Organizations have become much more confident about its significance and have learnt to use it as an effective tool in their work. Its importance has come to be appreciated by both politicians and civil servants.

The second important strand is coping with balancing acts. One interviewee described their job as 'walking on a tightrope'. Working with government, for instance, and perhaps even more with the pharmaceutical industry, involves some collaboration but also avoiding loss of identity and capture. As I learnt when Chief Executive of the Long-term Medical Conditions Alliance, as opportunities increase, this becomes a real challenge.

Collaboration between health consumer bodies forms the third strand. People outside the voluntary sector, when learning of the work of alliances, used to express surprise that very different organizations could want, and were able, to work effectively together. This study clarifies how organizations' shared values underpin joint work and lead to the formation of alliances. Both formal and informal alliances emerge as an effective way of influencing policy.

This is not a dry study but one which readers, from whatever constituency, can use to understand the complexities of the relationships they need to manage. A wide variety of readers will find it illuminating. Current advocates for change, especially those new to the field, will learn what works and what to avoid. They should be able to gain insight into how politicians and civil servants see their role. Government and professional bodies will understand more of the pressures on organizations, particularly those arising from limited resources, when offered a seat at the table. Politicians, civil servants and professionals should also be able to better understand the strong motivation of health consumer bodies, often driven by altruism, to bring about change. The pharmaceutical industry should read it too and might well consider how to develop guidelines for their work with patient organizations.

There were inevitably some omissions. One identified by the authors, arising through limitations on time, is the lack of interviews with individual pharmaceutical companies. I would have liked to learn more from them about their motivation for investing in liaison and support for the sector. There is also a scarcity of data about influence on primary care, probably because the research was undertaken at a time of transition. With the crucial importance of primary care trusts, this could well be an area for future research.

As the authors comment, one can never quite disentangle cause and effect. There are numerous and interrelated factors that affect the policy process. Baggott, Allsop and Jones conclude that health consumer bodies lack 'heavyweight', informal political contacts, contrasting them with the medical profession. There is however evidence of many changes which owe much to the work of health consumer bodies.

As I write, the White Paper *Building on the Best: Choice, Responsiveness and Equity in the NHS* (Cm 6079, 2003) has just been published. It was strongly influenced by patients, users and carers and their organizations. The White Paper confirms the need for continued development of the National Health Service as a service that listens to their views and responds to their needs. Health consumer groups have come a long way on their journey. This study makes an invaluable contribution to continued debate on their role and the challenges that will still face them.

JUDY WILSON, OBE

Acknowledgements

The Economic and Social Research Council (Grant Number R000237888) funded the research for this book and we are grateful for their support. We owe particular thanks to those people from the voluntary health sector who filled in the questionnaire, who agreed to be interviewed or who provided us with information about their organization. Our thanks also go to the politicians, civil servants, ministers, health professionals and other health care stakeholders who talked to us about their experience of working with health consumer groups.

We are indebted to Val Billingham, Christine Hogg, Simon Lawton-Smith, Phillip Lee, Stephen MacKenney, Barbara Meredith and Bruce Wood who were members of our project advisory group. They willingly shared their expertise with us and gave wise advice. We also wish to thank Judy Wilson, whose contribution to the health consumer movement is referred to at a number of points in the book, for agreeing to write the foreword; Professor Joe Collier of the Department of Pharmacology and Clinical Pharmacology at St George's Hospital Medical School for his comments on Chapter 8 and the two reviewers who suggested amendments to the draft manuscript.

A number of colleagues at De Montfort University provided advice and support and we appreciate their help. Pete Lowe and Professor Martyn Denscombe gave assistance with the questionnaire analysis. Dr Merrill Clarke, Professor Vivien Lowndes, Dr Lawrence Pratchett, Dr Lorraine Culley, Dr Simon Dyson and Professor Mark Johnson all contributed to the development of our ideas and advised on areas where they had a particular expertise.

Thanks to Dr Dwijen Rangnekar and Dr Mark Duckenfield at University College London, for permission to cite from their paper on *Drug Development and Patients Groups* in Chapter 8 and from Andy Brown editor of *PMLive.com*, for permission to quote from articles on *www.pmlive.com* also in Chapter 8.

Throughout the project, we relied heavily on the skills, good humour and patience of Katherine Hooper, the administrator of the Health Policy Research Unit, and her predecessor, Tracey Dodman. They gave us assistance through the various stages of the project and lightened our task considerably. Our editor at Palgrave Macmillan, Jon Reed, and his assistant, Magenta Lampson, have also given us support and encouragement throughout. However, the responsibility for the work remains ours.

ROB BAGGOTT
JUDITH ALLSOP
KATHRYN JONES

Abbreviations

ACHCEW	Association of Community Health Councils in England and Wales
ABPI	Association of the British Pharmaceutical Industry
AIMS	Association for Improvement in the Maternity Services
ARM	Association of Radical Midwives
BCPA	British Cardiac Patients Association
BLAR	British League Against Rheumatism
BMA	British Medical Association
CERT	Campaign for Effective and Rational Treatment
CHC	Community Health Council
CNA	Carers National Association
CPPIH	Commission for Patient and Public Involvement in Health
DoH	Department of Health
EDM	early day motion
GMC	General Medical Council
IDDT	Insulin Dependent Diabetes Trust
LMCA	Long-term Medical Conditions Alliance
MIND	National Association for Mental Health
MP	member of parliament
MS	multiple sclerosis
NCT	National Childbirth Trust
NHS	National Health Service
NHSE	National Health Service Executive
NICE	National Institute for Clinical Excellence
NCVO	National Council of Voluntary Associations
NRAS	National Rheumatoid Arthritis Society
NSAID	non-steroid anti-inflammatory drug
NSF	National Schizophrenia Fellowship
NSPCC	National Society for the Prevention of Cruelty to Children
ONS	Office for National Statistics

PCG	primary care group
PCT	primary care trust
PIN	Patients Involved in NICE
PQ	parliamentary question
RCOG	Royal College of Obstetricians and Gynaecologists
SANDS	Stillbirth and Neonatal Death Society
SANE	Schizophrenia A National Emergency
TAB	Transition Advisory Board
TAMBA	Twins and Multiple Births Association
TNF	Tumour Necrosis Factor
UKBCC	UK Breast Cancer Coalition
UKFSMA	UK Federation of Smaller Mental Health Agencies
VHO	voluntary health organization
WHO	World Health Organization

Introduction

This book is about the role of health consumer groups in the policy process at national level in the United Kingdom. It draws on research undertaken at De Montfort University between 1999 and 2003. That research, funded by the UK Economic and Social Research Council (ESRC),[1] aimed to investigate the characteristics of health consumer groups and their internal and external relationships, in particular how they worked with other interests in the health arena and with government. As well as including the findings of that study, called here the De Montfort study, the book aims to consider their implications for government policies related to patient and public involvement in health; the voluntary sector; the representation of interests in health care politics and the workings of the policy process.

The research context

The promotion and representation of health consumer interests is an important research topic. As a tax-funded, centralized and paternalistic service, the NHS has long been seen as having shortcomings by virtue of being a monopoly supplier, and as suffering from a 'democratic deficit' (Cooper *et al.*, 1995; Coulter, 2002). There have been few opportunities for those using health services or for the wider public to act as consumers or citizens. Consumer choice has been impeded by poor information, restrictions on direct access to services, and a failure to offer alternatives and options with regard to treatment. Moreover, systems of accountability have been weak, independent scrutiny of health services has been under-resourced and limited, and mechanisms for redress and complaint have been difficult to access (Wallace and Mulcahy, 1999; Allsop and Mulcahy, 2001). In terms of exercising democratic rights, user and carer involvement in decision-making has been slow to develop, leading to accusations of tokenism and professional or managerial control (Hogg and Williamson, 2001). Similarly, the advocacy role of health consumer groups has been limited despite their efforts to expose the shortcomings of services and their demands for greater accountability, openness, and responsiveness to user and carer perspectives.

The dominant theoretical paradigm in health care politics has attributed political supremacy to professional interests, particularly medicine (Alford, 1975). Although medical dominance has been challenged by government efforts to exert greater control over the cost and quality of health services, the scale and impact of this has been disputed (Johnson, 1995; Harrison, 1999). Indeed, consumer interests are still assumed to be weak relative to government, management and the medical profession, and consequently organizations representing these interests have been characterized as lacking influence over policy (Hogg, 1999; Wood, 2000; Salter, 2003).

However, over the last decade or so, a number of developments have challenged the assumption that health consumers and their representative organizations are weak and have little influence on the policy process. Since the early 1990s, governments have introduced policies that have, at least symbolically, championed the patient. For example, the *Patient's Charter* (DoH, 1991) set out what patients could expect from the health service and, more recently, the commitment to create 'patient-centred' services in the *NHS Plan* for England (Cm 4818, 2000) proposed a new statutory framework for patient and public involvement. It also appeared that health consumer groups – including patient associations, user groups and carers' organizations, had become more active as policy advocates for their particular client group, though this had not been investigated systematically. Previous studies tended to focus on the self-help role of groups, on specific conditions, or on activity at the local level (Trojan, 1989; Weeks *et al.*, 1996; Barnes *et al.*, 1999). In contrast, the De Monfort study aimed to investigate the activities of a range of groups across different condition areas and types of groups operating at the national level.

In the study, health consumer groups were seen as one of a number of interest groups in the health care arena. Such groups

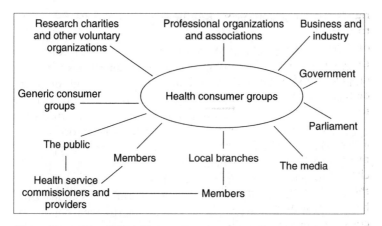

Figure 1.1   The policy arena of health consumer groups

develop relationships within, and outside, the health consumer group sector to promote and represent the interests of their constituents. Figure 1.1 illustrates how the policy arena within which health consumer groups operate was conceptualized by the research team.

A further reason for undertaking this research was the resurgence of interest in civil society and the contribution that voluntary associations, including those concerned with health issues, can make to social capital and to enhancing the democratic process. As voluntary forms of association, health consumer groups may generate particular social and political resources and may even, as Putnam (1995) suggests, contribute to good governance. Furthermore, according to Hirst (1994, 2002) associations can play a vital role in the rebuilding of democracy and the strengthening of welfare provision and public services. In addition to this, groups raise funds from the public and some receive grants from government. Researching the activities of health consumer groups provided an opportunity to explore these issues and furnish evidence about the contribution of the voluntary health sector to civil society. The research has been timely in that since 1997, Labour governments have been seeking to introduce policies that will allow a more open and productive relationship between government departments and voluntary sector organizations to develop (Cm 4100, 1998; Plowden, 2001).

Definitions: why 'health consumer group'?

For the purpose of the De Montfort study health consumer groups were defined as 'voluntary sector organizations that seek to promote and/or represent the interests of users and/or carers in the health arena ~~at national level~~'. This definition focused attention on those organizations that were primarily concerned with speaking for patients, users, and carers in the policy process.

The choice of the term 'health consumer' was based, in part, on a rejection of the term 'patient' on the grounds that many people represented by groups in the health sector either do not see themselves as being ill, or believe that 'patient' gives an inappropriate medical, and externally imposed label to their condition. For example, an expectant mother is not necessarily 'ill'. Similarly, many people who self-manage their long-term chronic conditions reject the notion of dependency that the term 'patient' implies.

The term 'service user' also presents problems. What about those who are not current users, but may become so in the future? What about people who are *former* service users, who are often members of groups and have strong views about services, rooted in their own experience? The term 'health consumer' is broad enough to incorporate all these people. It also embraces carers and relatives, as well as patients and users. Carers and relatives often act as service users, both directly and as 'proxy users' when caring for someone incapable of making certain choices and decisions for themselves.

On the other hand, it has been argued that to call those who use health services 'consumers' is misleading. The first objection is that the term is too closely associated with an individualized market model of health care. As Deakin and Wright (1990, p. 9) comment in the context of public services generally:

> The language of consumerism, with its focus on the position of individuals in a market-place of goods and services, has obvious limitations in relation to services which are essentially organized on the basis of collective provision for common needs and not as responses to individual consumer demands and power in the market.

Others have argued that the term 'consumer' defines service users too narrowly. In particular it has been criticized for reducing the role of service users to that of passive recipients rather than active participants (Potter, 1988; Long, 1999). From this perspective, the notion of 'health consumer' is alien to the concept of an active citizenry engaged in collective action to establish rights to services.

The term 'consumer' is regarded by some as particularly inappropriate to health care in the UK setting because, as noted earlier, there is limited choice, and because users of health care do not engage in the kind of consumerist behaviour found in commercial settings (Shackley and Ryan, 1994), even in the private health sector (Calnan, Cant and Gabe, 1993). The term may be particularly inappropriate to mental health, and other situations where treatment may be given without explicit consent for example, in certain accidents or emergencies. As Rogers and Pilgrim (2001, p. 112) have observed with regard to mental health:

> A consumer model can only retain coherence if the supply of a service is regulated by demand from those wishing to use that service. But many psychiatric patients do not ask for what they get: it is imposed upon them.

Similar arguments may also apply where individuals feel they have been damaged by treatment. Here the term 'victim' may be more appropriate, but this too is disliked by some groups. On the other hand, when people have completed a prolonged episode of effective care they may not wish to be identified as consumers or users but as 'survivors', a term used both in cancer and in mental health (Rogers and Pilgrim, 2001).

Against this, it can be argued that health consumerism is a reality. Health care, like other spheres of life, is increasingly commodified (Edwards, 2000; Henderson and Peterson, 2002). Furthermore, to see health consumerism as purely a commercial phenomenon, is, as Williamson (1992) has noted, a narrow and limiting perspective. It is far more useful to see consumerism in health care as representing a distinct interest. Individuals who use health services are becoming more assertive. They are more likely to obtain information from the internet and other sources; more willing to complain about poor service; have high expectations of what services they should receive and wish to exercise choice, particularly in terms of rapid access to services (Allsop and Mulcahy 2001; Kendall, 2001; de Lusignan 2003). They may also come together to defend existing services, to demand service improvements or to secure greater choice and greater accountability (Hugman, 1994). In short, it should be recognized that consumers are also citizens and may use 'voice' as well as 'choice' to articulate their views and preferences (Hirschmann, 1970). A further point is that the UK government has increasingly championed the notion of patient choice. This culminated in a key policy statement in late 2003 proposing new ways of extending patient choice in the NHS (Cm 6079, 2003).

One remaining problem with the term 'health consumer', is that users and carers also produce health care, through self-help, self-management, and caring for others (Stacey, 1976). While this is certainly the case, it is not a sufficient reason to discard the term. Indeed, it will be argued in the various chapters of the book that both individual health consumers and health consumer groups 'produce' important services and resources. Indeed, their role as service providers and producers of social and political resources is critical to their ability to speak for their client group and the wider public.

In summary, the authors accept that the term 'health consumer' is contested (Henderson and Peterson, 2002). In the sense that it is used in this book, it incorporates the notion that people may have rights as citizens in relation to health services, whether publicly or privately provided. They engage in collective action and may seek to influence the formation and implementation of public policy. Following Williamson (1992), the 'health consumer' is seen as an interest rather than a commercial entity, with health consumer groups seeking to promote and represent a broad constituency of patients, users and carers. Indeed, in countries such as Holland and Australia, where there is substantial state involvement in health care, 'health consumer' is widely accepted. In Holland, the Federation of Patient and Consumer Organizations is the main representative body for patients, while the key national patients' body in Australia is called the Consumers' Health Forum (Dekkers, 1997; Bastian, 1998).

The structure of the book

The De Montfort study aimed to describe the characteristics of a sample of health consumer groups in Britain in the period

1999–2001; to examine their internal dynamics; and to analyse how they engaged with each other, and other interests, in order to promote their concerns and represent the interests of health consumers within the health policy process at national level. This book reflects these aims and is structured in the following way.

In Chapter 1 the main concepts, theories and models used by the study are outlined. In Chapter 2 the recent development of government policy in two distinct but related areas affecting the operation of health consumer groups is explored: (1) patient and public participation in health and (2) policies relating to the voluntary sector. Chapter 3 discusses the policy context of the various condition areas in the study. Chapter 4 presents data on the characteristics of health consumer groups, their financial and human resources, and the similarities and differences between them; and Chapter 5 analyses their social and political resources. In Chapter 6 the networks and alliances that exist between groups are described along with the rationale for collaboration. Chapter 7 shows how health consumer groups engage with health professionals and their associations and presents data on how each views the other; and Chapter 8 discusses the links between health consumer groups and the pharmaceutical industry. The relationships between health consumer groups, government ministers and civil servants are explored in Chapter 9. In Chapter 10, the ways in which groups network with and lobby parliament are discussed, while in Chapter 11, the interface between health consumer groups and the media is analysed.

In Chapter 12 these findings are drawn together to assess the impact that groups have made on the policy process and to address the question of whether particular types of group or those that focus on particular conditions are more influential than others. This final chapter also sets out the contribution of the De Montfort study to theoretical debates about the policy process, while assessing its wider implications for the politics of consumer and citizen involvement in health.

Health care politics and the policy process: concepts, theories and models

In setting up the research, a 'multiple-lens' theoretical approach was used to aid understanding (Sabatier, 1999). The main theoretical starting points are outlined here, while other concepts and theories that help explain the behaviour of groups and institutions are introduced throughout the book where relevant. Three main areas of theory were used. First, the literature on structural interests in health care and social movements informed interpretation of the macro-political forces that shape health policies. Second, theories of policy networks and pressure group politics helped to focus on how interests operated within the institutional framework of the state. Third, normative theories of representative and participatory democracy suggested how groups could claim to speak for service users, carers and the wider public in decision-making.

Structural interests

Alford's model

In devising a model that proved influential in interpreting the health policy process in the UK, Alford (1975) identified three main structural interests in health care: 'the professional monopolizers', 'the corporate rationalizers' and 'the community interest'. He argued that as a consequence of legal and institutionalized control, professionals, and in particular the medical profession, constituted a dominant interest. There was wide acceptance by society, in government and within the health care system, of their status and knowledge, and the supremacy and indeterminacy of biomedical knowledge has shaped the understandings and preferences of others (North, 1995). The corporate rationalizers consisted of health planners and managers who were seeking to rationalize health care and improve efficiency. They were not without influence, but although they challenged the dominant interest, they could not master it. Meanwhile the community interest, which consisted of community groups, was repressed within the institutional structure and could only exert influence if they were able to mobilize 'extraordinary' political resources (Alford, 1975).

Alford's model was set in a US context and written over thirty years ago, but is still regarded as useful (North, 1995; Harrison, 1999). Although governments in the UK have become increasingly directive and managerialist in relation to the NHS (Paton, 1993; Klein, 1995; Appleby and Coote, 2002; Greener, 2003), the medical profession is far from supine and continues to exert considerable influence over policy and service delivery. This is reflected not only in terms of decision-making, but also in shaping the political agenda, and, in Lukes' terminology (1974, p. 24), the 'perceptions, cognitions and preferences' of others.

The research provided an opportunity to explore whether there has continued to be an institutional bias towards incorporating the medical profession as a dominant partner at the national level. As Chapter 9 will show, government has increasingly consulted with health consumer groups. This raises some interesting questions. Has this increased access equated with influence over policy? If so, has this enhanced role for health consumer groups been at the expense of other interests, such as the professions? Finally, where is 'influence' being exerted: over decisions, agendas, preferences, or in all these areas?

Health care consumers and new social movements

As suggested, there is evidence of rising expectations among individual health care consumers, who have become more critical of the biomedical model while demanding rapid access to good quality medical care. This has been matched in the realm of collective action, where there is a long tradition of voluntary groups seeking to influence policy and service provision through consumer advocacy. People have also taken action to provide each other with mutual support and to campaign for improved services. As Hogg (1999) has observed in relation to the UK, this began in some areas of care during the 1960s and 1970s, notably in maternity services with calls for a more 'woman-centred' approach to maternity. People with mental health problems and those with disabilities also have been active in campaigning for more responsive and appropriate services (Campbell and Oliver, 1996; Barnes *et al.*, 1999; Crossley, 1999; Beresford and Holden, 2000; Rogers and Pilgrim, 2001). Similarly, people with HIV/AIDS have demonstrated considerable capacity to provide both support and campaign (Weeks *et al.*, 1996). Groups have also been formed to protest about poor standards of health care, as in the events which led to the Bristol Inquiry[1] (Cole, 2001).

Collective action has been framed and explained in different ways. For example, the concept of a 'new social movement', has been used by both political scientists and sociologists to describe some areas of collective organization. According to Byrne (1997, p.11), 'new social movements...are amorphous entities which resist neat classification'. However, he goes on to note a number of features common to most new social movements: their adherents are motivated by expressive considerations. That is, they have fundamental values which they express in both political and 'non-political' arenas. Participation in a new social movement is also seen as an expression of identity rather than simply a reflection of self-interest or preference.

New social movements are not necessarily organized, although they may contain specific organizations. They are largely autonomous and have mass membership or mass support. They tend to pursue unconventional approaches to politics, such as protest and direct action, though this does not prevent them also employing more conventional tactics (Byrne, 1997). They often seek to mobilize marginalized communities or unconventional values and are in many cases 'rights-based', seeking to increase the rights of a marginalized section of the community, or to extend the rights of all citizens. Furthermore, new social movements pose a challenge to existing forms of knowledge, particularly those that dominate social and political processes. This is believed to be the case particularly with regard to new social movements which operate primarily at the symbolic level and which are embedded in adherents' sense of identity and within the networks of everyday life (Melucci, 1995; Martin, 2001).

Giddens (1991) saw such movements as facilitating deliberative democracy and in turn building trust as dominant forms of expert knowledge weaken. Habermas (1984, 1991) placed emphasis on the role of self-help groups in developing an experiential knowledge based on the 'life-world' of people's experiences, and the actions that could confront systems of expert knowledge (in this case, medicine) that have colonized it. He too argued that social movements are important in shaping identities and generating courses of action. In this way, they may impact on policy and service provision (White, 2000; Martin, 2001).

In this book, the concept of new social movements is relevant to our examination of the formation and internal dynamics of health consumer groups in Chapters 4, 5 and 6. In the final chapter, the question about whether, and in what sense, there is a 'health consumer movement' is considered.

Policy networks, pressure groups and institutional processes

The theories that enable us to comprehend societal and structural forces facilitate an understanding of the broader influences that shape the interaction between health consumer groups and the state. Important though they are, such macro-level theoretical frameworks are less helpful when trying to examine highly specific interactions within the policy process. It is at this level, where health consumer groups operate within the institutional framework of the state and the wider political system, that data has been scarce. The conventional wisdom has been that groups representing patients lack the capacity, and in some cases the will, to engage politically (Hogg, 1999; Wood, 2000). However, these conclusions were based largely on assumptions about the structural power of other interests and observations about groups' financial resources, their internal structures and their formal aims and objectives. There was little data on how the groups actually behaved within the policy process and how they interacted with other interests and with government. It was this gap that the De Montfort study sought to address, by examining their engagement in the national policy process; their strengths and weaknesses as policy actors; their contribution to policy-making; and their alliances and relationships with other health care interests.

This empirical focus raised important questions, such as: what representation did groups have on decision-making committees? How did they interact with government and other interests within these fora? What impact did health consumer groups have on the agendas and decisions of these bodies? How well-networked were health consumer groups with key decision-makers and opinion formers? Were some groups more closely involved than others in policy-making, and if so, why?

These questions raised theoretical issues of a different kind from those mentioned above. Two approaches in particular lend themselves to this analysis: policy networks and pressure group analysis. The policy networks approach focuses on the relationships between interest groups and government. Policy is influenced by the continuous interaction between groups, government departments and agencies within networks and at the same time reflects the status and power of the various interests (Rhodes, 1997). The process of interaction is 'two-way', with interest groups and government influencing each other. This reflects a general feature of modern governance identified by Kooiman (1993, pp. 250–1) that: 'interests are not "given" but are moulded – as are the structures of interest – in the process of governance itself'.

Policy networks

The literature on policy networks is extensive. The concept developed out of a growing interest in 'private interest government' or 'group sub-government' in the USA (McConnell, 1966; Lowi, 1969) and in Europe, the study of inter-organizational relations and corporatism (Hanf and Scharpf, 1978; Schmitter, 1979). Richardson and Jordan (1979) applied the concept to the British policy process, using the term 'policy community' to describe the relationships between government departments and interest groups through which the detail of policy was developed and implemented. Subsequently, Jordan (1981, p.105) clarified the terminology by reserving the term policy community for: 'that comparatively small circle of participants that a civil servant might define as being of relevance for any particular policy'. Later, Marsh and Rhodes (1992) identified two ideal types of network: 'policy communities', stable and highly integrated and interdependent communities of organizations and 'issue networks', a looser collection of organizations that exhibited instability and a small degree of interdependence.

There is disagreement among political scientists about the theoretical utility of a policy network. Some see it as a metaphor of the policy process or a way of thinking about interactions between government and groups (Dowding, 1995; Richardson, 2000). Others, notably Marsh and Rhodes (1992) and Smith (1993), view it as a theoretical device linking micro-level politics – specific interactions on policy – with broader theories of the state. For the latter, changes in the nature and composition of policy networks can bring changes in both the policy process and in policy outputs. Notwithstanding this debate, the policy networks approach is useful in focusing attention on relationships between groups and government and on the relative status of the players. One of the aims of the De Montfort study was to establish the status of health consumer groups within policy networks and to explore their relationships with other stakeholder interests and with government.

The study also reflected on other approaches that focus more specifically on the resources of groups within the policy process. Saward (1990), for example, identified six resources that could be held by groups co-opted by government as advisers or informants in decision-making. These were: non-positional authority, generated by the group's skills, competence, expertise or status; the group's size; its cohesiveness; its control of capital inputs; its control of labour inputs and the salience of its values, that is, the extent to which the group's values are supported by society. Saward hypothesized that co-option based on expertise, particularly when combined with cohesion, placed groups in a strong position within respect to government. A key factor is that expert groups are often in the position of assisting government with policy implementation, as well as providing and disseminating information and that consequently their participation can strengthen the legitimacy of a particular policy. Saward identified the medical profession as an example of a group which had comparative strengths in the provision of expertise (while maintaining sufficient cohesion, despite the potential for division). In contrast, groups representing consumers of health care were seen as lacking in cohesion and expertise and also did not have a broader public appeal. However, Saward noted that the weakness of such groups was not necessarily permanent. Their role in the policy process could become stronger and they could, as a result, exert more influence over policy.

While co-option is an important feature of access to the policy process, others have focused on the barriers that restrict access to policy fora and how these may be overcome. In a US setting, Baumgartner and Jones (1993) sought to explain how groups challenged existing ways of agenda setting and decision-making. According to these authors, institutional structures create participatory arrangements that include some groups and exclude others. Associated with these institutional arrangements are powerful 'buttressing ideas' connected to core political values. The net result is that 'policy monopolies' dominate and remain in place for long periods making it difficult for those with different views and values, who are excluded from this process, to influence policy. However, such monopolies may be challenged by previously excluded groups, who set new agendas and redefine problems. These challenging groups choose arenas where their resources, skills and expertise have greatest value. If successful, institutional changes lead to the incorporation of groups and their values within a new policy monopoly.

These various approaches to the policy process were helpful in highlighting ways in which groups, particularly those excluded from institutional arrangements, may begin to shape the structures and networks of policy-making. The importance of this approach also lies in its identification of factors and activities that may strengthen the position of challenging, or repressed interests, such as patients, users and carers.

Pressure groups

Finally, the literature on pressure groups gave insights into how health consumer groups might interact with policy-makers and opinion-formers. It suggested how and why groups adopt particular strategies and tactics and why some have greater status and credibility than others in the eyes of policy-makers. The literature also suggests why some groups may be more influential than others (Jordan and Richardson, 1987; Baggott, 1995). Furthermore, the 'typologies' adopted by pressure group analysts were used to inform the study design and data analysis (see Appendix 1).

Pressure group analysis is often based on classifications of groups, which are in turn based on features believed to affect policy influence. One of the best known is Grant's (1995) distinction between 'insider' and 'outsider' groups. Insider groups are regularly consulted by government and have most influence over policy, while outsider groups are less well connected with (and in some cases excluded from) government. Grant developed this simple model further by identifying other sub-categories. He noted that some insiders are relatively weak, being dependent on government, while others, 'high profile insiders' are strengthened by adopting broader strategies aimed at generating public support. Meanwhile, other insiders are 'low profile', relying on their good links with the executive to maintain influence over policy. Outsiders are also divided into three categories: 'outsiders by necessity' have nothing to offer government and lack influence. 'Ideological outsiders' do not wish to be tainted by involvement with government. However 'potential insiders', the third category, are able to build a relationship with government and may become insiders in the future. Grant's model is therefore dynamic and makes us consider factors that may lead to the inclusion of previously excluded groups into the executive decision-making process.

Grant's typology has been both praised and criticized for its simplicity. One of the main criticisms has been that the insider/outsider dichotomy conflates strategy and status; another is that access should not be equated with influence (Maloney, Jordan and McLaughlin, 1994). To remedy some of the shortcomings of Grant's typology, Whiteley and Winyard (1987) in their study of the poverty lobby suggest a four-dimensional classification system based on the following:

1. Groups either pursue an 'open strategy' (lobbying a range of political actors and institutions) or a 'focused strategy' (concentrating mainly on the executive or government institutions).
2. Groups are either 'promotional' (speak on behalf of a group of people) or 'representational' (are comprised of, and speak for, a group of people).
3. Groups are either 'accepted' by government or are 'not accepted'.
4. Groups are classified as either 'lobbying' (their primary purpose is to lobby policy-makers) or 'service providers' (their main purpose is to provide services for a particular client group).

Although groups fell into several categories based on various combinations of these characteristics, two profiles predominated: OPAL (Open, Promotional, Accepted and Lobbying) and FRAS (Focused, Representative, Accepted, Service Provider). The OPAL profile was more common among groups formed in the 1960s and 1970s and these were identified by Whiteley and Winyard as the most effective. More specifically with regard to strategy, they observed that groups with a high media profile, who did not concentrate their efforts on Whitehall (and to some degree parliament), tended to be the most influential.

Meanwhile, Maloney, Jordan and McLaughlin (1994) also sought to clarify the distinction between insider/outsider *status* and insider/outsider *strategy*. 'Strategy' is to a degree determined by the group (though other constraints, such as group resources and the structure of government, are regarded as important). 'Status' is conferred by government, though group characteristics (notably their resources) will have an influence over how they are regarded. Bearing this in mind, Maloney, Jordan and McLaughlin identified three types of insider. 'Core insiders' are seen by the executive as important sources across the range of a broad policy area. 'Specialist insiders' are highly regarded within smaller and more detailed policy arenas, while 'peripheral insiders' have limited access to the consultation process and have marginal influence over policy. They went on to identify two types of outsider: 'outsiders by ideology' (whose goals are ideologically incompatible with those of the government) and 'outsiders by choice' (which do not wish to become ensnared in the processes of government). For these researchers, the key question is not why some groups are outsiders and others insiders; but rather, why some groups are more highly regarded by policy-makers and what determines core as opposed to peripheral insider status. They argue that research should focus on 'making distinctions about the influence of groups once they have met the minimal requirements for insider status' (Maloney, Jordan and McLaughlin, 1994, p. 37), an issue which the De Montfort study sought to pursue.

The various theories and models discussed above were used to structure the analysis of the De Montfort study, particularly with regard to discussions about status and strategy in Chapters 9, 10 and 11. They raised important questions about the nature of relationships between groups and government, groups' strategies and tactics and the resources they could bring to bear in the policy process. They also raised the possibility of linking these factors to policy influence.

Democratic theory, representation and participation

In the introduction to this book, it was stated that one of the longstanding problems of the NHS has been a democratic deficit. Indeed, this criticism has been levelled more generally at contemporary government and is linked to concerns about the decline in participation in civil society and the consequences for governance (Putnam, 2000). The extent to which a democratic deficit persists is a broad question which this study can only partially address. Nonetheless, the effectiveness of health consumer groups in representing their constituency and their involvement in national level decision-making sheds some light on the current state of democracy, representation and participation in the NHS.

The case made by participatory theorists is that if ordinary citizens engage actively in politics, the quality of democracy will improve (Pateman, 1970; Macpherson, 1973; Barber, 1984). These writers reacted against the conventional view that political representation and the task of governing were matters for elites, subject only to indirect democratic control. This led to greater interest in ways in which individuals might become engaged more actively in political debate and decision-making. In particular there are those who endorse discursive or deliberative democracy (Dryzek, 1987) as an approach to addressing social problems, political institutions and policy issues. This involves replacing instrumental rationality (selecting effective means to clearly-defined ends) with discursive rationality (where free collective discourse produces mutual understanding through argument and persuasion). This perspective endorses those institutions that extend public participation and which incorporate 'discursive designs' to encourage communicative rationality among all interested parties. It also links democracy with the rise of the new social movements discussed earlier, seeing them as contributors to the establishment of free discourse and confronting established authority.

Meanwhile, others have focused on devising practical forms of group representation to improve democracy. While acknowledging that groups vary in power and resources, it has been argued that changes can be made to political processes that provide equality between participants or at least 'a level playing field' (Mansbridge, 1992; Cohen and Rogers, 1995). However, Schmitter (2001) sees such participatory forms of governance as a method for dealing with a broad range of problems and conflicts, using negotiation and bargaining to produce mutually satisfactory and binding decisions. He sees organizations, represented by particular persons, as 'holding' the interests of particular constituencies and as accountable to them. He sets out a number of principles for this to operate successfully, including: decisions based on consensus; participants' acceptance of the 'rules of the game'; the openness of participants to argument, and their nominal equality. Schmitter takes a positive view of the role of organizations in promoting good governance. Such forms of governance can be introduced by governments themselves, or be built from below, by the democratization and decentralization of institutions and the encouragement of voluntary self-governing associations (Hirst, 1994, 2002).

However, questions have been raised about the extent of internal democracy in voluntary associations. Critics suggest that internal divisions, a lack of internal participation and a tendency towards elite decision-making, leads to a misrepresentation of interests (Baggott, 1995; Waldegrave *et al.*, 1996). More specifically it is possible for leaders to set their own agenda and subvert the expressed interests of the rank and file (Jensen and Froestad, 1988). In addition, as Cigler and Loomis (1995) argue, powerful interests can create the illusion of public support, which they term 'astroturf', in contrast to genuine grassroots support.

Against this, it can be argued that groups representing service users and consumers are actively developing internal participatory practices. For example, Campbell and Oliver (1996) noted that organizations representing disabled people were becoming more democratic and accountable, giving increased scope for participation. It is also possible for groups to develop participatory skills and experience, as Barnes *et al.*, (1999) observed in their study of user groups and community care:

> Participation provides experience of the potential of collective action for social change as well as a forum in which personal experiences can be theorized and new knowledge developed. User

groups contribute to action within civil society through which both welfare and government can be democratized. (Barnes *et al.*, 1999, p.101)

The findings from the De Montfort study provide the opportunity to investigate these issues. Groups may have the potential to play an important role in promoting democratic participation. But they can also undermine it, if they distort preferences, misrepresent views, or reinforce existing elite domination. These issues are explored further in Chapters 4 and 5 and elsewhere in the book and are returned to in the concluding chapter, where the contribution of health consumer groups to a more responsive and inclusive form of policy-making is assessed.

Research design and methods

The research was undertaken in four phases. In late 1999, a semi-structured postal questionnaire survey was undertaken, which achieved an effective response rate of 66 per cent (n=123). The questionnaire, which posed questions about the activities of groups and their interaction with government and other stake-holders, was sent out to health consumer groups in five condition areas: namely, arthritis and related conditions; cancer; heart and circulatory disease (focusing on heart disease and stroke); maternity and childbirth; and mental health. Together these conditions are responsible for a large proportion of morbidity, mortality and health service expenditure in the UK. This selection also reflected the need to cover as diverse a range of user and carer experiences as possible, including life-threatening illness, long-term chronic conditions and life-changing events (see Chapter 3). In addition, mental health was included to ensure that the focus was not wholly on physical conditions. The aim was to include conditions that were currently high on government's list of stated priorities (cancer, heart disease and stroke, mental health) and others (arthritis, maternity/childbirth) that were not. It should be noted that by limiting the study to these condition areas, the activities of some significant health consumer groups, such as the Multiple Sclerosis Society and the Parkinson's Disease Society, were not included in this study.

The sample also included groups concerned with a number of conditions; such as those with a general interest in patient/carer welfare (such as the Patients Association) or with the specific interests of population groups, such as elderly people or children (for example, Age Concern or Action for Sick Children). Another category was 'umbrella' groups, whose membership included other national groups, such as the Genetic Interest Group and the Long-term Medical Conditions Alliance.

The focus of the research was on groups promoting or representing health service user/carer interests, and to retain this we excluded research charities and professional associations. Other organizations excluded were: general consumer organizations (as they had a much broader remit than health) and disability organizations (which had already been extensively researched). Local and regional groups and statutory organizations (such as the now defunct Community Health Councils in England) were excluded too, as were organizations whose sole function was to provide a help or advice line (as they did not seek a significant role in the policy process). However, some professional groups, general consumer organizations, research charities and statutory health consumer bodies were interviewed in the third phase of the research in their capacity as policy actors representing key interests.

In the second phase of the research, which took place in 2000, semi-structured interviews were undertaken with key informants from 39 health consumer groups[2]. These groups were selected to ensure a mix of characteristics such as size, condition area, date of formation and type of group. The interview sample was chosen to reflect the features of the Whiteley and Winyard (1987) classification of pressure groups, mentioned above. The third phase, undertaken in 2000/01, consisted of semi-structured interviews with 31 key policy actors (civil servants, MPs and individuals from professional associations, research charities, the pharmaceutical sector and general consumer groups). The aim of the second and third phases was to develop a theory of the internal and external relationships of health consumer groups in the policy process grounded in their own accounts. A final round of interviews, undertaken in 2002/03, with former ministers and other key participants and observers was used to test initial interpretations. Details of the interviews undertaken are provided in Appendix 2.

It should be noted that during the course of the research a number of the interviewed groups changed their name, for example the National Schizophrenia Fellowship was renamed Rethink (Severe Mental Illness) in 2002. In this study the original name of the group is used, although the name changes are referenced in Appendix 2. Further details of the methods and analysis are given in Appendix 1.

Categorizing health consumer groups and data analysis

On the basis of the questionnaire analysis, a typology of groups was developed, which will be referred to throughout the book:

Condition-based groups – representing people with particular conditions (such as cancer or heart disease).

Population-based groups – groups representing all patients, carers or a specific population sub-group within the health arena at national level, such as carers, elderly people, children or people from ethnic minorities.

Formal alliance organizations – national groups whose membership includes other autonomous national organizations.

The rationale behind this classification was that it allowed comparisons to be made between types of group as well as between condition areas.

Interpretation: assessing influence and impact

The main purpose of the De Montfort study was to understand the role and influence of health consumer groups in the national policy process. However, assessing the influence of any interest group presents problems because of numerous and interrelated factors that affect the policy process (Baggott, 1995; Grant, 2000). Indeed during the course of the research, interviewees from health consumer groups acknowledged that success in policy terms depended greatly on others outside the organization. It is not possible to disentangle the influence of health consumer groups from others. This difficulty is compounded by the level of secrecy surrounding both the policy process and the role of various actors (Whiteley and Winyard, 1987).

Another problem is that groups may be unsuccessful in influencing policy in the short term, yet may secure important policy changes in the long run. Any judgement about their influence will therefore depend on when an assessment is made. Moreover, influence on one issue may be part of a much bigger game. As Grant (2000) suggests, it is sometimes difficult to determine what government priorities really are and government may purposefully give way on some issues in the short term to gain on others in the long term. A further point is that much of the literature on policy influence is focused around questions of access and influence over central government. However, political contacts with the media and Parliament can also shape the political agenda and policy-making and must not be ignored.

The research explored health consumer group influence over other health policy stakeholders, including politicians, civil servants and professionals, and their impact over policy. The assessment of influence in the De Montfort study was based on both subjective and objective measures. The questionnaire data revealed details about frequency of contact with other policy actors. These variables were used to establish characteristics of different groups, along the lines of the Whiteley and Winyard (1987) typology described earlier, and an assessment of how these characteristics related to policy success was undertaken. In interview, group respondents were asked to identify instances where they believed they had influenced, and had difficulty influencing, policy and these areas were explored in greater detail. Civil servants and other stakeholders were also asked to identify where they believed groups had influenced policy. Documentary evidence was also used to identify examples of influence, enabling 'self-reported influence' to be corroborated by other data.

Conclusion

As noted in the Introduction, health consumer groups had been relatively neglected as a research topic. Previous research had not focused upon some key aspects, in particular the role of health consumer groups within the policy process at national level. This book aims to fill these gaps by exploring the internal dynamics of groups, their social and political resources, their relationships with other policy actors and with each other. It also explores the relationships between groups and government, parliament and the media. It does so within a clear conceptual framework outlined in this Chapter. However, before analysing these aspects in depth, we outline the policy context within which these groups have operated.

The policy context

The role of health consumer groups cannot be understood without reference to broader 'policy streams' (Kingdon, 1995) in health and welfare policy. Ideas about improving patient and public involvement, and extending the role of the voluntary sector in policy-making and provision, are particularly relevant. These have been associated with policy developments that appear, on balance, to have strengthened the legitimacy of health consumer groups and created opportunities for them to engage in policy networks and to influence policy. This chapter examines the impact of these policies on the broad relationship between government and health consumer groups. Data have been drawn from several sources: government policy documents, studies of the voluntary sector and interviews undertaken as part of the De Montfort study.

Patient and public involvement

Government policies on patient and public involvement have been part of wider efforts to improve health services and make them more responsive to the needs of patients, users and carers. They have also been related to initiatives to strengthen consumerism and citizen engagement within the public sector. The *Citizen's Charter*, introduced by the Conservative government under John Major, focused on entitlements and what individuals could expect from public services (Cm 1599, 1991; Connolly, McKeown and Milligan-Byrne, 1994; Wilson, 1996). The reasoning was that if people could not exit from a publicly-provided service, or directly exercise choice, then these services should be monitored against explicit performance standards. In addition it was argued that there should be clear information about entitlements and improved systems for voicing concerns and obtaining redress. In a parallel development the introduction of the *Patient's Charter* set out a range of rights, expectations and standards for the NHS (DoH, 1991). However, these mechanisms were criticized for providing levers for managers rather than empowering health service users (Harrison *et al.*, 1992).

The *Citizen's Charter* was superseded by an approach which retained elements of the consumer ethos, while placing greater emphasis on consulting with the public and service users, and involving them more extensively in the process of service improvement (Cabinet Office, 1998; Office of Public Services Reform, 2002). This shift engendered greater interest across government in obtaining the views of organizations claiming to represent the public and service users. At the time of the De Montfort study, a section of the Cabinet Office had a remit to promote good practice in user involvement across government departments. Its role was sustained through research, surveys, policy documents, inter-departmental seminars and by working through designated departmental 'consumer champions'. The Treasury also had an interest in user perspectives across government, having a cross-departmental brief through its Public Services Directorate to monitor the activities of individual departments and major spending programmes. It was primarily concerned with measuring the input of resources against outcomes, to meet the objectives and targets set out in performance agreements. In connection with this, service users were seen as having a legitimate role to play in giving feedback on the effectiveness of services and public expenditure.

In interviews undertaken by the De Montfort study, both the Cabinet Office and Treasury respondents endorsed the role of voluntary organizations and health consumer groups in representing service users in policy-making. While this acknowledgement created a favourable climate, it was clear that neither the Treasury nor the Cabinet Office could compel departments to engage with groups, nor would they necessarily seek to do this. At the time of the research, it was left to each individual department to determine their own particular arrangements.

The 'democratic deficit' in the NHS

Turning more specifically to health policy, developments in the 1990s reflected a long-standing concern about the perceived democratic deficit in the NHS. The importance of representing health service users, other than through the lay membership of NHS boards, was first recognized by health ministers in the late 1960s. In 1974, Community Health Councils (CHCs) were introduced in each local area to represent the interests of local people. CHCs had a statutory right to be consulted on substantial service changes and provided a source of advice and information for local people (Klein and Lewis, 1976). Many had also developed roles in relation to advocacy, campaigning and providing support for people wishing to complain.

During the 1980s under Conservative governments, both health service reorganization and the introduction of general management were used to drive change in the NHS (Social Services Committee, 1983). Patients were thus reconceptualized as customers. As Milewa *et al.* (1998) suggested, the vocabulary of the policy documents stressed managers' accountability for improving the 'quality' and 'responsiveness' of services, as seen by patients. However, despite the rhetoric, as Harrison *et al.* (1992) found, the real policy driver in this period remained cost-containment. This primary objective was also enshrined in the 1990 reforms, which although headlined as *Working for Patients* (Cm 555, 1989), in fact focused on creating competitive pressures to constrain costs and improve service quality by introducing an internal market. In principle, purchasers with fixed resources contracted with local providers to deliver services, though in practice the market was highly regulated and competition was limited (Le Grand, Mays and Mulligan, 1998). Genuflexion towards greater public involvement was subsequently made through an injunction to purchasers in *Local Voices* (NHS Management Executive, 1992) to consult with local communities in reaching purchasing decisions. In the following year, the Health Secretary called on health authorities to seek public participation when establishing priorities and later asked for details about how they were achieving this. Research, however, shows that there were considerable barriers to achieving participation at the local level (Allsop and Taket, 2003).

Although various mechanisms to involve local communities were suggested, these were not systematically developed, tested or evaluated and, perhaps most important of all, resources were not targeted towards this objective. CHCs, who might have contributed more to this process, were put in a difficult position.

Their boundaries did not always coincide with those of purchasers, they were under-resourced and lacked expertise. They also feared that their role as consumer watchdogs could be compromised by contributing to the purchasing process (Cooper *et al.*, 1995).

In summary, during the 1980s and early 1990s, policy initiatives introduced to engage health care users were high on rhetoric, but ultimately achieved little because they contravened the political realities of the health care system. In addition, there was little evidence about the efficacy of various approaches to patient and public involvement. Techniques to operationalize these policies were also underdeveloped. This is not surprising, as Jenkins-Smith and Sabatier (1993) have argued, since policy changes of this order take decades to accomplish. Nevertheless, the 1990 reforms were a watershed in the relationship between the dominant medical profession and the state (Klein, 1995; Salter, 1996). The largely informal 'negotiated order' on which health service policies were based began to be replaced by a different approach, where explicit aims and objectives were imposed by government, where managers sought a greater role in determining local priorities and where performance was more closely audited and monitored. This process continued to develop under New Labour with reforms of clinical standards and governance (Walshe, 2003).

The response of health consumer groups to the Conservative reforms

Although the impact on user involvement in the NHS was initially limited, the Conservatives' reform plans had an unintended effect on health consumer groups. *Working for Patients* (Cm 555, 1989), mentioned earlier, and its 'sister' White Paper *Caring for People* (Cm 849, 1989), which set out policies for community care, were turning-points for many groups concerned with health and welfare. The White Papers proposed major policy shifts, the consequences of which were uncertain. For voluntary groups providing health and social care services, there was the prospect of a more competitive environment of contracts with new and poorly understood procedures. Within groups, leaders feared adverse consequences for their particular constituency. Added to these concerns, as the reform process got underway, group leaders were asked to respond to a tide of consultation documents from government. Interviews undertaken for the De Montfort research show that groups were expected to produce measured responses within a tight timetable – a task which drew heavily on their scarce resources, but to which they felt bound to respond. One strategy developed for dealing with these pressures was to seek allies. This led to a strengthening of informal networks between health consumer groups, coalitions with professionals, and in some instances, the formation of new alliance organizations, such as the Carers Alliance UK, the Patients Forum and the Long-term Medical Conditions Alliance (LMCA).

The Carers Alliance UK

Around 1990, a number of groups with interests in carer support began to meet as the Carers Alliance UK, co-ordinated by the Carers National Association (now Carers UK). These included the Residents and Relatives Association, Contact a Family, Crossroads and the Alzheimer's Disease Society (now the Alzheimer's Society) as well as Age Concern, the Royal National Institute for the Blind and Macmillan Cancer Relief. Meeting formally two or three times a year, their common agenda was to campaign, not only for a specific cause, but for the whole constituency of carers. The group continued to meet through the 1990s and in particular, lobbied collectively on specific legislation.

In the view of one interviewee in the De Montfort study, this grouping was the basis for a 'carers' movement' and succeeded in making 'a private trouble into a public issue' (Interview, si24, see p. 306). Following the 1990 NHS and Community Care Act, a Private Member's Bill reached the statute book as the 1995 Carers (Recognition and Services) Act. Jill (now Baroness) Pitkeathley and Francine Bates, both at that time of the Carers National Association, were acknowledged in Hansard as prime movers behind the Bill (Hansard, 1995a). Other health consumer groups, such as the Alzheimer's Disease Society, Contact a Family and Scope were also recognized for their contribution to the debate (Hansard, 1995b). One interviewee commented that the role of carer was acknowledged for the first time in the Act and that significant resources for carers, through additional carers' allowances and grants were generated as a result (si12). There was, of course, parliamentary support for these developments, notably from Malcolm Wicks, MP, who successfully piloted the Bill through the House of Commons.

The Patients Forum

The initial base of the Patients Forum was the Patients Association, which formed in 1963. In later years it had been led by Dame Elizabeth Ackroyd, assisted by two part-time staff. Dame Elizabeth was a former senior civil servant. She became a leading member of a number of voluntary bodies and was very much an establishment figure with good Whitehall connections. In 1988 Linda Lamont, who had been active in CHC work, took over the administration of the Association.

The proposed health service reforms generated a major increase in requests to the Patients Association for media interviews and for responses to various consultation documents. Within a small central staff, the demands became increasingly difficult to meet. One way of coping was to draw on existing networks with other consumer stakeholders, including leading members of other organizations such as the Association of Community Health Councils of England and Wales (ACHCEW, the national body for CHCs), the Consumers' Association, the National Consumer Council and the College of Health. At the same time, attempts were made to meet with the medical establishment, which was also concerned about the implications of the reforms.

The idea for a national network that would act as a link between patients' groups developed from these meetings. Consequently, the Patients Forum was established in April 1989. The aim was to share information on policy and pool information on those willing to speak for the patient on various bodies and at conferences and seminars. The Patients Forum continued to meet on a regular bi-monthly basis, organized by the Patients Association, with around 26 full members. In 1996, the Patients Forum became a freestanding organization with a constitution, a steering group and a chairperson drawn from member organizations on a rotating basis. There was full membership for patients' organizations and associate membership for professional and other groups. The aim was to facilitate communication between organizations and provide information on policy changes. Subsequently, the Patients Forum became a vehicle for improvements in co-ordination between health consumer groups at national level. In 1998/99 it became very active in seeking to amend certain clauses in the 1999 Health Bill (see Chapter 10). In 1999, the Forum received a grant from the Department of Health to develop its role as a national co-ordinating body for health consumers and to help create a framework for more effective representation at national (and regional) level for patients' and carers' interests.

The Long-term Medical Conditions Alliance (LMCA)

The 1989 White Paper *Working for Patients* (Cm 555, 1989) also caused concern among health consumer groups associated with chronic illness, such as the British Diabetic Association (now Diabetes UK) and Arthritis Care, as patients with chronic illnesses would be viewed as 'expensive' in the internal market, due to the long-term costs of treatment. As Jean Gaffin, the then Chief Executive of Arthritis Care commented:

> Many of us had a concern that the patient/doctor relationship would change with the internal market as the cost of treating a patient could enter the doctor's mind when deciding on that treatment. Patients with chronic illnesses might become undesirable. (Quoted in LMCA, 1999a, p.1)

Informal meetings began to take place and in 1992 the LMCA was launched, funded by the groups themselves. The following year the National Council for Voluntary Organizations (NCVO) provided funding, and staff seconded from the Department of Health, provided the basis for organizational development (LMCA, 1999a). In 1995, additional resources were provided by a range of bodies, including the Department of Health, NHS Executive (NHSE) (formerly the NHS Management Executive), the King's Fund and six health authorities, to fund the LMCA's action research project, *Patients Influencing Purchasers*. A project officer was appointed to find a model for health authorities to work with patients to commission quality health services for people with long-term conditions within the NHS internal market (Lewthwaite and Haffenden, 1997). In 1996, with further funding and a membership of 60 organizations, the LMCA appointed its first chief officer.

These new organizations later became heavily engaged in calling for improvements in patient and carer representation in the NHS. Initially however, this was not their main concern, as they were preoccupied with responding to the government's NHS reform agenda. Nonetheless, partly in response to government initiatives to persuade health authorities to take into account public views in the commissioning process, a national strategy for patient and public involvement began to take shape.

The development of a public and patient involvement strategy

In response to specific demands from ministers and from the NHS for clearer guidance, policy officers within the NHSE began to develop a strategy for patient and public involvement. The NHSE had been established as the headquarters of the NHS in the late 1980s and at this time, as Day and Klein (1997) point out, there were important differences in the culture of the health service managers working within the NHSE and career civil servants working for the wider Department of Health.[1] The former had 'hands-on' experience of the NHS and 'street credibility' whereas the latter emphasized the traditional 'Whitehall' values shaped by the requirements of working for ministers. Compared with the career civil servants, those with a health service management background were more willing to take risks, were outcome-rather than process-oriented, focused on individual rather than collegial values and emphasized verbal rather than written skills. This distinction is useful for interpreting the approach of the health service managers during this period as they attempted to build coalitions and develop policies for user involvement in the policy that became known as the Patient Partnership Strategy (NHSE, 1996).

The Patient Partnership Strategy

During the early 1990s, the NHSE had responsibility for monitoring policy on the *Patient's Charter*, CHCs and complaints. Within the NHSE the key section was the Quality and Consumer Branch, established in the early 1990s. This branch was responsible for developing and implementing policies where there was a strong consumer or patient interest. It also had a brief to co-ordinate activity on consumer and public involvement by working with other parts of the NHSE. Later, responsibility for developing policies in this area was given to one of the NHSE board members, Barbara Stocking.

In the De Montfort study interviewees from both health consumer groups and from those working in the NHSE at the time commented on the Patient Partnership Strategy. These accounts, although from different perspectives, concurred with each other. In their view, policy development had been encouraged by several factors, not least the recognition by senior personnel in the NHSE that the health service must become more responsive to users and patients. Ministers, though sympathetic to moves to push the NHS in this direction, were not the main drivers of policy development, as one civil servant noted:

> I think it's fair to say that it did emerge as much as a managerial initiative within the NHS Executive rather than something that was a Ministerial imperative or 'must do' in those sorts of terms. (Interview si19)

A major impetus for the Patient Partnership Strategy was the difficulty encountered with the implementation of the 1992 *Local Voices* initiative (NHS Management Executive, 1992). Intended to encourage health authorities to involve local communities in planning, its mechanisms remained under-developed. By 1994, the NHSE saw that a broader strategy for 'partnership' with patients was needed and this was reflected in the 1995/96 *Priorities and Planning Guidance for the NHS* (NHSE, 1994).

In April 1995 a workshop on patient partnership, 'But Will it Work Doctor?' was held at Warwick University. The workshop was attended by representatives from the health service, the professions, and user and carer groups. It was, according to one interviewee, 'really the genesis of the Patient Partnership Strategy' (si29) and was followed by the setting of a medium-term objective in the 1996/97 *Priorities and Planning Guidance for the NHS* to:

> Give greater voice and influence to the users of NHS services and their carers in their own care, the development and definition of standards set for NHS services locally and the development of NHS policy both locally and nationally. (NHSE, 1995, p. 5)

Resources, though limited, were allocated to policy development in this field and staff were appointed within the NHSE specifically for this purpose. In 1996, *Patient Partnership: Building a Collaborative Strategy* (NHSE, 1996) was published to provide a framework for further development at various levels of provision from doctor/patient interaction, through local level bodies, to the national level. It outlined four aims for patient involvement: to promote user involvement in their own care; to encourage informed choice; to make the health service more responsive to the needs and preferences of users and to support the effective involvement of users. The strategy emphasized the importance of professionals and patients working together and identified areas where additional work was required to deliver the aims. These included the production and dissemination of information for health service users and representatives; the creation of structures, organization and resources for skill development and support for users and staff associated with the programme; support for all staff in achieving an active partnership with users, and research and evaluation of these new processes.

A Patient Partnership Steering Group, to which a number of user and carer representatives were appointed, helped draw up the document. The group remained in place for a short while afterwards to monitor progress, before being replaced by a Patient Partnership Overview Group. This latter body, which met two or three times a year, included representatives from the NHS, professional bodies, user and carers, and NHSE staff. In addition, each NHS region appointed a lead to take the patient partnership agenda forward. Specific activity at national level included the launch of the Centre for Health Information Quality and several conferences to publicize the strategy. Funding of over £250 000 was provided for three years with a staff member appointed to develop and co-ordinate activity.

Those interviewed from both the NHSE and health consumer groups said that from 1995 to 1999 policies evolved slowly, as NHSE officials attempted to build bridges between different interests and involve leaders in the medical and other professions, ACHCEW, general consumer bodies and specific health consumer groups. Those interviewed from the NHSE said they were taken by surprise by the extent of collaboration between groups in the sector and were also keen to support alliances. According to one senior official: 'We really needed to have some umbrella groups that could...be seen to represent other groups' (si16). Dunning, Needham and Weston (1997) also comment that particular groups, such as the Patients Forum and ACHCEW and, subsequently the LMCA, were seen by the NHSE as particularly useful in embedding the strategy.

However, the NHSE's concern to develop a strategy did not always square with what individual health consumer groups wanted. Some interests were highly specific and groups preferred to pursue detailed issues that were more closely related to members' immediate and pressing concerns (for example, regulations about the provision of wheelchairs). Consequently, such groups were less interested in strategic matters relating to public and patient involvement. However, groups that did take an interest were often critical of the Department's approach. They told civil servants that the 'good practice' being developed by the NHSE was at odds with their experience of dealing with government and that civil servants were seen as relatively inaccessible and difficult to work with.

A further barrier to participation was a shortage of people suitable, willing and able to act as health consumer representatives at national level. There was no list of potential candidates for these positions and the result was multiple committee membership by the few who had become in effect 'professional consumers' or in the terminology used by some interviewees, the 'usual suspects'. According to one of the civil servants interviewed:

> [This] was so ridiculous because we had got…this big user movement, some very good people there, really quite experienced people. We weren't drawing on the range of them at all actually within the Department. (si16)

Nonetheless, as a consequence of working with the health consumer groups, further policies did develop. For example, an initiative was launched within the Department of Health called Practice What We Preach. The presumption was that users should be involved in the work of the Department unless there was a very good reason for not doing so. This policy was, in the parlance of the time, 'cascaded down' through different sections of the Department. A lead was given by the then chief executive of the NHS, Alan Langlands, who met formally with leading health consumer groups two or three times a year.

However, support from ministers was variable. Civil servants mentioned in interview that they were sometimes unsure about ministerial support for engaging with health consumer groups. As one senior civil servant put it: 'Some ministers are very keen to talk to user groups, very happy to talk to them, and some of them don't want to touch them with a barge pole' (si16). This added to the atmosphere of uncertainty and created hesitancy in some departmental sections. In others, it reinforced civil servants' fears and reluctance to work with groups.

Even where civil servants had no such reservations, interaction was required to develop mutual understanding. Some groups were seen as not appreciating the 'rules of engagement'. Civil servants gave examples of where this had resulted in meetings that focused on the 'wrong' issues and were therefore less than productive. They assumed that groups were adequately resourced and were surprised to learn how limited resources sometimes were, thus failing to acknowledge the burdens of the consultation process. As one interviewee commented:

when we did suddenly start involving them, it put a heck of a burden on them. Because they just didn't have the capacity. After years of asking to be involved they obviously had no idea of what it would mean for their organization to suddenly have this huge bureaucratic machine latching onto [them]. (si29)

At the time, NHSE officials were also attempting to build informal networks with health service managers, the medical profession and health consumer groups. Their view was that there had been little change at the level of the doctor–patient relationship, which remained paternalistic despite support from leading figures in the medical establishment for change (Irvine, 2003).

By the time that the Labour government came to office in 1997, a policy with several strands had emerged. First, within the NHS, health authorities were expected to have in place local policies to involve patients, users and carers. Second, the Department of Health had begun to be more proactive in engaging with health consumer groups and was involving them more in policy discussions and consultations. Third, it was recognized that these groups could represent the interests of patients, users and carers at local and national level, but that they needed support in order to perform this role. Overall, the strategies adopted in the mid-1990s were not led from the top-down but developed laterally across organizational boundaries (Colebatch, 1998).

Patient and public involvement policies under the Labour Government 1997–99

The strategy to encourage greater partnership with service users was carried forward by the incoming Labour government in 1997. However, it was 're-badged' (as one civil servant interviewee put it) by pushing forward the concept of user involvement across all NHS services and activities. It was also renamed as the Patient and Public Involvement Initiative. The 1997 White Paper *The New NHS: Modern, Dependable* (Cm 3807, p.11) set out six key principles, one of which was 'to rebuild public confidence in the NHS as a public service, accountable to patients, open to the public and shaped by their views'. Health authorities were charged with involving the public in service planning and priority setting, the new primary care groups were expected to develop arrangements for public involvement. There was also a greater emphasis on measuring levels of satisfaction with services, including a new national survey of patient and user experience.

In 1998, the NHSE published a document, along with the Institute of Health Services Management and the NHS Confederation, entitled *In the Public Interest*, which offered advice and guidance on good practice in consultation. This publication provided clear support for consulting with voluntary organizations, including user and carer groups. In the context of local level consultation it was suggested that:

Together these groups offer the NHS enormous experience and expertise; about how diseases and conditions are actually experienced; about how treatments and services are actually received, and what the real priorities and issues of concern are for health service users and their families. Incorporating these groups into decision making has major benefits for the service in terms of meeting real instead of perceived need, targeting and focusing on areas of neglected need, and monitoring quality and performance. (NHSE/IHSM/NHS Confederation, 1998, p.10)

This document noted the drawbacks of direct involvement by such organizations, including the difficulties faced by smaller, less well-organized groups in getting their voices heard and the tendency of most groups to be dominated by white middle-class people. The report also recommended additional resources for weaker groups and those representing ethnic minorities.

At the national level, other opportunities arose for health consumer groups to engage with government and other stakeholders. Health consumer groups sat alongside the professions as members of the advisory groups, set up to develop national standards and plans (known as national service frameworks) for key condition areas and client groups. They were also represented on various consultative and advisory bodies under the aegis of the National Institute for Clinical Excellence (NICE), a new organization established to review the cost-effectiveness of treatments to be funded by the NHS. The Commission for Health Improvement – introduced to monitor health service standards and oversee the implementation of the new system of clinical governance – also drew on the expertise of members of health consumer groups.[2] Finally, as Chapter 9 will show in more detail, health consumer groups became more closely engaged in discussions about policy across a range of issues within the Department of Health.

Despite civil servants' fears and uncertainties about ministerial support, there was some reassurance when the Labour government allocated important health portfolios to individuals with previous experience of the voluntary sector or health consumer groups. For example, Baroness Jay, health minister in the House of Lords was founder director of the National AIDS Trust and had been involved with other voluntary health organizations. She took an active part in promoting the Labour government's plans for patient involvement. This support continued when Baroness Hayman, who had also been previously active in the voluntary sector, took over Baroness Jay's role in 1998. The public health minister in this period, Tessa Jowell was also supportive of closer links with health consumer groups, having formerly served as assistant director of MIND (the National Association for Mental Health).

The new strategy for patient involvement
Eventually, in 1999, the Labour government produced its own strategy – *Patient and Public Involvement in the New NHS*

(DoH, 1999a). This emphasized that public and patient involvement should not be an 'add on' task but integrated in the work of NHS organizations. It called for action in several areas. NHS trusts and particularly, primary care trusts, were urged to incorporate patient and public involvement and make special efforts to engage with minorities and socially-excluded people. Patient and public involvement was identified as part of clinical governance, and was to be led by a senior person, and assessed through the review process (DoH, 1999b). In addition, skills in patient communication and partnership were to be built into peer reviews, appraisals, proposed revalidation schemes and clinical education and training. Finally, NHS organizations were expected to provide resources and support for patient and public involvement, including administrative support, training and expenses, as well as fees where individuals or groups were involved as consultants.

This document was regarded by health consumer groups as a statement of good practice, but not in any way radical. The document said little about the role of groups in policy-making at the national level. Its action points focused mainly on promoting research, information and training. The need for additional resources to facilitate a policy role for groups was not addressed. Some of the groups interviewed commented that momentum had been lost, and few believed that the revised strategy had much impact on their activities.

In some respects, the strategy was overtaken by events: in particular the bed shortages, cancellations and waiting list problems in the NHS that resurfaced in the winter of 1999/2000, and the Bristol Royal Infirmary Inquiry referred to above. Following widespread public and media criticism about a lack of resources, a full-scale review led to the *NHS Plan: A Plan for Investment, A Plan for Reform* (Cm 4818, 2000), which contained new proposals for patient and public involvement. This was reinforced by the Bristol Inquiry report (Bristol Inquiry, 2001, p. 438), which argued for a more accountable, patient-centred NHS where patients must be regarded 'as equals with different expertise'.

Meanwhile, another agenda was being quietly pursued, which also emphasized the importance of a patient-centred service. The *Expert Patients Programme* announced in September 2001, aimed to give people suffering from long-term medical conditions a greater say and control of their own treatment. Groups such as Arthritis Care and the Manic Depression Fellowship were at the forefront of developing the self-management programmes which would enable people living with chronic illness to have a greater say in their treatment.

The NHS Plan and the new statutory framework for patient and public involvement

The *NHS Plan* (Cm 4818, 2000) arose out of a perception of crisis. In an attempt to identify possible ideas for reform, the government appointed six committees known as Modernisation Action Teams. Appointees were drawn from NHS management, the health care professions, and the voluntary sector, including health consumer groups. The latter included individuals from the Alzheimer's Disease Society, the Carers National Association, the College of Health, Diabetes UK, LMCA, Patients Forum, and the Stroke Association. Civil servants from the Department of Health and the Treasury were also involved, and all but one of the committees were chaired by a health minister (the other – on prevention and inequalities – was chaired by the Chief Medical Officer). Each Modernisation Action Team explored a particular area of policy: Partnership (in the health and social care system); Performance and Productivity; Professions and the wider NHS workforce; Patient Care (empowerment); Patient Care (speed of access) and Prevention and Inequalities.

The discussions on patient empowerment fed into the proposed new statutory framework for public and patient involvement contained in Chapter 10 of the *NHS Plan*. New advisory forums at local level were proposed to enable the public to have a voice in determining health priorities and policies. Patient forums in each NHS trust and primary care trust were to represent patients and the public at local level, Patient Advocacy and Liaison Services (later renamed Patient *Advice* and Liaison Services – PALS) were to deal with patient queries and concerns, and new powers were to be given to local councils to scrutinize health services. Controversially, the *NHS Plan* also proposed the abolition of CHCs. In addition, a commitment was made to increasing lay and citizen involvement in professional and regulatory bodies and on key government bodies, including the new Modernisation Board, established to oversee the implementation of the *NHS Plan*, which drew a third of its membership from citizen and patient representatives.

Eventually, and after much controversial debate, new legislation emerged. In particular there was strong resistance to the government's plans to abolish CHCs. These bodies lobbied the Department of Health to alter the proposals and secured support from the media, backbench MPs and many health consumer groups. As a result important changes were later secured to the detail of the legislation, notably additional roles for those Patient Forums in primary care trusts.

A new statutory duty was introduced in the Health and Social Care Act of 2001 on Strategic Health Authorities (StHAs), primary care trusts and NHS trusts to involve and consult health service users and the public in service planning and changes to services. Later, the NHS Reform and Health Care Professions Act (2002) paved the way for the abolition of CHCs in England,[3] and ACH-CEW. This legislation also enabled the creation of patient forums in every trust and primary care trust. These bodies, later renamed Patient and Public Involvement Forums, operated under the auspices of a new national organisation, the Commission for Patient and Public Involvement in Health (CPPIH). This statutory body was given a wide range of functions, including: advising health ministers about arrangements for public involvement and consultation regarding the health service; advising on the provision of Independent Complaint and Advocacy Services, representing the views of the local level forums and voluntary organizations, providing staff for the forums, and advice and assistance to other forums; facilitating the co-ordination of their activities; advising and assisting providers of complaint and advice services; setting and monitoring quality standards on complaint and advocacy for the local level bodies; reporting on issues relating to the safety or welfare of patients to regulatory bodies, raising matters from the various annual reports, and promoting public involvement in health service decision-making.

The statutory functions of the CPPIH specified a role in representing the views, not only of patient forums, but of 'those voluntary organizations and other bodies appearing to the Commission to represent the interests of patients of the health service in England and their carers'.[4] While this did not guarantee a role for health consumer groups, it placed some responsibility on the new organization to work with them. In this regard, the process of appointment of the commissioners of the CPPIH became an important consideration. An earlier scoping exercise recommended a membership organization with some drawn from the voluntary sector, including by implication, health consumer groups (Hogg and Graham, 2001). Subsequently, a Transition Advisory Board (TAB), established to advise the Department of Health, recommended that innovative ways of selecting Commissioners should be considered at a later stage, including the election of a proportion of Commissioners (TAB, 2002a). This raised the possibility that members of health consumer groups and other voluntary organizations might secure appointments to the Commission. To begin with, however, Commissioners were appointed by ministers on the recommendations of the NHS Appointments Commission. Of the ten initially appointed, five had previous health consumer group experience, although the Commissioners were appointed as individuals in their own right. The Transition Advisory Board produced two reports (TAB, 2002a, 2002b). These recommended that the CPPIH should work closely with national voluntary organizations, especially in its policy development role and when advising on how to target 'hard to reach' groups. It also suggested a reference group, including patient and carer group representatives, to act as a sounding board for policy (TAB, 2002a). At the time of writing, the new system of patient and public involvement in the NHS is in the implementation phase.

Further changes also occurred in the Department of Health with regard to patient and public involvement. In 2001, the Department was restructured to clarify responsibilities in this area.[5] In addition, it committed itself to systematic patient, user and public involvement in policy development and implementation. Subsequently, a Director ('czar') of Patient Experience and Public Involvement was appointed. The first post-holder, Harry Cayton, was previously director of the Alzheimer's Disease Society. One of the key tasks of this post is to facilitate links between the Department of Health and voluntary groups in the health sector and to bring the user and carer perspective to decision-making at senior level within the Department. One of his key tasks was to facilitate the consultation process on patient choice, which led to the introduction of the policy document, *Building on the Best: Choice, Responsiveness and Equity in the NHS* (Cm 6079, 2003), based on extensive consultation with health consumer groups.

Policy developments in the wider voluntary sector

Health consumer groups are part of the voluntary sector and are subject to the constraints of regulation and the dynamics of policy in this sphere. Over the last few decades the voluntary sector has grown in size and significance, due partly to changes in the welfare state and broader debates about the role of the state (Passey, Hems and Jas, 2000). From the early 1980s, Conservative governments introduced policies to reduce direct state service provision through statutory agencies. The ideological impetus was to secure reductions in state expenditures and devolve responsibility through a more competitive mixed economy of welfare. State agencies could contract with voluntary agencies to provide services allegedly bringing gains in both efficiency and effectiveness by linking the voluntary ethos with market testing and quality management (Waine, 1992). This also promoted the notion of an 'enabling state' which would fund and oversee the delivery of services provided by other agencies (Osborne and Gabler, 1992).

These developments provided opportunities for voluntary organizations, promising a greater role in service provision and additional resources to expand their activities. However, constraints were also imposed. Government clearly saw the need to tie resources to government priorities (Home Office, 1990), which was seen as an attempt to alter the priorities of voluntary organizations and limit their ability to innovate. It also created a new 'contract culture' under which organizations had to either broaden or expand their activities to ensure funding (Lewis, 1999). Others pointed out how greater dependence on government for resources could have adverse implications for the voluntary sector's campaigning activities and in particular its role as an independent critic of policy (Taylor, 1999).

The funding and regulation of the voluntary sector

The voluntary sector faces a complex system of funding and regulation. Within central government, several departments provide funding and give support to the voluntary organizations that operate within their area of activity. For example, 'Section 64' grants given by the Department of Health provide a funding source for many health consumer groups.

The operation of the voluntary sector is also affected by charity law, even though not all organizations are registered as charities. In England and Wales, the charitable sector is regulated by the Charity Commission, a non-governmental organization that reports to parliament. Charities are registered by the Commission and thus qualify for tax advantages, but are also bound by its rules. These include restrictions on activities such as fundraising or campaigning and additional administrative requirements, such as financial audit. The Charity Commission has responsibility for ensuring that charity trustees operate within the law. To this end, it offers guidance, information and advice; maintains a register and monitors the annual report and accounts that must be produced under the Charities Act 1993. It investigates complaints and also gives advice on good practice (Charity Commission, 2001). This dual role was referred to by the Deakin Commission on the voluntary sector (Commission on the Future of the Voluntary Sector, 1996, p. 33) as being both 'policeman and friend'.

A closer relationship?

In the mid-1990s the Deakin Commission's report, *The Future of the Voluntary Sector in England* (Commission on the Future of the Voluntary Sector, 1996, p. 21) extolled the benefits of an independent third sector as social critic and innovator. It argued that the independence of the voluntary sector could be compromised and recommended clear rules of engagement between the state and the sector in the form of a concordat. This idea was rejected by the then Conservative government. However, the Labour Party supported the proposal (Michael, 1997) and once in office, began to promote the voluntary sector with a series of key policy initiatives (Kendall, 2000).

The Labour government encouraged partnership between national and local government agencies and the voluntary, not-for-profit sector in tackling poverty and social exclusion. This provided the basis of a number of new programmes such as: Sure Start, New Deal, Education Action Zones, Health Action Zones and Healthy Living Centres. In addition, the government initiate a review of charity taxation and relabelled and strengthened the unit responsible for the voluntary sector, the Active Community Unit, which was relocated to the Home Office. Voluntary sector liaison officers were also placed in other Departments. This was an attempt to 'join-up' activity in this area, a reflection that other key departments, including the Cabinet Office, the Treasury, the Department for Education and Skills, the Department of Culture, Media and Sport and the Department of Health, had major links with the voluntary sector.

In 1998, separate compacts on the relations between the state and the voluntary and community sector in England, Scotland, Wales and Northern Ireland were drawn up, their individual style and content reflecting differences in approach between the various countries within the UK. The compacts emphasized the importance of both large and small, local and national voluntary organizations in contributing to a more democratic, socially inclusive society. They explicitly linked the voluntary, not-for-profit sector to policies for increasing public participation and the wider government agenda on strengthening civil society. The compacts were not legally binding but set out 'shared principles'. For example, the English Compact (Cm 4100, 1998) included statements about the importance of partnership and accountability and set out a range of principles, including integrity, objectivity, openness, honesty and leadership. The English Compact also included undertakings by government to: recognize and support the voluntary sectors' independence; consult it; support its infrastructure; and respect the confidentiality of information it provided.

For its part, the voluntary sector undertook to use its infra-structure to encourage participation in government consultations, agreeing: to co-operate with each other through intermediary bodies and networks to streamline the consultation process; to define and demonstrate how they represented their stated con-stituency by stating clearly who they were, what groups or causes in society they represented and how they involved these interests in forming their policies and positions; and, when responding to the consultation itself, to give their constituency feedback on the outcome of consultation and, wherever possible, consult their constituency directly, including service users, volunteers, members and supporters.

The Compact promised codes of practice on funding and consultation, which were published in 2000 (Active Community Unit, 2000a, 2000b). The latter contained several undertakings, including to involve the sector in consultations at an early stage, be sensitive towards the additional resource implications of involvement in consultations, and provide feedback on consultation. These codes were followed by others, including one on ethnic minority groups and another on volunteering (Active Community Unit, 2001a, 2001b).

Morison (2000) placed the development of the Compact at the heart of the 'Third Way' agenda to strengthen institutions between the market and the state. He suggested (p. 131) that a common language and explicit criteria have emerged and argued that, for government, the compact is a means of 'influencing, allying with, and co-opting the voluntary sector as a resource that they do not directly control' and that for the sector, their contribution and independence is acknowledged. Indeed, a Treasury report (HM Treasury, The Public Inquiry Unit, 2002) supported the argument put forward by Billis and Glennerster (1998), in relation to the social welfare sector, that voluntary organizations had a comparative advantage in terms of service supply given their specialist knowledge and skills; could involve users in service delivery and/or promote self-help and could be more innovative and flexible. This gave 'added value' which was augmented by their ability to use volunteers. On the basis of this, the report supported building the organizational and technical infrastructure; the community capacity of voluntary organizations and proposed additional funding to develop relationships between the sector and government.

Divided responsibilities within central government

At central government level there are overlapping roles between Departments and a coherent strategy has yet to emerge. Within Whitehall, the Home Office's Active Community Unit has responsibility for overseeing guidelines and developing capacity. However, Plowden (2001, p. 11) has commented on the lack of an overall strategy from the Home Office, despite an increase in the numbers of staff and resources, saying that the Active Community

Unit has: 'plainly proved incapable of enforcing any kind of consistency in the multifarious relationships between different parts of Whitehall and the voluntary and community sector'. From 1997, devolution brought further complications with increasing divergence between the governance structures in the separate countries of the UK.

The impact on health consumer groups

It would appear that voluntary sector organizations are now considered as stakeholders in a policy process. While funding may be used to further broaden policy objectives within particular departments, there is some negotiation on policy priorities and the policy agenda through both consultation and the representation of user interests. Policy continues to evolve. Indeed, a Charities' Bill to clarify the terms of engagement in relation to the status and funding of charities has been proposed for the 2004 legislative programme.

Despite the relevance of voluntary sector policies, the De Montfort study found little direct evidence that health consumer groups had so far benefited from these wider voluntary sector policy initiatives. Although the Compact was introduced before the fieldwork for this study was undertaken, few of the groups referred to it. One interviewee did note that ministers expected civil servants to have consulted with the voluntary sector but this may not have been directly the result of the Compact. This lack of awareness may have been because the Compact was at an early stage of implementation. Or perhaps it was not seen as directly relevant to health consumer groups as their links were chiefly through the Department of Health, which had already adopted its own ways of working with voluntary organizations. Indeed, as one senior advisor to the Department of Health on patient and public involvement put it, the Compact did not make 'one jot of difference' to the voluntary health sector (si12). Osborne and McLaughlin (2002) have suggested that the Department of Health initially took little interest in the Compact, though it has been recently revived and the Department now recommends following the Compact's guidance and is promoting the formation of local compacts (DoH, 2002a).

Conclusion

In summary, the two policy streams discussed in this chapter are relevant to understanding the expanding role of health consumer groups in the policy-making process – the first directly, the second indirectly. Health consumer groups, and particularly the formal alliances, were eager to gain access to policy-makers and their influence. Government increasingly recognized the need to include them as it sought to develop its reforms, and later its modernization agenda in the NHS, and acknowledged their role as representatives of patients, users and the wider public interest. This built on earlier linkages made horizontally between policy actors in the NHSE and health consumer groups, rather than being established from above. During the same period, it should be noted that similar relationships were being developed between health consumer groups and medical organizations (see Chapter 7).

Interviews with senior civil servants indicated that by the late 1990s there was an awareness of the barriers to building a different policy process that included health consumers. These included a lack of capacity; the problem of 'consultation fatigue'; the recognition of a dilemma for organizations that wanted to participate but lacked resources to do so; an absence of a clear leadership structure within the sector and the possibility of a split between insider groups who were consulted and outsider groups who were not.

The problem of who should represent the health consumer was also emerging. Several different categories were mentioned: people who were current service users; those who had personal experience of services and also considerable experience of the policy process, and 'proxy' consumers – those who ran organizations specializing in information provision, developing good practice in consumer involvement or providing services for particular groups. As will become clear in later chapters, this was an area of varied practice where, in the absence of a clear set of rules or policy, it was recognized that a 'broad church' principle should be adopted. Alternatively, personal politics could drive who was or was not seen as a 'legitimate' representative. The entry of these groups was, nonetheless, based on specific claims about legitimacy and representation. The strength of these claims depended on internal arrangements within groups. Chapters 4, 5 and 6 explore this in greater depth. Before doing so, however, further context is needed. The next chapter sets the scene for the various condition areas inhabited by the groups in the De Montfort study.

3 The condition areas

As noted in Chapter 1, the De Montfort study aimed to explore the differences between groups in five condition areas: arthritis and related conditions, cancer, heart and circulatory disease (focusing on heart disease and stroke), maternity and childbirth, and mental health. This approach was based on a hypothesis that the activities of these groups might be shaped by factors specific to each condition area. The conditions were chosen because they had different impact on the population; had different priority status within government policy; varied in their media and public profile and were embedded to a greater or lesser extent in the medical model. This provided a basis for comparison and enabled the study to assess two issues. First, whether groups in popular and/or priority areas were more or less influential and second, whether groups acted differently in areas where the medical model was strong or weak; where illness was mental or physical; or where health problems were long-term or short-term.

In addition, this approach explicitly acknowledged the possibility of micro-political environments affecting group activities and policy outcomes. Each condition area had a particular configuration of groups and other stakeholders, including government. They could be seen as a distinct policy 'sub-network', each of which might harbour a particular pattern of policy-related activities, a distinct approach to political alliances and specific policy outcomes.

As a prelude to the analysis, this chapter explores the characteristics of each condition area in order to establish the similarities and differences between them. It also provides some important background information about each condition that will assist the reader in later chapters.

Arthritis and related conditions

Arthritis covers a wide range of musculoskeletal conditions (approximately 200) including rheumatism. There are four main types: inflammatory arthritis (inflammation of joints or tendons); osteoarthritis (wearing away of the joints); soft tissue rheumatism; and juvenile chronic arthritis. The last condition aside, arthritis disproportionately affects older people – around half of arthritis sufferers are over 65. But perhaps more importantly, it is widely perceived and portrayed as a condition of old age. Estimates of the extent of arthritis and related conditions vary, largely because there is no agreed national system for monitoring musculoskeletal health (in contrast to cancer and heart disease), reflecting its low status within medicine and health policy. Nonetheless, arthritis is a widespread health problem and one that is likely to increase with an ageing population and rising obesity rates. According to self-reported health surveys, around 16 per cent of the adult population have experience of musculoskeletal conditions (ONS, 2000a). In the UK, eight million adults (just under a fifth of the adult population) visit their general practitioner every year for arthritis or a related condition.

The impact on individuals and society

The cost of arthritis-related conditions is high.[1] In 1999, prescriptions for musculoskeletal and joint diseases cost the NHS £341 million. A further £405 million was spent on hip replacements. The total cost to health and social services was estimated at £5.5 billion. After mental health disorders, arthritis is the second most common reason for taking time off work and 206 million working days were lost as a result in 1999/2000 (at a cost of £18 billion). Half of all people with rheumatism and arthritis stop working within five years of diagnosis. Arthritis-related conditions are major causes of pain and disability, and substantially affect quality of life. Indeed, many arthritis sufferers are in constant pain. People with arthritis also face increased living costs (Hansard, 1999). Arthritis can increase mortality risk through vulnerability to infections and some conditions such as rheumatoid arthritis are linked to a shorter life expectancy (Ashcroft, 1999). However, it is rarely mentioned as a cause of death: in 2000 only 3242 deaths in the UK were so attributed, less than 1 per cent of the total.

Key policies and issues

The key issues in the arthritis field are: self-management; access to new treatments and therapies, and service standards and entitlements. All have drawn health consumer groups more closely into the policy process. Self-management is based on an increasing recognition by professionals, users and government that people with long-term medical conditions have a vital role to play in managing their own health. In 1997, the Department of Health funded a self-management pilot project in England *Challenging Arthritis*. Promoted by the organization Arthritis Care, the programme was user-led and training in self-management was delivered by volunteers. In the following year, the Department of Health, along with GlaxoWellcome (now GlaxoSmithKline) and The King's Fund, funded the Long-term Medical Conditions Alliance's Lill Project to increase knowledge and share expertise on the potential of self-management. In 1999, in recognition of lay expertise in chronic illness, an Expert Patients Taskforce was established to 'look at the role which those affected can themselves play as experts in managing their chronic disease' (Cm 4386, 1999, p. 39). A number of health consumer groups, including Arthritis Care, were represented on the taskforce, which reported in 2001 (DoH, 2001a), leading to the *Expert Patients Programme* (see Chapter 2).

Most treatment programmes for arthritis-related conditions alleviate symptoms rather than provide a cure. Drug regimes are of secondary importance in treating osteoarthritis. Instead, life-style changes such as weight loss and exercise are recommended and, ultimately, surgery. (Youngson, 1998, p. 22). For inflammatory arthritis, however, drugs are central to the management of the condition, and access to treatment has been a major issue. In recent years, new drug regimes have been developed and it has been claimed that these reduce the side affects of traditional treatments. COX-2 specific inhibitors, a new generation of non-steroidal anti-inflammatory drugs (NSAIDs) aim to minimize the risk of damage to the stomach and digestive system. In 2001, the National Institute for Clinical Excellence (NICE) recommended that these new NSAIDs should be used for patients at high risk of developing gastrointestinal problems. NICE also approved other drug regimes, notably biological response modifiers/anti-TNF alpha (such as remicade/infliximab; enbrel/etancercept) which slow the process of inflammation in rheumatoid arthritis. Issues of access have also been raised with regard to surgery. Waiting times for joint replacement surgery have often been a cause for concern. In addition, arthritis groups have called for better access to new surgical techniques, such as 'metal on metal' hip resurfacing.

As noted in Chapter 2, national service frameworks, which set out national standards and action plans, have been established in several condition areas, including heart disease, cancer and mental health, and for particular client groups, such as children and older people, but not for arthritis. Although calls to include arthritis standards in the Older People's national service framework were rejected, osteoporosis was specifically included and both Arthritis Care and the National Osteoporosis Society were represented on the relevant external reference groups (DoH, 2001b).[2]

The politics of arthritis

Although a significant cause of morbidity and disability, arthritis has a low political and media profile and has struggled to get on to the policy agenda. Moreover, within medicine, rheumatology is not a glamorous specialty. Arthritis is not a priority for the NHS. It is perceived as irreversible, rarely fatal and associated with old age (Woolf and Akesson, 2001). In 1988, although the European Region of the World Health Organization identified arthritis as a priority, many governments, including the UK, failed to respond accordingly. To the disappointment of those in the field, the White Paper *Saving Lives: Our Healthier Nation* (Cm 4386, 1999) did not adopt back pain, rheumatism and arthritis as a national priority. Unlike heart disease, mental illness and cancer, where a national clinical director (or 'czar') has been appointed to oversee policy implementation, there is no counterpart for arthritis.

The low priority of arthritis is reflected in its failure to attract government funding for research. In 2001/02, the Medical Research Council spent only £5.5 million on research into arthritis and rheumatology, compared to over £75 million on cancer research. However, the arthritis field does boast one of the largest medical research charities in the UK. With an annual income of £26 million in 2001/02, the Arthritis Research Campaign is the fourth largest medical research charity in the UK.

The arthritis sector is dominated by three organizations: the Arthritis Research Campaign; the British Society of Rheumatology, a professional association; and the health consumer group, Arthritis Care. All three organizations are members of the British League Against Rheumatism (now called the Arthritis and Musculoskeletal Alliance), which brings together professionals, research charities, health consumer groups and other voluntary health organizations. Working relationships between the various organizations in the field of arthritis and related conditions have been fairly harmonious. Given the diversity of conditions within arthritis, particularly with the number of relatively rare conditions, there is the potential for fragmentation and rivalry. Yet, the common problems faced by groups, such as the low political profile of the condition, have helped bring about co-operation in the sector.

Another possible explanation for these generally co-operative relationships is that as a long-term condition, arthritis requires a close and continuous relationship between clinician and patient (Barlow, Turner and Wright, 1998; Thorne, Ternhulf-Nyhlin and Patterson, 2000). Although treatment is medicalized and clinicians remain dominant (Wilson, 2001), they nonetheless depend heavily on patient self-management and compliance with treatment regimes.

Cancer

Cancer is a generic term relating to malignant growth in the body. It is not therefore a single disease: indeed there are over 200 different forms and it can develop at different sites in the body. As a consequence, treatments differ according to the site and type of cancer. The effectiveness of treatment also varies, with some cancers being more responsive than others. There are wide variations in survival rates. For example, five years after treatment 70 per cent of women survive cancer of the uterus and 90 per cent of men survive testicular cancer, while only 5 per cent of men and women survive lung cancer.

Cancer is not confined to a particular age or social group although two-thirds of cancers are diagnosed in people over 65 and three-quarters of the deaths from cancer occur in this age group. This means that the experience of the disease and treatment affect a cross-section of different people. However, there are important gender differences in the prevalence of cancer, as several of the high risk sites for cancer are gender-specific (cervix, prostate, testicle, ovary, female breast).

The impact on individuals and society

Cancer places a heavy burden on both individuals and society. Around a quarter of deaths in the UK are caused by cancer. The biggest cancer killer is lung cancer (around 33 000 deaths in the UK annually), followed by bowel cancer (around 16 000 deaths) and breast cancer (13 000 deaths). Morbidity levels are also high, with around 40 per cent of the UK population being diagnosed at some point in their lifetime with cancer. Approximately 200 000 new cases of cancer are diagnosed every year and cancer was responsible for over 1.3 million in-patient episodes in England in 2000/01, over 10 per cent of the total (DoH, 2002b). The cost of cancer to the NHS is large and is increasing. In 2002, it was estimated that cancer services accounted for £2.5 billion of NHS funding (Wanless, 2002). Recent policy initiatives, discussed below, have pledged increases in spending of at least another £1 billion by 2005/06. The wider economic and social costs of cancer, in terms of disability benefits and losses to the economy, are also high.

Key policies and issues

Cancer has a high political profile. It attracts considerable media coverage (see Chapter 11) and directly, or indirectly, affects large numbers of people. Cancer also has a high 'fear factor'. Although most diagnoses are among elderly people, it can affect younger and middle-aged groups as well and is perceived as a disease that can strike people down in their prime. Cancer has been a stated priority since the early 1990s, when it was identified as one of the key targets for a reduction in death rates by the Conservative government's *Health of the Nation* strategy (Cm 1986, 1992). This was followed by the Calman-Hine report of 1995, which represented a pioneering attempt to set national standards for cancer services (DoH, 1995a). It outlined a blueprint for the provision of cancer services and recommended that dedicated cancer units should be set up in district hospitals to manage the commoner cancers. Specialized cancer centres would provide expertise in the management of both common and rare cancers, and at the primary care level better systems of cancer detection and referral would be put in place. The report also emphasized the need for a multidisciplinary approach to the management of cancer with a higher level of integration in the work of cancer units and closer co-operation between secondary and primary care providers.

Under the Labour government, the political profile of cancer rose even further. In 1999, the prime minister, Tony Blair, took a close interest in the issue and indeed chaired a cancer summit at Downing Street. Cancer was reaffirmed as a key priority in Labour's health strategy, *Saving Lives* (Cm 4386, 1999). A target was set to reduce deaths from cancer by 20 per cent in people under 75 (between 1996 and 2010) and along with heart disease and mental health was one of the key government priorities mentioned in the *NHS Plan* (Cm 4818, 2000).

In 1999, the Department of Health established a Cancer Action Team for England, 'to raise the standard of cancer care in all hospitals' (Cm 4386, 1999, p. 68) and later that year, Professor Mike Richards was appointed as the National Cancer Director or 'czar' to oversee the development and implementation of cancer services. The Cancer Services Collaborative was set up to develop local good practice in order to improve the experience and outcomes of care for people with cancer. A National Cancer Research Institute was also established to co-ordinate voluntary and statutory funding for research.

In 2000, the Government published a *National Cancer Plan for England* (DoH, 2000a). The plan – which was the equivalent of the national service frameworks in other areas – brought together all aspects of cancer care: prevention, screening, diagnosis, treatment and care for cancer and outlined the level of resources needed to deliver improved services in terms of improved staffing, equipment, drugs, treatments and information systems. The plan also announced new smoking cessation targets, treatment and diagnosis waiting time targets, and further funding for hospices and specialist palliative care. Even before this, targets had been set for cancer screening (some dating back to the previous Conservative government) and for specialist referrals. The latter included a two-week waiting time for urgent referrals to a specialist for suspected breast cancer.

This was extended to other cancers and it was stated that from 2005, no one should wait for more than two months from an urgent general practitioner referral to treatment. However, in spite of these targets, and the additional resources allocated to cancer, concerns remain.

Criticisms of a lack of access to effective treatments, and of unacceptable variations in access, known as 'post-code prescribing' have continued. NICE, established to provide an evidence-base for decisions about the availability of treatments, has evaluated a number of cancer drugs (for example, for breast, ovarian, brain, bowel, lung, pancreatic cancer and leukaemia) and recommended their use within the NHS. It has also made recommendations about surgical interventions, such as laparoscopic surgery. Even so, cancer groups continue to complain that individuals face difficulty in accessing treatments in some parts of the country. Inequities are not confined to drug therapies. Studies have found a wide variation in the quality of cancer services (NCEPOD, 2001) and 'often striking variations in provision both across geographical areas and between patients with different types of cancer' (Commission for Health Improvement and Audit Commission, 2001, p. xi).

Despite the fact that additional resources have been committed to cancer, the House of Commons' Select Committee on Science and Technology (Science and Technology Committee, 2002) found that funds had been diverted to other services. Subsequently, a survey by CancerBACUP (2002) found that half the cancer networks established to achieve co-ordinated planning and common treatment standards received less money in 2002/03 than expected, undermining their ability to modernize cancer services.

A major stumbling block to service improvement is the relatively low numbers of trained oncologists in the UK compared to numbers in other countries. Prior to the *Cancer Plan* there were only 365 full-time-equivalent oncologists: one for every 500 new cases of cancer every year. The ratio of oncologists to new cases at this time in Norway was 1:75; in Belgium 1:100; in Germany, 1:140 in Austria; 1:150; and in France, Spain and the USA, 1:200 (Bower and Boseley, 1999). It was also argued that other countries adopt more effective drug regimes and spend more than the UK on cancer medicines (UK £1.01 is spent per head annually; Italy £1.24; Germany £2.31; France, £2.93; USA, £4.93)

(Bower and Boseley, 1999). There is also a shortage of specialist cancer nurses (DoH, 2000b; Commission for Health Improvement and Audit Commission, 2001). The *Cancer Plan* aimed to increase capacity substantially, both in terms of staff and equipment, but the long lead times for the production of new oncologists remains a cause for concern.

The politics of cancer

The politics of cancer is highly complex. Overall, its high profile guarantees the attention of policy-makers, gives it priority and attracts resources. But cancer is also a highly fragmented field where different interests, various types of cancer and numerous organizations compete for public attention, political support and funding.

It is generally assumed that doctors are very powerful in the cancer field, a point made very clearly in the De Montfort study interviews (see Chapter 7). The dominance of clinicians was reflected in the appointment of a cancer 'czar' with a medical background and the strong representation of doctors on cancer planning teams. It may also reflect the continuing development of biomedical knowledge in cancer and the increasing effectiveness of cancer treatments. However, there are indications that the views of users, traditionally weak and vulnerable in this field, are being more carefully considered. Indeed, there has been a concerted effort, particularly over the last decade, to improve communication and engagement with users, a move supported by leading clinicians.

The major research charities are also highly influential organizations. However, in the past their efforts have been limited by fragmentation and rivalry. In 2002, the two largest charities, Imperial Cancer Research Fund and Cancer Research Campaign, joined forces to form Cancer Research UK. But there remains a large number of fundraising research charities related to specific forms of cancer, for example, Breakthrough Breast Cancer, which has also developed an important role in raising awareness about the disease and campaigning for improved services. Other prominent voluntary organizations in the field include service providers such as Marie Curie Cancer Care and Macmillan Cancer Relief, which are highly regarded by government. Added to these, are a host of health consumer groups, both general and specific, some of which have a high profile, such as CancerBACUP. Some types of cancer are heavily represented by groups, notably breast cancer. Some have a single organization (for example, bowel cancer), while others, such as skin cancer or bone cancer, have no dedicated national organization representing their interests.

The extent of collaboration between groups varies, with some larger organizations providing financial support to smaller ones, for example by sponsoring services or funding specialist staff. However, the complexity and diversity of groups has inhibited joint campaigning and lobbying. In 1999, the chair of the All-party Group on Cancer, Ian Gibson MP, called for cancer organizations to lobby jointly for improved services rather than separately (Kent, 1999, p. 874). Whilst there have been mergers, as well as regular joint meetings between groups and co-operation on some issues, such as the provision of information about cancer, the cancer field still tends towards fragmentation.

Heart and circulatory conditions

Heart and circulatory conditions include a range of cardiovascular diseases and disorders, including coronary heart disease and stroke. In coronary heart disease the arteries supplying the heart become narrow, leading to chest pain (angina), and may ultimately become blocked, leading to a heart attack. Even if the patient survives, he or she may eventually suffer from heart failure. Other types of disease affect heart rhythm, the heart valves and the cardiac muscle. There are also congenital heart diseases, where people are born with heart defects. A stroke is a cerebrovascular accident – where blood flow in the brain is impaired by a haemorrhage (known as haemorrhagic stroke) or by a blockage by embolism or thrombosis (ischaemic stroke). Should the patient survive, there is usually some loss of brain and physical function including paralysis, which may be temporary or permanent.

The impact on individuals and society

Heart and circulatory diseases are a major cause of mortality and morbidity. In the UK around 40 per cent of total deaths are attributed to heart disease, stroke and related conditions (British Heart Foundation, 2002). Although overall death rates from heart and circulatory disease have declined since the 1970s, it remains the main cause of death for both men and women. Around one in ten of the population (a higher proportion of males) reported a longstanding disease of the circulatory system in 1998 (ONS, 2000a). In 2001/02 diseases of the circulatory system were responsible for over a million in-patient episodes of care in England, a twelfth of the total (DoH 2002b).

Currently around 1.4 million men and 1.2 million women have experienced coronary heart disease (British Heart Foundation, 2002), which is responsible for around half the deaths from cardiovascular disease (124 000 in 2000). Coronary heart disease is one of the main causes of death among the elderly, although it significantly affects other age groups (17 000 coronary heart disease deaths in the UK in 2000 were among people aged under 65). It is therefore a significant cause of premature death. It also has a class gradient, with unskilled working men being three times more likely to die prematurely from the disease than men in professional or managerial occupations. In 1998 the National Heart Forum, an alliance of professional and health consumer groups, published a research report that indicated that these health inequalities are increasing (National Heart Forum, 1998). It should also be noted that certain ethnic groups, notably men originating from the Indian subcontinent, have a higher risk of heart disease. The cost of treating coronary heart disease is high, around £1.7 billion in 1999 (Liu *et al.*, 2002), accounting for over 2.5 per cent of NHS hospital spending and almost 2 per cent of expenditure on primary care (Cm 4386, 1999, p. 19). There are additional costs through absence from work, amounting to around £5.3 billion per year (Liu *et al.*, 2002).

Stroke is also a major cause of mortality, accounting for 60 000 deaths in 2000 in the UK (British Heart Foundation, 2002) and less than 10 per cent of deaths are in people aged under 65. Deaths from stroke are more common in women than men. The direct health care cost of stroke was over £1.6 billion in 1999 in the UK (British Heart Foundation, 2002; Liu *et al.*, 2002) and over 4 per cent of NHS spending. It also accounts for 7 per cent of community health and social care expenditure. This is largely because strokes are a major cause of disability. Indeed it has been identified as the single biggest cause of severe disability (Wolfe, Rudd, and Beech, 1996). Among the over-75s, 3 per cent of men and 4 per cent of women report experience of stroke (ONS, 2000a).

Key policies and issues

Heart disease has been one of the main government priorities since the 1980s. In 1992, formal targets for the reduction of coronary heart disease and stroke were included in the Major government's *Health of the Nation* Strategy (Cm 1986, 1992). Waiting time targets for patients requiring coronary artery bypass grafts were also set during the 1990s. The importance of coronary heart disease and stroke was recognized by the incoming Labour government, which included new targets in its public health strategy, *Saving Lives*, launched in 1999 (Cm 4386, 1999). The government aimed to reduce the death rate from heart disease and stroke by at least 40 per cent for people under the age of 75 between 1996 and 2010. Tackling heart disease was re-emphasized in the *NHS Plan* of 2000, where a commitment was made to improve services by: increasing the number of cardiologists (physicians who diagnose and treat patients with heart disease, but who do not conduct open heart surgery) by half within four years and by expanding services such as rapid access chest pain clinics. Targets were also set to improve ambulance response times and access to thrombolysis (clot-busting drugs). Government plans also included increasing the number of revascularization procedures and improved access to effective medicines after heart attack (aspirin, beta blockers and statins). In addition, there was a commitment to reduce the waiting times for treatment, including a maximum wait of six months for routine cardiac surgery by 2005 and three months by 2008. In 2002, this was augmented by giving patients waiting longer than six months for heart surgery the choice of where to have their operation, including the private sector, or even abroad.

Most of the new initiatives, set standards and targets established by the *National Service Framework for Coronary Heart Disease*, published in 2000 (DoH, 2000c). This was formulated with the assistance of an external reference group that included clinicians, scientists, epidemiologists, health service managers, voluntary agencies and patient and carer representatives from the British

Cardiac Patients Association (BCPA). The framework established standards for reducing heart disease in the population; preventing coronary heart disease in high-risk populations at primary care level; treating heart attacks, investigating and treating angina; revascularization; managing heart failure, and cardiac rehabilitation. The framework also set out the actions required to meet these standards including the establishment of local networks for cardiac care. Models for service delivery were outlined, as well as methods for audit and evaluation. The Labour government also appointed a national clinical director, or 'czar', for heart disease and an implementation group to oversee the programme. The *National Service Framework for Coronary Heart Disease* excluded stroke, but subsequently, specific standards for stroke prevention and care were included in the *National Service Framework for Older People* (DoH, 2001b). These related to the identification and treatment of people at risk from stroke, improved care and treatment of patients immediately following a stroke (including performing a brain scan within 48 hours and treatment by a specialist stroke team) and early and continuing rehabilitation and long-term support.

Despite the high priority given to heart disease and stroke, concern remained. In coronary heart disease, doubts continue that the government's ambitious targets will be met, even with the infusion of additional resources announced in the *NHS Plan* and subsequent budgets. As with cancer, the production of additional trained clinicians is a long-term process and depends crucially on the supply of individuals willing to train and work in the UK as specialists. Prior to the 1990 reforms the UK had fewer specialist staff and undertook fewer procedures than many other European countries. In the late 1990s, the UK had approximately 16 heart surgeons per 100 000 population compared to 30 in France and 42 in Germany. The number of consultant cardiologists in this period (630), was half that estimated to be required (*Heart*, 2002). Around 1995, fewer pacemakers were fitted in the UK than in other comparable European countries: 232 per million people compared to 438 in Germany; 602 in France and 678 in Belgium (Rayner and Peterson, 2000, p. 42). Out of 28 European countries, the UK ranked eighteenth in the rates of coronary bypass surgery adjusted for coronary heart disease mortality (Rayner and Peterson, ibid.).

It remains to be seen whether the increased investment in coronary heart disease care and treatment will improve services significantly. However, by 2003 waiting times for routine heart surgery had fallen in line with targets set out by the Department of Health. There has been particular concern about the poor response to the framework standard on managing heart failure (Siddall, 2002). Complaints about the lack of availability of drugs have continued, including evidence that older patients with coronary heart disease were not receiving cholesterol-lowering drugs such as statins (Whincup *et al.*, 2002). Other issues of concern have related to the quality of heart surgery, particularly in children, arising from the Bristol Royal Infirmary Inquiry (Bristol Inquiry, 2001) and prescription exemptions for people with long-term heart conditions. Complaints about inequities in treatment have also continued, notably with regard to allegations of poorer standards of care for women and ethnic minorities (Clarke, *et al.*, 1994; Lear *et al.*, 1994).

The criticism of stroke services has been greater. Although stroke is officially a priority, clinicians, patients and carers believe that in practice it lacks priority status. Despite the targets, it is alleged that stroke patients do not receive appropriate care and treatment. In its audit in 2001/02, the Intercollegiate Working Party on Stroke found that only a third of stroke patients spent any of their hospital stay in a specialist stroke unit (Gulland, 2002; Intercollegiate Stroke Working Party, Royal College of Physicians, 2002). The report also indicated that there was a shortage of full-time stroke doctors and therapists. However, it noted some improvements: the majority of hospitals participating in the study now had a stroke unit, also a majority of patients received brain imaging and were receiving the recommended anti-thrombolytic medication.

The politics of heart and circulatory disease

In terms of the internal politics of heart and circulatory disease, the field is inhabited by many different organizations. The clinicians operate through general associations and professional bodies (such as the Royal College of Physicians and the Royal College of Surgeons). There are a number of specialist groups including the British Cardiac Society, which includes cardiologists and many cardiothoracic surgeons. Other professions, including nurses and technicians, are also affiliated to this body. The main specialist organization for heart surgeons is the Society of Cardiothoracic Surgeons.

As in cancer, doctors are strong relative to other interests. This again reflects the nature of doctor–patient interaction at the individual level in this field, which has a strong paternalistic tradition. However, there have been recent efforts to strengthen relationships with patients and focus greater attention on their needs. A recent joint initiative led by the British Cardiac Society and the British Heart Foundation brought together patients and professional representatives in order to explore how communication can be improved (*Heart*, 2002, p.10).

The British Heart Foundation is the main research organization in the heart field. Initially this body focused on fundraising for research, but has since diversified into other areas, including training in emergency life support skills for the public and professionals; educating the public and professionals about heart disease, and providing support and information for patients and their families. It funds specialist posts for cardiac liaison nurses and also supports a number of local self-help groups, whose members include patients and carers.

There are several health consumer groups at national level, including the BCPA, which arose out of the activities of other local support groups. Other national groups include the Children's Heart Federation, the Cardiomyopathy Association, and with regard to stroke, the Stroke Association and Different Strokes. Most health consumer groups did not appear to have a particularly close relationship with the professional and research organizations, although an exception to this occurred in 2002, when the Family Heart Association merged with the research charity, the British Hyperlipidaemia Association, to form Heart UK. There were also signs that organizations in this field might be willing to co-operate more closely in the future.

Another organization, the National Heart Forum, includes a range of interests: professional groups, lobbying groups, research bodies and a small number of health consumer groups. It therefore has the potential to co-ordinate all these interests. However, it is geared mainly to campaigning on prevention, which reduces its appeal to organizations whose interests focus on treatment and care. It also relies on funding from the British Heart Foundation, which would be unlikely to appreciate any encroachment within its field of expertise, should this arise.

In summary, the heart disease field is quite fragmented, though not perhaps as much as that of cancer. Relationships between the principal organizations have not been as close as might be expected. The medical specialists and the research organizations are strong politically and there is some recognition of the importance of health consumer groups. Relationships in the stroke area are closer, this is largely because of the co-ordinating role played by the Stroke Association, which accommodates both clinical and patient/carer interests.

Maternity and childbirth

The Audit Commission (1997) identified three key differences between maternity services and other NHS services. First, the women who use these services are not like other service users, they are generally healthy and hold strong views about their care. Second, there are differing views about how maternity services should be delivered. For example, one school of thought advocates medical surveillance for all women on safety grounds. Another sees the mode of childbirth as a matter of choice, with most women needing support and care rather than medical intervention. Third, unlike some other specialities, there is a long tradition of evidence-based practice in maternity care. Notably, obstetrics and paediatrics were among the first to introduce systematic reviews, such as the *Confidential Enquiry into Maternal Deaths* and *Confidential Enquiry into Stillbirths and Deaths in Infancy.*[3]

The impact on individuals and society

Every year over 600 000 women use maternity services in Britain. These services account for 5 per cent of the NHS hospital and community health services budget. In the UK, most pregnant women seek care within the NHS – less than 1 per cent of births take place in a private hospital. However, most births take place in hospital rather than at home, and hospital births increased from 25 per cent of the total in the 1940s to around 97 per cent by the late 1990s (English Nursing Board, 2000). Nevertheless, much antenatal and postnatal care is community-based (Garcia *et al.*, 1998).

Antenatal care and delivery have changed as a result of the introduction of various technologies, most of which are used routinely. The proportion of all hospital deliveries occurring spontaneously has fallen in recent decades. Just over half of women (53 per cent in 2000/01) have a spontaneous onset of labour and delivery with no use of induction, instruments, or caesarean section. In the early 1970s, less than 5 per cent of deliveries were by caesarean, by 2001 this had risen to 21 per cent (Thomas and Paranjothy, 2001). This has caused concern in government, as well as among health professionals and health consumer groups.

Critics have often commented that childbirth has become increasingly 'medicalized' (Oakley, 1986). This criticism goes beyond the use of caesareans to include the routine use of drugs, episiotomies,[4] instruments and ultrasound (Tew, 1998, pp. 129–30). It has been suggested that there is insufficient knowledge of the possible consequences and side effects of such technologies, despite the tradition of evidence-based medicine in this field (Kitzinger, 1987; Beech, 1991).

Meanwhile, maternal deaths, stillbirths and perinatal (the time preceding, during and shortly after birth) mortality have all declined dramatically since the early years of the last century. Nonetheless, in 2001 over 3000 families suffered a stillbirth in England and Wales. The *Confidential Enquiry into Stillbirths and Deaths in Infancy* found that sub-optimal hospital care was still a major factor in a fifth of cases examined (CESDI, 1999). Meanwhile research into compliance with evidence-based recommendations in obstetrics revealed that in spite of a massive shift in practice in line with evidence, many units still had substantial room for improvement (Wilson *et al.*, 2002). By the mid-1990s maternal deaths in the UK had fallen to around seven per 100 000 maternities. In the early twentieth century this figure was around 400 per 100 000 (Tew, 1998). Even so, the *Confidential Enquiry into Maternal Deaths* suggests that further improvements in maternity care are possible and necessary, as well as efforts to tackle the socioeconomic factors in maternal deaths, notably social deprivation and ethnic minority status (DoH *et al.*, 1998).

Key policies and issues

The attention of policy-makers has focused on improving access to an adequate range of services and improving safety for mother and baby. Policy-makers have also responded to pressure from health consumer groups. However, there have been tensions between the concerns of maternity and childbirth groups to increase choice and the concerns of some obstetricians to maintain and improve safety. In practice, services vary considerably, with some providers and practitioners positively supporting home births by making facilities available, while others fail to do so. In reality there may be a limited choice. In one survey, women reported that they were given little option, with less than one in five claiming that they were offered a home birth (Garcia *et al.*, 1998).

Several professional groupings are involved in maternity care – general practitioners, community midwives, consultant obstetricians and their junior doctors, and hospital-based midwives. In some areas there are also independent midwives in practice. Most babies are delivered by midwives in hospital (under the authority of consultant obstetricians). However, doctors are more involved in deliveries now than ten years ago, largely because of the rise in surgical intervention and particularly caesarean section. In 2000/01 a third of deliveries were conducted by hospital doctors compared with a quarter in 1989/90, with midwives responsible for the remainder (DoH, 2002c).

In the 1980s and 1990s pregnancy and childbirth became a site of competing discourses and power struggles between professionals and lay people, represented through health consumer groups and the lay representatives on local maternity service liaison committees (Tew, 1998). The central question was control: who should make the key decisions throughout pregnancy and childbirth, and where and how should they be made? These arguments entered the policy arena through the 1992 Health Select Committee inquiry into maternity services chaired by Nicholas Winterton (Health Committee, 1992). Declerq (1998) suggests that these debates occurred for several reasons: in 1989, the National Perinatal Epidemiology Unit[5] had published authoritative data on the rising rate of hospital births (Chalmers, Enkin and Keirse, 1989); the 1990 health reforms had led to a rethink about how maternity services should be commissioned in the new 'quasi-market';

politically, there was a powerful alliance between health consumer groups and certain professional groups such as the Royal
College of Midwives.[6] Furthermore, members of the Health
Committee were strongly committed to change – they had direct
or indirect personal experience of childbirth which brought both
an 'ordinary' and 'policy-analytic' interpretation of evidence.

In response to the recommendations of the Winterton report,
an Expert Maternity Group was established in 1993 by the
Department of Health, to draw up an action plan.[7] The Group,
using what Declerq (1998, p. 845) called 'classic bureaucratic
strategies' included a range of interests and by now there was a
wide degree of consensus between interested parties. For example,
in 1994, a report from the Royal College of Obstetricians and
Gynaecologists (RCOG) had argued that for most pregnancies
and births, the use of sophisticated technologies in childbirth was
unnecessary (Chamberlain and Patel, 1994). The Expert Maternity
Group's (1993) report, *Changing Childbirth*, laid down guidelines
for policy development, emphasizing choice; women-centred
care; access to information and continuity of care. In the 1994/95
Priorities and Planning Guidance for the NHS, the NHS Management Executive stated that health authorities should review their
maternity services in light of these recommendations and the then
Conservative government set a five-year implementation target.
An important feature of these policies was that they reflected the
objectives of the dominant health consumer groups within the
childbirth arena.

By the late 1990s, there was disappointment that the strategy
had not achieved more. A review by the Audit Commission
(1997) showed continuing widespread variations in practice.
Other research reported a lack of change in attitudes on the part
of health professionals and managers in trusts, and a high use of
technological interventions (Tew, 1998). However, doubts were
also raised about the policy itself. Allen, Bourke-Dowling and
Williams (1997) looked at new models of delivery, based on mid-
wife-led practice, and warned that reorganizing services along these
lines could have consequences for effective working partnerships
with the medical profession. They also argued that user empowerment and choice should not jeopardize safety considerations.

Recently, in addition to continuing debate on medicalization
and the rising caesarean rate, maternity and childbirth groups

have criticized government plans to close smaller maternity units and have drawn attention to the shortage of midwives. The Royal College of Midwives reported that a quarter of hospital midwifery posts lie vacant for three months or more, 80 per cent of maternity units have vacant posts and only one in three trained midwives are currently in practice. In 2000, the *NHS Plan* set a target to recruit an additional two thousand midwives for the NHS.

In the earlier stages of the De Montfort study, there was a feeling among health consumer groups and professional organizations that maternity and childbirth issues had drifted off the political agenda. However, in 2001, a national service framework for children was announced. An external working group on maternity services, which includes representatives from health consumer groups, will set standards for antenatal, delivery and postnatal services as part of this process. Also, in 2003, the Commons Health Committee produced a series of reports on the provision of, and access to, services as well as the extent of choice offered in maternity services (Health Committee, 2003a, 2003b, 2003c).

The politics of maternity and childbirth

Maternity and childbirth issues have a high profile. The majority of the population are affected in some way by childbirth issues during their lifetime and giving birth is an important life-experience for most women. Furthermore, childbirth, children and mother-hood is a popular topic in the media and there are strong voluntary organizations in the sector that have campaigned vociferously for improvements in the design and quality of services. A number of organizations exist in the sector, representing various inter-ests. Medical interests are represented by the Royal College of Obstetricians and Gynaecologists, the Royal College of General Practitioners and the British Medical Association. Midwives are represented by the Royal College of Midwives and a smaller body the Independent Midwives Association. There are also research charities such as Tommy's Campaign and the Foundation for the Study of Infant Deaths, who have a high media profile.

A number of longstanding health consumer groups inhabit this sector, including the Association for Improvements in the Maternity Services and the National Childbirth Trust, which were established over forty years ago and were at the forefront of the consumer movement in health (see Chapter 4). Other health consumer groups exist which support women who have particular complications during pregnancy, such as pre-eclampsia, or who have experienced miscarriage. However, traditionally, the medical professions have dominated the sector (Oakley, 1986; Donnison, 1998). Paradoxically, medicalization has if anything become stronger in recent years, yet there does appear to be a new climate of co-operation between professional and consumer groups which is discussed in more detail in Chapter 7.

Mental health

Mental health is a broad term that concerns the psycho-social well being of individuals, families and communities (DoH, 2001c). The term mental illness, however, focuses more narrowly on mental disorders. An Expert Committee set up to review the Mental Health Act (1983) argued against a precise definition on the grounds that concepts of mental illness are constantly changing. It adopted the Law Commission's broad definition of a mental disorder as: 'any disability or disorder of mind or brain, whether permanent or temporary, which results in an impairment or disturbance of mental functioning' (DoH, 1999c, p.38). Mental illness is usually subdivided into several categories: neurotic disorders, which disrupt daily activities and cause distress. These include anxiety, depression, obsessive disorders, phobias and panic disorders. Psychoses, which disturb thinking and distort perception, including organic psychoses, such as dementia and Alzheimer's disease, and functional psychoses, such as schizophrenia and manic depression. Finally, there are personality disorders which develop in adolescence or early adulthood and which bring changes in patterns of behaviour.

The impact on individuals and society

One in six adults aged 16–74 in Britain suffer from some form of mental illness at any time. Around one in ten experience a mixture of anxiety and depression (ONS, 2000b). It has been estimated that more than half of all women and a quarter of all men will report some form of depression before the age of 70 (Rorsman *et al.*, 1990). Neuroses should not be regarded as necessarily less important than psychotic conditions. Indeed neurotic conditions can have very serious consequences for the sufferer and for their families. For example, depression is a major factor in suicide, which is the cause of death of around 4000 people a year in England.

Mental health problems vary according to age and gender. Women report higher rates of mental illness than men (ONS, 2000b). However, suicide rates in men aged under 35 have risen in recent years and it is now the second largest cause of death in this age group. At the other end of the age range, the number of people over 65 suffering from mental health problems is expected to rise substantially. One quarter of those aged over 85 develop dementia, some of whom will require constant care or supervision (Audit Commission, 2000). There is also variation by ethnic group. Afro-Caribbean people have a higher incidence of psychotic illnesses, such as schizophrenia, than the rest of the population, though this may be due to diagnostic bias (Cope, 1989; Sashidaran and Francis, 1993; Nazroo, 1997).

The links between mental health problems and social exclusion are increasingly acknowledged (ONS, 2000b). Separated, divorced and bereaved people have higher rates of anxiety and depression. Unemployed people are more likely to report a mental health problem. There is a class gradient in the suicide rate (for males in Class V the rate is four times that of Class I, DoH, 2002d). Mental health problems are also more common in the prison population (Singleton, Meltzer and Gatward, 1997) and amongst homeless people (Social Exclusion Unit, 1998).

The cost of mental health problems is high. The annual total cost in England for 1996/97 was estimated at £32 billion (Patel and Knapp, 1998; MIND, 2002) – or around £40 billion in 2004 prices. Mental health accounts for approximately 12 per cent of total NHS costs – as well as costs to local authority social services, the criminal justice system and social security payments. There are also costs to informal carers, and loss of income through unemployment. Employment losses make up over a third of the total cost, reflecting estimates that mental illness accounts for around 80 million lost working days per annum (DoH, 1998a). Mental health problems in children also have wide implications.

It has been estimated that one in every five children has a mental health problem, which has a significant knock-on effect on educational and social services, as well as on criminal justice authorities (Mental Health Foundation, 1999).

Key policies and issues

Although mental health was always considered a 'Cinderella' issue, neglected by policy-makers, this assessment is no longer accurate. Mental health is now one of government's stated priorities. Efforts to prioritize mental health date back to the 1970s, with the publication a statement of intent in the White Paper *Better Services for the Mentally Ill* (Cmnd 6233, 1975). This highlighted the importance of mental illness as a major health problem and endorsed the policy of 'care in the community'. Although it raised expectations about the pace and direction of mental health policy, little was achieved in practice (Peck and Parker, 1998; Rogers and Pilgrim, 2001). Instead, there followed a review of mental health legislation, culminating in the Mental Health Act of 1983, which, according to Butler (1993, p. 52), 'did little to address the fundamental issues of fragmented services and chronic under-funding'. The 1983 Act provided statutory grounds for compulsory hospital treatment of patients without their consent, though with additional safeguards. These safeguards, such as the Mental Health Act Commission to monitor detention powers and standards of care, and greater access to review tribunals, were ineffective in protecting patients from harm (Rogers and Pilgrim, 2001). More-over, the whole approach of the 1983 Act was criticized as inappropriate. It was, as Peck and Parker (1998, p. 242) observed, 'a resurgence of the legalistic approach which had so dominated mental health care in the preceding 150 years' and ignored 'the fact that most mentally ill people are treated voluntarily outside hospital'.

Despite this activity, mental health did not attract much attention until the following decade, when several high-profile incidents occurred, highlighting poor standards of care, death and injury. Three cases in particular caused enormous public concern and had a major impact on policy (Peck and Parker, 1998; Rogers and Pilgrim, 2001). These were: the killing of a social worker, Elizabeth Schwartz, by a patient with mental health problems in

1984; the death of Jonathon Zito, in 1992, killed by a man diagnosed with paranoid schizophrenia, and, shortly afterwards, the mauling of Ben Silcock, a person with schizophrenia, who climbed into the lion's den at London Zoo. The media interest in these stories, coupled with genuine concern from the public, professions and voluntary organizations about the threats to public safety posed by community care, provoked a government response. In addition, inquiries into such incidents produced authoritative recommendations both in terms of policy and practice as mental health ascended the political agenda.

In 1993, the Conservative government issued a ten-point plan aimed at strengthening the legal framework for mental health, improving the delivery of care to patients, and the development of new processes to support services (Peck and Parker, 1998). In the meantime, mental health became a public health priority under Major's government (Cm 1986, 1992). This involved a commitment to improving the health and social functioning of mentally ill people. A target was also set to reduce the number of suicides in England by 15 per cent between 1990 and 2000.

Under the Labour government, mental health has continued as an official priority. In its White Paper *Saving Lives,* a target was set to reduce deaths from suicide and undetermined injury by 20 per cent by 2010 (Cm 4386, 1999). This was followed by a National Suicide Strategy (DoH, 2002d) that set out goals and interventions to reduce the suicide rate, particularly in high-risk groups, such as young men. In 1999, the Labour government also unveiled its Mental Health national service framework, which set out standards and service models across a range of services for adults up to 65, including mental health promotion, primary care, access to services, effectiveness of services, carers and preventing suicide (DoH, 1999d). The over-65s were covered by the *National Service Framework for Older People*, published two years later. These built on an earlier policy document on mental health services (DoH, 1998a), which announced additional funding for mental health services and emphasized three key aims: *safe services*, protecting the public while effectively caring for mentally ill people; *sound services*, ensuring that patients and carers have access to an appropriate range of services when needed, and *supportive services*, working in partnership with patients, users, families, carers and communities. At the same time, mental health was deemed a shared priority between the NHS and social services (DoH, 1998b) and a review was launched into the 1983 Mental Health Act.

As in other areas of policy, efforts were made to improve the implementation of policy. This was to be achieved through mechanisms of clinical governance in the NHS. In 2002, a national clinical director (or 'czar') for mental health in England was appointed and a Mental Health Taskforce was set up to oversee implementation of policy.[8] In a further attempt to improve standards in 2001, a National Institute for Mental Health was established in England. Its tasks were to create: a mental health research network to improve the evidence-base for mental health interventions and a service development network to advise on the introduction of national service framework initiatives.

Despite the higher profile of mental health, and its status as a health priority, a number of problems remain. Concerns persist that the government's agenda is dominated by considerations about public safety. This is linked to a belief, particularly among groups representing service users, that the civil liberties of mentally ill people are not protected in law. This issue formed the basis of a campaign against proposed changes to mental health legislation that were announced by the Labour government in 2000. This campaign, led by health consumer groups and professional organizations is discussed later in the book.

Mental health organizations have continued to claim the sector fails to attract the necessary resources merited by the scale of the problem as they campaign on access to effective care and treatment. However, since it was established in 1999, NICE has approved new drugs (atypical antipsychotics) for schizophrenia. It has also stated that people with schizophrenia must be involved in all decisions about their care and should be offered psychological as well as drug therapies, and has recommended restrictions on controversial treatments unpopular with user groups, such as electro-convulsive therapy.

NICE decisions, as in other areas, have not had an immediate impact on practice. Mental health groups have complained that access to effective drugs is still limited, a problem not confined to the UK (WHO, 2001). Similar concerns have been expressed about the insufficient resources for the implementation of the Mental Health national service framework (Health Committee, 2000). Although many important early targets were met (500 additional secure beds, 170 assertive outreach teams and 320 '24 hour' staffed beds), many believe that improvements have been too slow and have pointed out that money earmarked for mental health was not being spent accordingly (Lewis, 2002). Other criticisms have included the relative neglect of acute inpatient mental health care (Eaton, 2002) and the over-emphasis on national targets at the expense of local priorities (Lewis, 2002) and users' needs (Carlisle, 2002).

The politics of mental health

Government policy strongly reflects the public perception, articulated by the media, that mentally ill people are inherently dangerous (Rogers and Pilgrim, 2001). Perhaps more so than in other areas, the media has played a crucial role in mental health politics. The coverage of mental health issues has been largely negative and this is why a major aim of the mental health user movement has been to challenge unhelpful stereotypes and the language used to describe mental illness. In so doing campaigners hope to generate a more sympathetic environment. People with mental health problems form a substantial minority of the population, yet many are reluctant to mobilize and campaign, perhaps because of the stigma attached to mental illness, while others are incapacitated by their condition.

Another reason why mental health has risen up the political agenda is that it has been a fertile ground for charities and lobby groups. These include self-help groups, user groups, carer groups and campaigning organizations, as well as charities dedicated to improving education, training, research, and services in the mental health field. In the past, there has been conflict between some groups due to their different focus and perspectives. An important fault-line has existed between carers' and relatives' groups on the one hand, for example, Schizophrenia A National Emergency (SANE), the Zito Trust, National Schizophrenia Fellowship (now Rethink) and user groups such as MIND (the National Association for Mental Health), Survivors Speak Out and the Manic Depression Fellowship, on the other. The former have placed stronger emphasis upon public protection and carers' concerns than the latter (Rogers and Pilgrim, 1991, 2001).

There has also been a history of antipathy between user groups and professionals, in particular psychiatrists (Rogers and Pilgrim, 2001). User groups have long campaigned against radical treatments such as electro-convulsant therapy and lobotomy, as well as some drug therapies approved by many psychiatrists. Challenges have come from other professional groups as well as users and carers. For example, within the mental health professions there are considerable variations in approaches to user involvement. Social workers and psychiatric nurses increasingly see themselves as advocates and may compete with each other to represent the patient perspective. There have also been boundary disputes between psychologists and psychiatrists (Rogers and Pilgrim, 2001). However, psychiatry has dominated mental health policy and practice, though its grip weakened to some extent with the advent of community care.

Within psychiatry there have been pressures to move away from a conventional biomedical model of disease. Indeed, psychiatrists increasingly accept the validity of social and psychological approaches to mental illness. They also accept that users have a role to play in their care and treatment. Even so, as Barnes and Bowl (2001) point out, the dominant discourse in mental health, underpinned by psychiatry, is not conducive to user involvement. This implies that the professional is competent, rational and emotionally detached, while the user is sick, non-rational, dependent and emotional. Practice of course varies between different psychiatrists. Some are highly supportive of engaging with users, but the paternalistic legacy is difficult to discard and remains a significant barrier to collaboration. Yet, despite the complexity of the internal politics of mental health, there are signs of greater co-operation both within the health consumer group sector, and between health consumer groups and the professions.

Conclusion

This chapter has shown that there are clear distinctions between each of the condition areas in terms of perceived policy problems and the configuration of interests. Arthritis is a condition which has been relatively neglected by policy-makers. It has a low media profile, despite affecting a great many people. It has also been an area where there is much co-operation and collaboration between different organizations, and they have tried to raise the profile of the condition in order to attract greater resources and receive priority status. Stroke, though part of the heart and circulatory disease area, shares many of the features of the arthritis field: close working and integration between organizations representing different interests; a focus on older peoples' health; and a perception that these conditions have a low political profile and deserve more resources and attention from policy-makers.

In contrast, maternity and childbirth was high on the health policy agenda in the early 1990s, in part because the government at the time was concerned about choice in public services and there was powerful support within both government and parliament from senior politicians sympathetic to the issue. However, maternity and childbirth issues waned and there were also major implementation problems at the local level. The low profile of maternity and childbirth in policy terms has now led to health consumer groups and professional organizations finding areas of common concern and the hostility related to perceived medical dominance has receded to a considerable extent.

In contrast, cancer and heart disease have been key priorities and there has been an avalanche of new initiatives in recent years. There are differences, with cancer health consumer groups being more numerous and more active politically than those in heart disease. In both areas, there is considerable co-operation between professionals and health consumer groups, but also tensions and fragmentation. The medical profession in these areas is renowned for its political influence and clinical dominance. But increasingly there appears to be an acknowledgement of the benefits of partnership and more acceptance of the role of users and carers as contributors to policy and service development.

Within the mental health sphere, the key priorities for health consumer groups and professionals are additional resources for community care. Although in certain areas, when bargaining for control of patterns of service, there are conflicts along the traditional lines of medically-dominated psychiatry and community service providers. Nevertheless, in campaigning terms, there is some common ground in opposing government proposals for increased restrictions on patients.

In all areas, there has been a shift towards greater self-care by the patient and, with the greater emphasis on partnership, a strengthening of the relationship between professionals and health consumer groups. Where new technologies and drug treatments can prevent further deterioration of a condition or alleviate symptoms, both professionals and groups representing patients have an incentive to lobby for additional resources. In connection with this, it should be noted that some condition areas have stronger interests than others in the pharmaceutical sector, in particular in relation to access to new treatments.

There have also been wider changes that have increased the opportunities for health consumer groups to engage with the policy process. These will be discussed in detail in later chapters. Before this, however, we must explore the formation and characteristics of health consumer groups, their internal dynamics, how they generate social and political resources, and how they work together.

4 Health consumer groups: formation and characteristics

This and the following two chapters focus on health consumer groups as patient-, user- and carer-focused organizations. The chapters draw on research data from both questionnaires and interviews. The questionnaire data provided a snapshot showing that health consumer groups were extremely diverse. Characteristics such as the period of formation; the aims and purpose of the founders; their current purpose and range of reported activities and the size of group in terms of membership, staffing and income, varied. However, underlying the diversity there were also similarities between groups in terms of why they had been formed; and their interest in representing and supporting patients, users and carers. The analysis of interviews with health consumer groups also showed that there were strong similarities in their norms and values, in the ways in which they worked with their membership, and what they saw as their strengths and weaknesses in terms of social and political resources.

The aim of this chapter is to point out the main lines of difference and similarity between groups in terms of formation and organizational characteristics, drawing on both the questionnaires and interviews. The following two chapters, 5 and 6, draw mainly on interview data. In the language of the now fashionable term 'social capital', Chapter 5 suggests the ways in which social capital is generated through the creation of social and political resources (Putnam, 1995; Kendall and Knapp, 1999; Putnam, 2000). Chapter 6 explores the networks between groups and the rationale for forging informal and formal alliances.

The interviews were undertaken with senior officers and post holders, paid or unpaid, and reflect their perspective and not that of members. In analysing them, the approach was to compare the interview accounts of the past and of current activities. We aimed to identify common themes in these accounts related to particular objectives, norms and values as well as networks of social relations with other groups and other stakeholders.

Some organizational characteristics of voluntary organizations

It has been argued that because people come together voluntarily for a common purpose, both trust and altruism play a larger part in social relations than in public or market sector organizations (Ware, 1989; Kendall and Knapp, 1999; Putnam, 2000). This has implications for organizational functioning. For example, Kendall and Knapp (1999) have suggested that although organizations may be more or less formally structured, high-trust relations allow a 'muddling through' to find solutions to problems and maintain organizational functioning. Furthermore, altruism, that is a concern to help others in the same predicament, rather than the pursuit of simply individualistic concerns for information and support may also be a factor that motivates both participation in, and public support for, specific health consumer groups.

Health consumer groups, like other voluntary organizations, are not only diverse but are able to change direction to suit new purposes (Evers, 1995). Typically, they carry out a wide range of activities and may consider these to be of equal importance. Activities shift over time due to both internal and external pressures, as well as to changes in leadership, but these may not be acknowledged or charted in a structured way. Billis (1993) has suggested that the use of volunteers and the more flexible decision-making structures in voluntary organizations lead to 'fuzziness and blurring' in who carries out activities – officers or members – and the boundaries between tasks. As a consequence, voluntary groups cannot be placed easily on a continuum in terms of elitist or participatory structures. There may also be 'stakeholder ambiguity' in the relationships between the various constituencies within voluntary organizations. An organization may have multiple stakeholders – trustees, board members, paid staff, clients, service users, volunteers, members – and a public that is, actually or potentially, perceived to be in need of services.

Kendall and Knapp (1999) have also referred to the 'tension field' within which voluntary organizations in the UK operate. One tension is between taking grants from government or commercial interests and maintaining a critical stance on policy while continuing to campaign on behalf of their constituency. Another is participating in government consultation exercises while continuing to provide services for members, the public and clients, whether under contract or otherwise. With limited funds and limitless possibilities for action, there are constant decisions to be made on priorities by those who lead voluntary organizations.

These concepts and insights were helpful in understanding the 'work-world' of those we interviewed and in interpreting the interview data. The interviews were with group leaders which, it could be argued, gave us an elite perspective. However, the line between officers, officials and members is often blurred. Paid officials had often suffered from a particular illness or had experience of caring for someone with an illness. Volunteers worked alongside paid staff. Rank and file members or clients took up leadership positions. This appeared to bring a particular empathy and commitment that made the sector a stimulating, if stressful, environment in which to work. However, further research on the internal dynamics of groups from the perspective of members, clients and those who do, and do not, join health consumer groups is required.

The characteristics of health consumer groups

The data sets and descriptive statistics

The definition of a health consumer group used in the data collection provided the basis of the identification of the data set within the condition areas (see Appendix 1). According to the typology developed in Chapter 1, the questionnaire data set consisted of:

- 11 formal alliance organizations with a mainly co-ordinating role;
- 14 population-based groups concerned with a range of issues related to a particular age, ethnic group or generic patient/carer activity;

- 98 condition-based groups which focused on a particular illness or condition: arthritis and related conditions, cancer, heart and circulatory disease, maternity and childbirth and mental health.

Most groups (92 per cent) were membership organizations. A small minority of groups provided services under contract to local providers or carried out client-centred research. These were mainly in the mental health field, where large and well established groups competed for contracts. A small number of groups within the population-based category received funding to support patient participation. Almost all groups were registered charities. Table 4.1 summarizes some of the key general differences between these groups identified from the questionnaire data.

Formal alliances tended to be London-based, which reflected their policy role, while condition-based groups were least likely to be based in London. It is probable that this also reflected the lower income level of many of the groups that focus on a particular illness. Table 4.2 summarizes some of the key characteristics of the interview sample.[1]

The formation of groups

The questionnaire data shows that most groups in the data set were of recent origin. As Table 4.3 shows, two-thirds of groups (n=77) had formed since 1981. This supports Wood's (2000, p. 36) claim that there has been a recent growth of groups concerned with patients and carers interests. The data are indicative rather than definitive as there is no reliable baseline information. Moreover groups form and disappear all the time.[2] Table 4.3 shows that formal alliance organizations are a relatively recent phenomenon. Almost three-quarters have been formed since 1981. Population-based groups have a longer history with a small percentage (8 per cent) formed prior to 1940 and 54 per cent before 1981.

A third of the condition-based groups were formed before 1981 and the remaining two-thirds over the past two decades. Within the condition areas, mental health and maternity/childbirth groups were formed earlier: 52 per cent of the mental health groups and 60 per cent of the maternity/childbirth groups were formed since 1981 compared to over 70 per cent of the arthritis (72 per cent), cancer (78 per cent) and heart/circulatory disease (77 per cent) groups.

82

Table 4.1   Dimensions of difference between types of group in questionnaire data set

	All groups		Formal alliance organizations		Population-based groups		Condition-based groups	
	n	(%)	n	(%)	n	(%)	n	(%)
Registered charity	110	91	8	80	14	100	88	91
Headquarters in London	47	38	10	91	9	64	28	29
Formed since 1981	77	66	8	73	6	46	63	68
Income £100 001 or over	49	47	6	60	8	67	35	41
Focused on single condition	92	75	6	55	none	none	86	88

Source: Questionnaire data set 1999.

Table 4.2   Differences between types of group in interview sample

	Formal alliance organizations		Population-based groups		Condition-based groups	
	n	(%)	n	(%)	n	(%)
Registered charity	8	100	9	100	20	95
Headquarters in London	6	67	7	78	12	57
Formed since 1981	7	78	3	33	10	48
Income £100 001 or over	5	56	8	89	15	71
Focused on single condition	6	67	none	none	20	95

Source: Questionnaire data set 1999.

Table 4.3 Breakdown of health consumer group formation, by type of group

Year group	All groups (%)	Formal alliance organizations (%)	Population-based groups (%)	Condition-based groups (%)
pre-1940	3	none	8	2
1941–1960	7	none	none	9
1961–1980	25	27	46	22
1981–date	66	73	46	68

Source: Questionnaire data set 1999. Due to rounding up some totals exceed 100.

Studies of the wider voluntary sector and sector-specific studies of the mental health and maternity/childbirth area, suggest that historical conditions have shaped voluntary group formation. Prevailing ideologies and perceptions of social problems at particular points in time can be linked to who forms a group and on whose behalf. Many charitable organizations were formed in the latter half of the nineteenth century, based on the principles of philanthropy, when a more leisured middle class set up charitable institutions for the, preferably deserving, poor. Some of these organizations are still in existence, although they have often changed their name and focus. For example, the Mental After Care Association was first established in 1879. The Stroke Association began life in 1899 as a charity to fund research into tuberculosis. In the early to mid-1980s, its interest expanded into other chest conditions, then into chest and heart conditions, and finally into stroke. In 1990 it was still called the Chest, Heart and Stroke Association but from 1991 became the Stroke Association, focusing solely on stroke and helping people affected by the condition.

Charitable groups aiming to support those in need were also formed following the Second World War to provide services and support for vulnerable people with particular illnesses or physical or mental disabilities. Arthritis Care (1947) and the Mental Health Foundation (1949) were first established to advocate, provide services and, in the case of the latter, to carry out innovative research. New groups may also form through amalgamation with others. For example, MIND (the National Association for Mental Health) was formed following the merger of three organizations in 1946[3] and in 1988 the Carers National Association was formed, following the merger of the National Council for Carers and their Elderly Dependants, and the Association of Carers.

Rogers and Pilgrim (2001) have argued that in the post-war period, new groups began to focus on campaigning for rights and an extension of state benefits and acted as pressure groups and advocates to pursue individual rights. This reflected the philosophy of welfare state provision and the gaps that became apparent within it. Another trigger for group formation in this period was where one voluntary organization perceived a gap in provision and, with the advantage of knowledge and experience, established another charity to fill it. Thus Help the Aged (1961) was established by Oxfam to facilitate the co-ordination of local groups concerned with elderly people while the Afyia Trust (1996), which seeks to develop community networks among ethnic minorities, was established with funding from the King's Fund.

More recently, group formation in the mental health field has been influenced by the rise of the new social movements referred to in Chapter 1. Such movements develop when an individual sense of identity associated with a minority status becomes recognized by people sharing that position, and networks develop as people are drawn together through a common commitment that is oppositional to dominant forms of status and power. Group membership provides a sense of belonging, reinforces identity and it has been suggested, fills the political vacuum left by the diminution of power of organized labour (Brown, 1984; Rogers and Pilgrim, 2001).

From the De Montfort study data, two trends can be observed in recent group formation. First, and most recently, the growth of formal alliance organizations. Second, within condition-based groups, the rise of groups established by service users themselves either to campaign or to provide mutual support, or both. Both these developments are important, supporting the claim for a 'health consumer movement'. Formal alliance organizations have the potential to create new structures for mobilization and engagement. Groups formed *by* people with particular conditions, rather than *for* people with those conditions, give a voice to new and previously marginalized constituencies.

The formation of groups by people who have experience of an illness or loss is not new but, from the interview data, their number appears to have increased across the condition areas. There is, however, a longer history of such groups in the maternity/childbirth area and in mental health. Tew (1998) describes how Prunella Briance, who had lost her baby and attributed this to technological intervention, went on to found the Natural Childbirth Association (1956), committed to the gentler methods then being promoted by Grantly Dick-Read. Renamed the National Childbirth Trust (1961), it has become the largest organization in the maternity/ childbirth sector. Another organization, the Association for Improvements in the Maternity Services (AIMS), formed in 1960, also committed to allowing women to assume greater control over childbirth and reducing technological interventions, gains active support from women who have had a poor experience of health care. Also within the sector, the Twins and Multiple Births Association (TAMBA) was formed in 1978 by parents who had had a multiple birth, and the Stillbirth and Neonatal Death Society (SANDS) was formed in 1981 by people who had experienced a stillbirth or neonatal loss. A common concern of founder members in all these groups was the lack of information, support and advice available and a wish to assist those in a similar position.

Within the mental health field a number of groups have been formed by those with personal experience of mental illness, as 'survivors'. Rogers and Pilgrim (1991) comment on the role of service users in the formation of groups such as Survivors Speak Out (1986) and the UK Advocacy Network (1990). Groups have also been formed by people as a result of their experience as carers. The National Schizophrenia Fellowship (1972) was formed after a carer shared his experiences of caring for someone with the illness in the letters page of *The Times* (see Levy, 1981). The Zito Trust provides a different example. It was established in 1994 by Jayne Zito after her husband was killed by a man with severe mental illness who had been discharged into the community. Her determination to get answers and explanations for her husband's death led to extensive media coverage. The Zito Trust was forged in the intense heat of media interest that surrounded the case and provided an opportunity for collective action to those seeking to prevent similar tragic events. The role of the media in group formation is discussed further in Chapter 11.

In the 1980s and 1990s a number of cancer organizations were formed as a consequence of personal experiences. In 1985, CancerBACUP was started by Vicky Clement-Jones, who was in her early 30s when diagnosed with ovarian cancer. She found that little information was available, so she set up the charity to provide this. As a doctor herself, but not a cancer specialist, she worked closely with a group of people, including her own oncologist, who took over as chair of the organization on her death (Clement-Jones, 1985). Other groups formed by people living with a condition or carers were Cancerlink (1982), the National Cancer Alliance (1994), Cancer Black Care (1995) and the UK Breast Cancer Coalition (1995). These organizations also sought to support people with cancer, for example Cancerlink supported the development of self-help groups, and the UK Breast Cancer Coalition developed a key role in lobbying for improvements in services.[4] For fuller accounts of group formation, see Revenson and Cassell (1991), McNeill (1997) and Watts (1997). Cartwright (1998) comments on the strength of community between women in cancer activism.

A number of small groups within the arthritis area were formed by patients with relatively rare conditions. An account given in interview by the founder member of one such group demonstrated the process of recognition, attribution and action which was repeated in other interviews with founder members. She said:

> In 1987 I'd been told I'd got...a rare condition and I met a girl called [name withheld] in hospital and found out that she'd got the same condition. [It] has got such bizarre signs and symptoms I honestly thought I was going doolally: psychiatric home, hospital next step. But having talked to her, I found she'd got all the same signs and symptoms, and just finding somebody who understood and didn't think I was going round the bend, it was so helpful. We said if it helps us to be able to talk to someone who understands, maybe it will help other people [too]. (gi15)

She went on to describe the early stages of running a group:

> We ran it with the help of our husbands for the first couple of years. We had to put our own money in and after about three years it was too big we couldn't cope and we got other people to help. (gi15)

And finally, she described the setting up a more formal organization when a litigation against a drug company supplying a drug associated with the condition began:

> Then, in 1992 when the [drug] litigation registration started and we were absolutely swamped. We had to get more and more people involved and [set up] a committee. (gi15)

By contrast, within the heart and circulatory disease area, only one group in the interview sample was formed by patients – the British Cardiac Patients Association (1982). Even here, the formation of the group was encouraged by doctors working at Harefield Hospital. The role of doctors in group formation for certain condition areas will be discussed further in a later chapter.[5] Other groups in the sector have been formed by patients, for example Different Strokes, established in 1996 by a group of 'younger stroke survivors who recognized and had experienced the then woeful lack of support and shortage of relevant information' (Different Strokes, 2003). Cardiac Risk in the Young (1995) was set up by a parent whose son was diagnosed with a potentially fatal heart condition and the Cardiomyopathy Association (1990) was established by a patient diagnosed with hypertrophic cardio-myopathy, a heart condition associated with 'adult sudden death syndrome'.

A common theme in the formation of condition-based groups is the movement from a personal pain and loss experience to political activity and group formation. The motivating factors, as hinted at in the example above, are often initial feelings of distress, anger and fear that constitute a threat to the self. This is compounded by a failure of the health service to meet people's emotional needs and their need for information. For example, a startling statistic in a national survey of 65 000 people who had had cancer was that 62 per cent had left the hospital after a diagnosis with no written information (DoH, 2000d). Finding others in a similar position appears to aid the processes of producing a narrative and biographical reconstruction (Bury, 1982; Charmaz, 1983; Williams, 1984). Borkman (1999) in a study of self-help groups in the United States, shows how shared experiences of particular conditions acts as a force to promote mutual aid.

Pain and loss experiences and the formation of condition-based groups

Why has there been an apparent increase in groups formed as a consequence of personal experience? Rogers and Pilgrim (2001, p. 109) link this to political forces: the demise of old labour movements; the rise and example of new social movements based on a sense of identity that provides 'a ticket of entry to the movement and an ongoing source of motivation and group solidarity'. However, unlike some new social movements, the new wave of health consumer groups do not tend to take direct action or open protest but use the more conventional channels of pressure group politics, such as lobbying and campaigning.

In another contribution to the debate, Jennings (1999) has drawn attention to the way in which life events such as illness, injury, or death may act as a catalyst for individual action, group formation and collective action within the public sphere. How blame and responsibility are allocated and the extent of social approval for both those living with a condition or loss, and the popularity of a cause, may aid, or inhibit, the consolidation of a group. The media can play a crucial role in both forming and reflecting public opinion. It can also act as a channel of communication for those facing a similar predicament or intending to join in collective action. Other factors that may aid group formation are the clustering of events, and social patterning, such as age, gender and ethnicity. Although considerable attention has been paid by sociologists to the impact of illness in renegotiating identity, this interest has not extended to an analysis of illness as a trigger to individual and collective action. However, studies of the formation of particular groups show that in a number of instances, an individual or like-minded individuals have responded to a traumatic life event by seeking explanations, finding common cause with others, forming a group and, as subsequent chapters will illustrate, engaging in political activity.

In the health and illness area, group formation may strengthen critical and challenging views of biomedicine, drug and medical technologies and the desire to take control of one's own body or alleviate burdens by seeking support from others in a similar position – a set of views that could be termed 'consumerist'. Interviews for the research supported Jennings' (1999) point that the media, and the extent to which a cause is socially approved, can affect the visibility of particular conditions. Letters to newspapers, television programmes and news coverage were frequently mentioned by interviewees as important pathways to group formation. A fit with existing political agendas is also important to the promotion of particular groups and causes. These factors will be discussed further in subsequent chapters.

So far, a working hypothesis from the questionnaire and interview data is that groups formed over the past two decades reflect increasing engagement by service users. This health consumer or 'service user' movement has not only affected group formation, but also the values and ways of working of groups formed earlier, when different values and traditions were prevalent. As will be shown in the next chapter, the internal dynamics of groups has shifted towards a greater orientation towards users.

The activities of health consumer groups

The groups examined by the De Montfort study spanned a variety of common and rare conditions and illustrated the diversity of aims and objectives. Some are concerned with patients, others with carers. In some condition areas there are groups that promote policies in opposition to each other. In mental health there are groups that favour community care and voluntary treatment while others, in the interests of public safety, prioritise hospital care and compulsory treatment in the community. In the maternity/childbirth field, some groups give greater emphasis to women's right to choose, while others actively promote home deliveries and non-interventionist methods. This 'consumer pluralism' has advantages for people who wish their views to be represented.

However, the questionnaire data indicated that most groups undertake a range of similar activities (see also Wood, 2000). Table 4.4 shows how 14 activities commonly undertaken by voluntary groups in 1999, were ranked in order of importance. This indicates that about three-quarters of the groups undertook service activities (information and support); policy-related activities (raising awareness, training and influencing national policy) and organizational maintenance activities, such as fundraising and recruiting members.

Table 4.4 Activities undertaken by health consumer groups, ranked by order of importance (all groups)

	Percentage of groups rating activities 'very important' or 'important'
Providing information	98
Publicity/raising awareness	97
Providing advice/support	96
Building networks	84
Fundraising	84
Promoting self-help	84
Influencing national policy	82
Education and training	76
Recruiting members	73
Patient/carer advocacy	72
Promoting research	72
Influencing local policy	63
Providing goods/services	57
Undertaking research	48

Source: Questionnaire data set 1999.

Providing information and support

Other health care stakeholders, both within and outside the voluntary health sector, commented that health consumer groups had a particularly valuable role in providing access to high quality information for the public. Leaflets, websites, internet chat rooms and member networks can be accessed by the public, sometimes for a small fee. Some groups publish leaflets on particular illnesses or conditions, which may also be available in different languages. Some groups also produce information on video. Eighty per cent of groups said they had help-lines and for some groups, such as Cancerlink and the College of Health, this was a major activity. At the time of the interview, the College of Health was receiving about 80 000 calls a year and these were used for policy development. As an interviewee said:

> Obviously we analyse those and the waiting list help-line...but we send a questionnaire out to every person who uses it. And we do annual surveys of people who listen to the help-line tape so we get

a lot of feedback about the problems that people are experiencing with the health service. And then obviously the actual research work, consumer audit qualitative research [that] feeds directly into identifying what people's problems are.

Another, from Help the Aged, commented:

We log all of the calls that come in. The advice team identifies calls on social policy forms, rather like CAB [Citizen's Advice Bureaux]... so that we are specifically collecting information about major problems like access to community care and we have a whole list of anony-mous examples of what people have experienced, the kind of issues which they face...and we publish that once a year. It is a devastating document, as you can imagine. Usually the majority of calls are around financial matters. But last year, for the first time, they were around access to community and residential care.

Support for members was often led by a group's local branches and is discussed more fully in the next chapter.

Politics and policy

Across the various types of group and condition areas, influen-cing national policy was regarded as important by the majority of health consumer groups. In the questionnaire, over four-fifths of all groups stated that influencing national policy was 'important' (21 per cent) or 'very important' (61 per cent). For some, such as the Maternity Alliance, policy activity was continuous as they covered a wide span of issues affecting the maternity rights of women. This consists of networking with civil servants, lobbying parliament, responding to enquiries from the media, and actively seeking publicity. Most groups take part in campaigns periodically and most health consumer groups have active media and political contacts and seek opportunities to put their point of view across. Party conferences provide another opportunity for making, and cementing, contacts. For example, in 1998, the National Heart Forum, Breakthrough Breast Cancer and the Family Planning Association gave a presentation at a fringe meeting at the Labour Party Conference to highlight common policy issues on women health. A number of groups launched national awareness weeks to highlight issues and attract people into the membership. For example, Arthritis Care, SANDS, Group Action into Steroid Prescribing (GASP) and the National Childbirth Trust (in relation to breastfeeding) had all sponsored awareness weeks. From the mid 1990s onwards groups also participated in professional conferences to present the user perspective.

Although almost three-quarters of groups saw promoting research as 'very important' or 'important', less than half undertook research or saw this as a priority. Whether these activities were undertaken depended on the mission of the groups and the resources available. Larger groups concerned with making a major impact on national policy undertook research on issues that were not necessarily current government priorities. For example, the National Heart Forum (1998) produced the report *Social Inequalities in Heart Disease: Opportunities for Action*, and the National Schizophrenia Fellowship (1999) launched *Picking up the Pieces* on policies for people with severe mental illness. In 2001, the Long-term Medical Conditions Alliance (LMCA) published *Making People's Voices Heard* (LMCA, 2001a). The aim of these documents was to raise awareness, improve knowledge and influence policy-makers.

Influencing local policy was regarded as important by a majority of health consumer groups, with 63 per cent stating that this was either 'important' or 'very important' in the questionnaire. Some groups focused on the local level as that was where they could make the most impact. For example, the National Ankylosing Spondylitis Society, an arthritis group, with support from local hospitals negotiated the use of physiotherapy departments 'out-of-hours' for their members. Both SANDS and TAMBA respectively work with local hospital departments to develop guidelines to help parents who have a stillbirth, neo-natal death or a multiple birth. This includes providing a help-line to their respective organizations. A main aim of the Afyia Trust and National Association for Patient Participation (NAPP) is community development and improving local practice, so they operate mainly at this level. The respondent from the Stroke Association commented that a significant proportion of their activity was

actually working within the NHS . . . and we also have our managers [who] are focusing very much on working with local NHS trusts, primary care groups and primary care trusts in trying to improve the services in their local areas.

The interviewee from National Childbirth Trust, which also provides training to enable members to represent the interests of women, also commented:

> We have been successful in getting user [representatives] onto multi-disciplinary maternity service liaison committees at local level and its the local work in many ways that we think is as important as anything else.

A comparison between different categories of group showed some differences between their activities. Formal alliance organizations undertook a more limited range of core activities (those that were rated as 'very important' or 'important' by three-quarters of groups). These were geared towards influencing policy and included: building networks, influencing national policy, providing information, publicity/raising awareness and influencing local policy. In contrast, both population-based groups and condition-based groups identified a broader range of activities. However, for the latter, member support activities were rated by a higher percentage of groups as 'very important' or 'important'. This reflects their significant role in helping people with illness and pain and loss experiences.

Services or policy

When asked to choose between whether their primary role was providing services for members, the public or their client group, or to influence policy or whether they were equally committed to both, there were differences between types of group, as shown in Figure 4.1.[6] As might be expected, a large majority of formal alliance organizations (82 per cent) said they were primarily concerned with policy while the majority of condition-based groups identified themselves mainly as service providers. Population-based groups tended to give no preference, with 46 per cent stating that they had an equal commitment to both.

Within the condition areas, mental health groups were more likely to identify policy as their primary purpose, although this was still a minority (17 per cent), followed by cancer groups (11 per cent) heart/circulatory groups (8 per cent) and maternity/childbirth groups (6 per cent). No arthritis groups stated that influencing policy was their primary purpose. Services for members

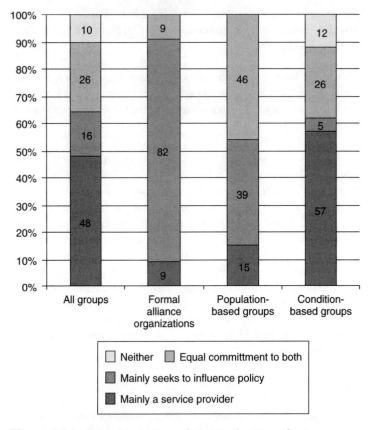

Figure 4.1   Primary purpose of groups, by type of group

Source: Questionnaire data set 1999.

could include (for a majority of groups) access to support groups and networks, special events and activities, and (for a minority) residential and community care facilities, access to buying appliances and products at less than retail prices, and access to training classes or counsellors. For example, the National Childbirth Trust provides access to locally-based breastfeeding and childbirth counsellors, and Arthritis Care runs four hotels, specially adapted for people with arthritis.

Issues not on the agenda

Reference should also be made to areas in which interviewees said they had little impact, or to which they did not refer to at all. Many interviewees said that primary care was important but they were uncertain about how to influence the practice of GPs and they were not represented on primary care groups or trusts. A number of groups expressed puzzlement about the direction of primary care reforms, which at the time of the interviews were in a transitional phase. Private sector health care was not mentioned at all by interviewees and serves to reinforce the point that health consumer groups focus predominantly on the NHS.

The financial and human resources of health consumer groups

Financial resources

Health consumer groups must raise the financial resources required to carry out their activities. Those that are registered as charities (91 per cent) are bound by the requirements of the Charity Commission, which aim to ensure their accountability, efficiency and effectiveness and provide guidance and support for both registered charities and those who wish to register. It is likely that those groups that were not charities did not register because they were too small or because they wished to maintain greater independence.

There has been an ongoing debate on whether the Charity Commission can both support and regulate the sector, and whether present arrangements are sufficient to prevent fraud and malad-ministration (Commission on the Future of the Voluntary Sector, 1996; NCVO, 2001).[7] Wood (2000), who looked at patient groups' annual reports and accounts, was scathing about the lack of proper accounting methods. In this research, one well informed interviewee commented that the current Charity Commission arrangements were 'fatuous' (si12). Concern has also been expressed about whether health consumer groups that receive public funding should be more accountable for how money has been spent and ensure value for money (see NCVO, 2001; Kendall

Table 4.5   Health consumer group income, by type of group

	All groups (%)	Formal alliance organizations (%)	Population-based groups (%)	Condition-based groups (%)
£10 000 or less	16	30	none	17
10 001–100 000	38	10	33	42
100 001–1000 000	33	60	33	29
1000 001–10 000 000	8	none	17	7
10 000 001 plus	6	none	17	5
Total	100	100	100	100

Source: Questionnaire data set 1999. Due to rounding, some totals exceed 100.

and Knapp, 1999). Table 4.5 gives a breakdown of income in 1998/99 by type of group.

The data show that only 6 per cent of health consumer groups have an income of £10 million or over per annum, with 16 per cent having an income of £10 000 or less. Most groups (87 per cent) have incomes of £1 million or less per annum.

Like the voluntary sector as a whole, a small minority of groups accounted for the vast majority of the sectors' income. The total income of the groups in the data set was approximately £206 million, yet six groups accounted for 77 per cent of this. The 54 per cent of groups with an income of £100 000 or less per annum shared less than 1 per cent of the total annual income recorded. However, in comparison to the voluntary sector in general, health consumer groups seem to have a broader spread of income. According to the Charities Aid Foundation 66 per cent of charities have an income of less than £10 000 per annum, yet this was the case for just 16 per cent of our questionnaire data set (Charities Aid Foundation, 2002). One possible reason for the difference is that health charities attract more public support than other charities (Parker, 2002). Another is that the charities' Register includes local and regional groups which were more likely to have smaller incomes.

In terms of the income going to various types of group within the data set, population-based groups received 38 per cent of the total income and condition-based groups just over 60 per cent. Formal alliance organizations accounted for less than 1 per cent of the total income. This is probably explained by their focus on policy, their lack of interaction with the public and that they may only have organizational members. Within the conditions areas, most arthritis groups (88 per cent) and around half the groups in the cancer, heart/circulatory disease, maternity/childbirth and mental health sector, had an income of £100 000 or less per annum. The range of incomes within each condition area varied, often considerably. For example, a fifth of mental health groups had an income of £10 million or over per annum, while a quarter of arthritis groups and 29 per cent of maternity/childbirth groups survived on £10 000 or less.

Human resources

Like the voluntary sector as a whole, health consumer groups both employ staff and draw on volunteers. The questionnaire data set showed that three-quarters of groups (76 per cent) had paid staff at headquarters. Conversely, almost a quarter of groups did not, with the implication that they were run by volunteers. Of those that had paid staff at headquarters, 38 per cent employed two or less full time equivalent members of staff. Only 20 per cent of groups employed more than ten people and 40 per cent had between two and ten members of staff. Less than a quarter of the groups had paid staff countrywide in branches, regions or within the countries that make up the UK. The voluntary sector has a tradition of unpaid staff working alongside paid staff. Half of the questionnaire data set said they had unpaid staff working at headquarters but half did not; 40 per cent said they had unpaid staff working countrywide. This figure is unlikely to reflect the full extent of volunteering, as 'staff' implies an administrative role and is unlikely to cover most member-led work.

As the research focused on the involvement of groups in the policy process, questionnaire respondents were asked if their organization employed specialist policy staff, such as policy or press officers. Although such staff were more likely to be paid, elected but unpaid post holders may also play a policy role. Again, the data showed there was considerable diversity with 29 per cent of groups having no paid policy staff. Of those groups having paid policy staff, 31 per cent had two or more and only one organization employed more than ten. Any voluntary organization wishing to influence policy and handle media relations effectively is likely to need such specialists, and for some groups this is a high priority. For example, one interviewee commented that in his organization the appointment of a policy officer took priority over a finance officer post. However, for many small groups, and this was more likely to be condition-based groups, limited resources did not permit a choice (see also Table 10.1). One member of staff was often responsible for all activity, including policy work. As the interviewee from one group said:

> Some of the very big organizations have actually got people employed to do lobbying. We're not even professionals... We are parents that are volunteering because there's a need... but the concern is that we just don't have the resources or the manpower. (gi34)

Poor staffing levels were acknowledged to be a barrier to influence and a matter for concern for nearly three-quarters of the questionnaire groups. As the official from one formal alliance organization said: 'You have got to be a certain size before your voice can be heard, you have got to have... back-up staff' (gi19).

One group, which had had a public relations officer but had not been able to renew the position because of financial difficulties, was torn between the awareness of the value of such a role and the need to provide other services. An interviewee said:

> We used to [have a PR officer] about five years ago... and it made a huge difference... but she left at a time when our funding was very uncertain and its always one of those jobs that unless you have that extra money, you can always cut back on, even though it is a very essential part of the organization. (gi18)

Sources of income

Questionnaire respondents were asked to select their sources of income. Figure 4.2 shows that two-thirds of groups received, membership contributions and public donations. Forty per cent derived income from charitable trusts. Sponsorship from the private

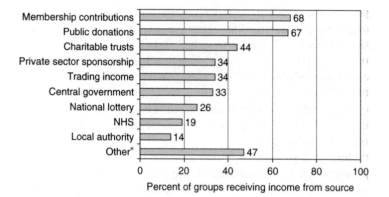

Figure 4.2   Sources of health consumer group income 1998/99
(all groups)

* includes fundraising and return on investment.

Source: Questionnaire data set 1999.

sector and central government was a source of income for about
a third of groups, and for a similar proportion, trading income.
A quarter of the groups said that the national lottery was a source
of income. Others received funds from the NHS and local
authorities. These findings probably reflect the national policy
orientation of the groups in the data set. Findings for local groups
would almost certainly have a different profile.

A breakdown of the data show that formal alliance organizations and population-based groups were more likely to report
income from statutory sources such as central government, local
authorities and the NHS. For example, half of the formal alliances had received income from central government, compared
to 40 per cent of population-based groups and just 30 per cent of
condition-based groups. Formal alliances were also more likely
than condition-based groups to receive funding from the private
sector. However, nearly three-quarters of condition-based
groups (72 per cent) received donations from the public, compared to half of the population-based groups and just 40 per cent
of formal alliance organizations.

Within the condition areas, over half of the mental health
groups received funding from central government, compared to
around a third of cancer (29 per cent) heart/circulatory disease

(33 per cent) and maternity/childbirth (28 per cent). No arthritis group said they received funding from central government. However, mental health groups were less likely to receive funding from the general public (57 per cent), compared to cancer (71 per cent), maternity/childbirth (72 per cent), arthritis (75 per cent) and heart/circulatory disease (83 per cent). This is perhaps due to the stigma attached to mental illness and is a tangible manifestation of the lack of social approval that some mental health groups referred to in interview.

Most groups sought funding from a number of sources. However, a few received a significant proportion of their funding from only one source. Four groups received over 60 per cent of their income from central government in 1998/99, including a population-based group which received 90 per cent from this source. A small number of groups received a large proportion of their income from other charities, indicating an element of cross-subsidy in the sector. One maternity/childbirth group and one mental health organization received over 95 per cent of their income from another charity, while two cancer groups and one population-based group received over 80 per cent from another charitable organization.

It has been suggested that in the UK the business sector has not had a tradition of generous charitable giving. In the USA charitable donations have been reported as averaging 1 per cent of pre-tax profits (*Guardian*, 2001, p. 19). Available data for the UK show that the top 100 companies gave only 0.4 per cent of their pre-tax profits to charity in 2000 (Murphy, 2001, p. 5). Information on sources of funding are hard to come by, as there is no standard format for reporting this information in annual reports. The topic warrants further investigation, particularly in relation to pharmaceutical company sponsorship (see Chapter 8).

As most health consumer groups have a variety of funding sources they have a degree of independence, unlike the situation in some European countries where, in the absence of government support, pharmaceutical companies play a larger role in funding patient groups. Indeed, in interview a few groups said they would not accept funding from certain sources as this might inhibit their freedom of action. A small number felt this way about accepting funding from government. For example, one interviewee commented: 'The moment you get funding, they start pulling the strings' (gi3).

Section 64 funding

Through the (Health Services and Public Health Act 1968) Section 64 scheme, the Department of Health provides a specific source of funding for the health and social care sector.[8] Section 64 grants are open to national voluntary organizations working in health and personal social services in England. A similar scheme exists from voluntary organizations in Scotland, Northern Ireland and Wales. For government, this provides a mechanism to support its policy objectives and the criteria for bids are set out annually (DoH, 1998c). For groups, it is seen as an important funding source as grants generally run for three years. Three types of grant can be awarded: core funding, capital grants or project grants. In 1998/1999, £20.8 million pounds was allocated through 620 separate grants to 440 voluntary organizations (DoH, 1998c, p. 13), indicating that some received more than one grant. From information provided by the Department of Health, data on Section 64 grants were extracted for groups in the questionnaire data set. As Table 4.6 indicates, in 1988/89, 32 were awarded. By 1993/94, this had risen to 64 and by 1998/99 to 106. By 1998/99 groups in the data set received around 10 per cent of all Section 64 monies available. The increase was mainly due to a large increase in project grants.

Data provided by the Department of Health indicates that there has been a change in the type of grants awarded. As shown in Table 4.7, over the period there was a significant increase in the total sum awarded for project grants and over a 50 per cent decline in the total sum awarded through core grants.

Table 4.6   Number of grants received by health consumer groups between 1988/89 and 1998/99, by type of grant

	1988/89	1993/94	1998/99
Core	24	26	35
Project	6	32	70
Capital	1	none	1
Not stated	1	6	none

Source: Calculated from Department of Health data.

Table 4.7 Amount of funding received by health consumer groups between 1988/89 and 1998/99, by type of grant

	1988/89 (£)000	1993/94 (£)000	1998/99 (£)000
Core	1 421	1 671	690
Project	110	835	1 968
Capital	10	none	10
Not stated	21	101	none

Source: Calculated from Department of Health data.

Financial position

However, despite additional sources of funding such as the National Lottery, a large majority of groups responding to the questionnaire (79 per cent) claimed that lack of money was a barrier to involvement in the policy process, while 83 per cent said that lack of staff was a key constraint. The condition-based groups were most likely to say that the lack of financial resources was a constraint, perhaps because there were more smaller groups in this area and they had a wider range of functions.

In interview, a concern about uncertainty in the flow of financial resources was highlighted by many groups. Most had to prioritize their activities continually as commitments outran resources. Considerable energy was spent in raising funds, and some interviewees believed that fund-raising was becoming more difficult. One interviewee commented that she spent most of her time 'sniffing around money' (gi5). The lack of funding was felt in both large and small organizations, as an interviewee from one of the largest groups in the study said: '[We would like] adequate resource[s] to deal with the variety and diversity of areas we're trying to cover. You tend to sort of jump from one thing to another and I feel that I'm not necessarily covering enough of them in enough depth' (gi30).

Particular concerns were that many funding bodies were reluctant to provide core grants for supporting organizational infrastructure. Even in instances when such funding was provided, this could be short-term and some groups argued that longer-term funding was necessary to help them build their organizational capacity. Project applications make considerable demands as they have to be tailored to specific criteria, take time and energy to prepare, and can distort longer-term objectives. They also take resources away from core functions, such as supporting members and the public, raising the group's profile, and planning for the future. These problems were particularly severe for small groups. Another problem mentioned was the levying of value-added-tax, which was seen as a drain on the resources of voluntary organizations.[9]

However, some interviewees suggested that the challenge of managing on tight resources was part and parcel of the voluntary sector environment and that their organizations provided good value for money. As one respondent from a cancer health consumer group said:

> We still are fighting for more influence and I think it's in part a resource issue. You know the professional organizations, and obviously the commercial bodies, have a lot more resources to spend on this kind of thing than we do and I think we actually do very well considering how small we are and how few resources we have. (gi31)

Groups recognized that applications for funding would be more likely to be successful if their agenda fitted with that of government. An interviewee from one mental health group believed that the renewal of their Section 64 grant had occurred partly because government needed their support. He said: 'I think it's a strategy...it's handy to keep having us around...they find it useful to have us as an organization, because we're actually supporting their reforms' (gi28). Raising funds, accounting for expenditure and the relationships that this involves is, as Kendall and Knapp (1999) comment, part of the tension field of voluntary sector/funder relationships. Organizations want to pursue particular goals while retaining as much freedom of manoeuvre as possible. Funding bodies, on the other hand, require accountability.

Members and membership

The size of membership

Most groups in the questionnaire data set (92 per cent) had some form of membership, this could be through individual membership

Table 4.8 Individual membership of health consumer groups (all groups)

	(%)
1–500	33
501–1000	23
1001–10 000	39
10 001 plus	6
Total	100

Source: Questionnaire data set 1999. Due to rounding up total exceeds 100.

(82 per cent) and organizational membership. Within the questionnaire data set, 41 per cent of groups included other organizations as members. Cross-membership facilitated the exchange of information and networking. In order to maintain a consumer focus, some groups restricted attendance at annual general meetings and/or voting rights to the individual or lay membership.

Among the groups with a membership, there was considerable variation in size. Table 4.8 shows that a third of the groups had an individual membership of 500 or less (and about half of these had a 100 or fewer individual members). About a quarter had between 501 and a thousand individual members and over a third between 1001 and 10 000. A small number of groups, about 6 per cent, were very large with over 10 000 members.

Individual membership could include both those with a condition or illness, and/or their carers and relatives. Some groups in the mental health field and those concerned with elderly people in residential care were composed mainly of relatives or carers. Almost two-thirds of groups (63 per cent) said they included relatives and carers as members. The extensive networking or health consumer groups with health professionals was demonstrated by the large number of groups that said they had health care professionals (68 per cent), or professional associations, (34 per cent) as members. This is discussed further in Chapter 7.

The internal structure of groups

There was considerable diversity in the internal structures of health consumer groups. This was inevitable given the variations in size. Some had boards of appointed trustees or a governing council that included sponsors and celebrities. Most groups (65 per cent) said they included patients or carers on their main decision-making body. A large majority of groups had some form of annual general meeting and elections to official positions. The direct involvement of service users themselves at a senior decision-making level has been a major trend in recent years. Those who have had, or have, a mental illness or who have been diagnosed as having arthritis, cancer or heart/circulatory disease are thus able contribute to decision-making. Charities from the older philan-thropic tradition of providing services for clients are nowadays more likely to have mechanisms for including those clients in decision-making through both formal and informal means. The interview data showed that a small minority of groups were run by a largely self-appointed committee, generally either because they were very small or because they wished to maintain freedom of action. However, these committees were often composed of activists with first-hand experience of the condition.

Nearly half of the health consumer groups in the questionnaire data set (49 per cent) said that their organization had a countrywide network of branches. For example, in 1999 Arthritis Care had a membership of 59 000 and 630 UK wide branches while the National Childbirth Trust had membership of 45 000 and 450 branches. It was slightly more common for condition-based groups to have branches (54 per cent) than population-based groups (43 per cent), although the latter often worked with local groups, helping to support and co-ordinate their activities. There seemed to be two types of arrangement relating to the degree of independence local groups had:

- 40 per cent of the groups that had branches stated that decision-making was undertaken at headquarters.
- 60 per cent said that local support groups were autonomous from headquarters. As long as they followed general guidelines set by the national organization, they were free to operate as they wished.

As many condition-based groups were relatively small and a number of larger groups have a local group or a branch structure, there is a level of operation in the health consumer group sector that is close to the grassroots. Olson (1965) has argued that smallness was an important factor is maintaining a high level of involvement and commitment in organizations. It became clear during the interviews that the maintenance of good relationships between the centre and the periphery was a major concern for headquarters staff, and is discussed below.

Health professionals were also involved at the decision-making level in many groups. Almost half of the groups said that doctors were represented on their decision-making body, although they did not always have voting rights. However, a small number of groups deliberately chose not to include doctors for ideological and political reasons, as they wished to be seen as user-centred and to determine their own agenda. Some population-based groups and formal alliance organizations did not include professionals because they were dealing with broader and less specialized issues.

The data supports the suggestion by Billis and Glennerster (1998) that a feature of voluntary organizations is stakeholder ambiguity. The clear defining of roles characteristic of bureaucratic organizations gives way to a blurring of roles. The fact that members, officials and board members may also be service recipients is one example. Many groups had volunteers who worked alongside paid officers, and there were also devolved management structures. The authority gap between office holders and users may thus be narrower in health consumer groups. A common concern to respond to user issues potentially overrides status differences. Voluntary organizations have been criticized for being undemocratic as they do not always have openly representative systems of appointment, but this is to apply a criterion from the sphere of state political and bureaucratic systems and may be inappropriate to more flexible and grassroots bodies such as health consumer groups (Fogarty, 1990). However, the De Montfort study did not seek to explore members' views and therefore further investigation of the internal dynamics of health consumer groups is merited.

Conclusion

The questionnaire data showed that health consumer groups are extremely diverse, not just in terms of their strategies, focus and scope, but also in their size, income, staffing and internal structures. In terms of formation, with some important exceptions, the mental health and the maternity/childbirth groups in general were formed earlier than groups in other condition areas. They led the way in terms of having a service-user focus. Size in terms of membership and income is an important variable, in that it affects the staffing and the range of activities a group can undertake. It has also been shown by Vincent (2002) that larger groups are more likely to have a greater influence on policy, a point considered further in Chapter 9.

However, the interview data showed that despite these differences, groups shared many of the same concerns and dilemmas, for example, the difficulty in maintaining resources and attracting funding. Moreover, the groups shared a common focus on patients, users and carers. This, it can be argued, helped to generate bonds of mutual trust within and between groups, discussed in more detail in the two following chapters.

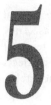

Health consumer groups: social and political resources

It has been claimed that voluntary forms of association are high on social capital: that is, they generate social and political resources that are not only beneficial to those involved, but also have a secondary benefit in contributing to civic society (Putnam, 1993, 1995, 2000). The aim of this chapter is to examine the values, knowledge claims and working practices of a cross-section of health consumer groups which the analysis of data showed to be widely shared. The chapter considers how group leaders generated the social and political resources that contribute to social capital, how network and trust relations were maintained. These provided the foundation for health consumer groups' claim to represent both members and the wider public interest discussed in later chapters.

The data were collected through interviews with senior officers and post holders from a cross-section of 39 groups. As the research was exploratory, a process of analytic induction was followed to identify recurring themes on the internal relationships within health consumer groups as they sought to maintain the group's activities and participate in the policy process (see Appendix 1 for further details). Interviewees made a number of claims relating to what they considered their strengths to be. These were remarkably consistent across the interviews, irrespective of the type and size of group. There were some exceptions, or negative cases, and these are referred to. It can be argued that exceptions serve to highlight a particular discourse, an underlying normative order and a culture shared by participants in this form of organization. Before presenting the data, some of the definitions and approaches to understanding the role of social capital in voluntary organizations in general, and the health consumer sector in particular, will be discussed.

The contribution of health consumer groups: a form of social capital?

Analyses of social capital are based on the claim that social interaction or sociability builds relations of trust and the capacity for collective action to resolve problems or put pressure on government to do so. Thus social interaction can lead to political engagement. However, definitions abound. In essence, these are based either on economic or social constructivist views of the world. For example, Coleman writes:

> The term capital, as part of the concept, implies a resource or factor input that facilitates production, but it is not consumed or otherwise used up in production... social refers in this context to aspects of social organization, ordinarily informal relationships, established for non-economic purposes, yet with economic consequences. (1993, p.175)

On the other hand Putnam defines social capital as

> features of social organization such as networks, norms and social trust that facilitate co-ordination and co-operation for mutual benefit. (1995, p. 67)

Similar definitions have been adopted by the World Bank and OECD and MacGillivray (2002). Distinctions have been made between different forms of social capital such as 'bonding' social capital – characterized by strong bonds such as kin or family networks; 'bridging' social capital that enables strangers to associate around a common interest or cause; and 'linking' social capital that links different power or status groups (Cabinet Office, Performance and Innovation Unit, 2002).

Although useful at a conceptual level, social capital through forms of association is difficult to measure. There is also a lack of clarity about the constituent components of social capital and therefore some circularity in the argument. This particularly affects the claim made by Putnam that voluntary association leads to stronger and more democratic forms of civic engagement (Almond and Verba, 1989; Putnam, 1995). The social capital thesis has been widely criticized and from a more sceptical European tradition it has been argued that voluntary associations inevitably involve those already more politically aware and relatively privileged in terms of social and political capital (Dahrendorf, 1993, quoted in Dekker and van den Broek, 1998.) In other words, such associations are more effective in creating bonding or bridging capital than linking capital. It should be noted, moreover, that voluntary activity may lead to networks that can weaken the social fabric such as criminal gangs and terrorist organizations.

Trust in voluntary associations

According to Coleman (1990, p. 302), social capital is not a single entity but facilitated by individuals within a social structure. He argues that: 'Like other forms of capital, social capital is productive, making possible the achievement of certain ends that would not be attainable in its absence... Unlike other forms of capital, social capital inheres in the structure of relations between persons and among persons.' Whatever the definition of social capital, trust relations appear to be central to the generation of social networks.

In a recent and useful theoretical contribution to the debate, Anheier and Kendall (2002) consider three approaches to explaining why national surveys show that the public place greater trust in voluntary associations. First, an economic and rational actor analysis suggests that voluntary organizations have supply-side advantages. People perceive non-profit organizations as less likely to take advantage of user vulnerability in the services they provide. This is enhanced by a high degree of stakeholder ownership where members or associates as participants have an interest in securing services or taking part in activities that suit their needs. Thus, trust is protected on both the supply and demand side.

Second, from a sociological or social constructionist perspective, theories on community have stressed the importance of the tacit agreements that prefigure contracts. Giddens (1990) has referred to trust as presumed reliability. People trust each other because they must. Trust is presumed and continues until shown by events to be misguided. This notion of trust begins to link with the social structures that encourage interaction and networks referred to by Putnam (1995). The important issue is therefore the reinforcement of trust through values, norms and ways of working that guide interaction, as suggested by Luhmann (1979). Anheier and Romo (1992), referred to in Anheier and Kendall (2002, p. 349), suggest that at least some types of voluntary organizations, particularly religious organizations are 'well positioned to draw on pre-existing trust that is unlikely to be questioned in the course of transactions', and indeed, such trust may be reinforced by ritual.

A third factor referred to by Anheier and Kendall (2002) draws on socio-psychological theories of motivation. Altruism, empathy and, for some groups, the need for action and redress can explain group formation. Health consumer groups more specifically give people opportunities for positive interactions with people who have a shared interest.

There have also been attempts to develop classifications of different forms of trust. 'Characteristic-based trust' is linked to the person and that person's cultural background. 'Process-based trust' is based on perceptions of past or the proven reliability of present exchanges while 'institution-based trust' is based on institutional credibility (Anheier and Kendall, 2002, p. 349). Other terminology used in relation to social capital has referred to 'thick' trust and 'thin' trust; the first being more deeply embedded in informal social structures such as family and kin and the latter relating to more casual social contacts (Putnam, 2000).

In the case of UK health consumer groups, there may be special factors at work that enhance trust. In the terminology of the economic model, supply-side factors may be enhanced by a tradition of altruism and possibly by the legal framework provided by the Charity Commission, however flawed. Furthermore, a high proportion, over nine-tenths, of health consumer groups are member groups. Many recently formed groups have some characteristics in common with new social movements as they are based on an identity shared as a consequence of a pain and loss experience. Shared needs, and a recognition of vulnerability, strengthen the psychological motivators for mutual trust and reciprocal support, and may lead to particular forms of thick trust, and bonding or even linking social capital. For example, the experience of the loss of child, or diagnosis of a serious and perhaps terminal illness can transcend gender, ethnic or class boundaries. Membership groups are freely joined, although not everyone with a particular disease or condition will wish, or be able to, join a group (Small and Rhodes, 2000).

In terms of theory, the mechanism for the development of values, norms and understandings is through the medium of language – the particular discourse which is a vehicle for conveying assumptions, goals, objectives and interests and is established through, and sustained by, face-to-face interaction. Bourdieu (1991) has argued that language both reflects and helps to produce social structure. It has been linked to social institutions, as people not only carry with them particular ways of perceiving and acting but groups and organizations may also have the authority to speak for, or represent, particular concerns. A particular discourse is therefore part of social and political practice and of power relations and struggles in particular fields. For Bourdieu and Passeron (1977) particular forms of discourse were also part of what was termed 'cultural capital', that is the knowledge, skills and other acquisitions, endowed by education and experience and the basis for defining communities.

As far as health consumer groups are concerned, not only are the assumptive worlds of participants demonstrated through the discourse found in interview, but also discourse has a role to play in forging collective group identity, maintaining trust and strengthening the organization as a community. Where values and understandings are shared across organizations within the same sector, or across international boundaries, then this again can generate the social and political resources necessary to maintain sufficient group activity to influence the political process.

Values, knowledge and ways of working

It has already been shown that although groups interviewed were diverse, there were also lines of similarity. In an analysis of the data set it was demonstrated that both providing services in the form of support or 'in-kind', as well as raising awareness and other forms of political activity, were carried out by all groups – a finding supported also by Wood (2000). The main lines of difference were in terms of the emphasis placed on research, training and education, and influencing local and/or national policy. Group size determined the range and depth of activities, while the type of group shaped the network of relationships they built.

The values and ethos of health consumer groups

The similarities in the activities carried out by health consumer groups are reflected in the values and ethos that drive these activities and which, in turn, reflect the UK political context.

First, all health consumer groups were committed to working within the NHS and to supporting the principles of equity in access to, and the distribution of, health services. For example, a number of group leaders interviewed referred to their concern about regional and local differences in the type and quality of service available; problems of access to new treatments; rationing by postcode; shortfalls in service; the difficulties of influencing developments in primary care, and the lack of joined-up policies for health and social care. Although a few groups said they were dedicated to more radical aims, such as identifying poor practice and exposing it, a large majority of interviewees wanted to work with health providers to improve services. No interviewee mentioned private health care.

A second core value was a concern to enhance the personal autonomy of clients or members in the face of illness, loss, or threats to personhood. In interview, many groups also referred to their concern to destigmatize conditions; prevent discrimination; redress disadvantage; and, more positively, build a sense of identity. For example, MIND's vision is set out as follows:

Mind has a vision of society where people with mental health problems are accepted and included – a society where their needs and ambitions are met and facilitated free from stigma and discrimination and within a legal framework of civil and human rights. (MIND, 2003)[1]

These concerns were related to a third value: empowerment. This was to be achieved by being non-judgemental, working with people's priorities, extending knowledge, informing people about conditions, services and choices, and promoting self-help. For example, an interviewee from a cancer group commented:

> We see our overall aim to empower patients through knowledge and information...[Patients] contact us once they've been diagnosed... it's an awful lot to take in...you receive a diagnosis and then at the very same time you're then offered a choice of treatments... people often will call our information service to discuss the issues involved. (gi31)

A fourth core value among respondents was a belief in the validity of personal experience and of a 'lay' knowledge. An interviewee in the cancer sector spoke for many when she said:

> Experience and knowledge of actually being a cancer patient or a carer is...really the vital part because its something that's a unique knowledge that doesn't exist anywhere else, you know... So what...we're saying [is] that the organization focuses on the value of experience and what patients and patient groups – particularly patient groups – have to offer is a collective knowledge about the experience of cancer and its management. (gi2)

These values were related to a fifth, concerned with process. Many groups referred to the values of inclusion and a concern to be consultative and encourage member or client participation. Some said they wanted to 'respond to members issues' and to work with agendas coming from below from members, clients, or the public in contact. Principles also affected practice: a majority of groups with a branch structure said they delegated authority to local groups as much as possible.

Groups also had particular beliefs about the 'representation' of the views of members and clients to other bodies. There was a general assumption that the role of leaders was to act as a voice for those they represented. Their concern was to 'gain acceptance' for the group and the condition and to draw attention to needs. This could only be done through a process that was consultative and participatory and gave a voice to those with knowledge of the condition. Groups implicitly saw themselves as the 'holders' of interests: as a conduit for expressing the views of those below. The term 'holders' of interests has been used by Schmitter (2001) to discuss forms of participatory governance and is discussed more fully later. An example of the general disposition towards an informal approach to representation was articulated by the interviewee from one mental health organization in terms of its history and development in the following way:

> We represented families. [Their] main concern was that the care of the person they were caring for should be made better. So therefore from day one, we've been campaigning around hospitals, medicine, homelessness, suicide etc. So we've become a bit of a broader church and we've also become a much larger organization as well. (gi23)

Another, smaller support group, said that they represented people at the grassroots. One interviewee commented:

> It's the grassroots... it's very much, meeting the needs of those people that [the organization] is supposed to represent... I think, what the government would have here is a group of people... that would represent a view of a special interest group and we wouldn't just be paid officials. (gi34)

Overall, the values outlined above could be said to constitute an 'ethics of caring' and may help to explain the network of internal and external trust relationships discussed here and in the chapter following. However, it is one thing to state values and produce mission statements and another to follow these in practice. The remainder of this chapter will draw on interview data to illustrate how, from the perspective of group officials, these values were accomplished in practice.

The knowledge base of health consumer groups

In common with all organizations as social structures, each health consumer group had a knowledge base related to their particular area of specialization. Lam (2000, pp. 492–93) refers to different forms of organizational knowledge as follows: 'embedded knowledge', that is based on shared values, norms and routines, which has already been discussed; 'embodied knowledge', that is individual, tacit, action-oriented, practical and context specific; 'encoded knowledge' that is based on codification and analysis of experiences; and 'embrained knowledge' that is based on a particular cognitive scheme.

Embodied knowledge

This knowledge comes from living with an illness, or caring for people who have had an illness. This was of fundamental importance to groups and often a criterion for group membership and inclusion. For example, many groups had volunteers with experience of an illness who could support people who had contacted the help-line or headquarters staff. Experience was seen to provide a unique insight that was accepted as valid and as representing a form of 'truth'. It was the basis of a claim to be heard. Where experiences between people were shared and shown to be similar, then this provided a form of bonding. For example, a member of one maternity/childbirth group said that a common denominator among activists was that they: 'become active after having their first child and see themselves as having been assaulted' (gi42). Thus 'naming' a condition and sharing accounts of experiences is part of a process acquiring an individual identity and, through interaction, developing a collective identity. Group interaction also allows for the identification of a shared knowledge. As an interviewee from one said:

> Yes, we've seen patients…We've seen new patients. We see existing [patients], we see patients who are facing their last year of their life. So we've got experience as far as experience is concerned. (gi41)

This approach was as true of alliances as it was of condition-based and population-based groups. For example, as one alliance group said:

> Obviously in the first instance and the bottom line is the experience of patients and their families…the 'on the ground', down-to-earth knowledge. That would be very relevant for things where there are health service issues directly to do with patients. (gi32)

Groups that were not made up of people living with a condition or their carers consulted with service users, co-opted them to positions within the organization, or provided employment. This is discussed further below.

Encoded knowledge

The leaders of health consumer groups drew on the experiences of their members to collect and codify their knowledge base. This was done in a variety of ways through networks of contacts, analysing help-lines, carrying out surveys, or collecting accounts of experiences. As an interviewee from a maternity/childbirth group said:

> What we value more than anything is the raw data. It's raw. It's not filtered consumer material... and it is putting that together and seeing how it fits in with what you've read in the journals that is important. (gi3)

One senior office holder in another maternity/childbirth group said that when she took the job on:

> I started going round branches and gathering information and doing surveys. I did several over the years to find out what women were wanting, what were their best memories and their worst memories, and what was good and bad about the care they had received. I was careful to collect both because if you're talking to a professional or whoever, it's good to be able to tell [them] what's good as well as bad. (gi37)

Larger health consumer groups had sufficient resources carry out systematic research. For example, in 2000 the Carers National Association (now Carers UK), concerned about financial hardship among carers, asked members to complete a questionnaire about financial issues as if they were writing to the prime minister. The questionnaire began 'Dear Tony' (CNA, 2000). They commented:

> We had over 2000 members respond to that and that's given us a very good sample and we have turned it into a report... It's tremendous because it actually comes directly from members and that's a very very powerful thing for us to have done.

In 1999, following reports of age discrimination in the NHS, Age Concern commissioned a large national survey to identify the extent of the problem and found that a significant proportion of respondents over 65 said they had been refused treatment (Brindle, 1999a). A similar proportion of those over 50 perceived attitudes towards them to have changed from when they were younger and believed they had received a poorer service.

A general population survey found that people believed that ageist attitudes were prevalent, particularly among doctors. On the basis of the findings, a report was presented to government with recommendations about combating ageist attitudes (Gilchrist, 1999).

Help-lines were a major source of information for virtually all groups and have already been referred to. Data were analysed to identify problems, issues and emerging needs. For example, one interviewee told us that the Alzheimer's Disease Society (now Alzheimer's Society) had become aware, from an analysis of their help-line, that there was an emerging constituency of younger people who had received a diagnosis of the illness. They not only required specific information about the illness but the prognosis and the genetic implications. They also wished to participate actively and, had opportunities not been made available, the respondent believed they would have formed a separate group.

Embrained knowledge

A fourth form of knowledge drawn upon by health consumer groups was embrained, or in this case, specialized clinical knowledge. Biomedical knowledge was most frequently referred to. This was acquired by active individuals. As one interviewee put it: 'It's funny; I didn't know anything about medical matters before. I reckon I could pass an exam now to be a doctor. You tend to self-educate yourself that much' (gi14). This knowledge then becomes part of the collective knowledge of the group. As another respondent commented:

> [Parents] often know a lot more than the professionals because they find out. They use the net and they are able to access links across the world to get information. For example, they may be in contact with US sources and with research data that may not be well known in this country. They are thus our source of information as well as what we can do for them. (gi40)

Evidence-based data sources, such as the Cochrane Collaboration and DIPEx[2], were widely used, as was a network of informal contacts with health professionals (Herxheimer, 2003). Answers to questions could be provided quickly and some groups could call on clinicians, who were honorary members and distinguished in their field, who would give advice directly to members of the public referred to them by the group. One interviewee whose group had this capacity claimed it was: 'a unique service and we just feel it's not recognized elsewhere, just how unique it is' (gi34).

Most groups produce a range of printed material for the public. Professional contacts are often used to check that the information provided is accurate and up to date. Typically, information leaflets provide a mixture of up-to-date biomedical and experience-based knowledge as well as contact numbers for help and support. Booklets are often produced in a range of languages and were deemed to be extremely important by groups themselves as well as other stakeholders interviewed. They provide a public service, helping to empower consumers both individually and collectively. The ability of health consumer groups to use specialized knowledge and contribute to issues of diagnosis as well as treatment has been discussed by Epstein (1996) in relate to HIV/AIDS.

Ways of working with members and clients

The ways in which groups work with their membership or client group is the basis for building and maintaining a community. Written communications, events and meetings, and particular employment practices provided channels of contact between leaders, members and clients.

Written communications

Newsletters and regular magazines were shown as a common form of communication. The questionnaire indicated that 94 per cent of groups had a newsletter and these were used to give information on policy issues; present recent research findings; keep members up to date on impending legislation; publicize support networks and activities; and give practical advice. For example, British Cardiac Patients Association's newsletter had discussed the case for automatic defibrillators in supermarkets and the self-monitoring of warfarin.[3] It recommended that its members should only use defibrillators with medical advice and explained the safeguards against incorrect use.

The following comment from the Carers National Association (membership 13 700) sums up the approach:

> The most obvious tangible way we involve members is that they receive a bi-monthly magazine called Caring Magazine. [This] carries what you might call soft information, which is sort of life-style information of gardening, general health tips, interviews with celebrity carers. But it also has hard information on benefits, quite leading information and any kind of news about events that are going on, also the events in parliament or fund-raising events that we've been running or things that are coming up.

In common with a number of other organizations, the Carers National Association commented that increasingly the magazine has been given over to members:

> So, there is a greater focus on what the reader wants to read rather than what we want to tell them or what we think they should know. And as a result of that we're getting a lot more correspondence and we are beginning to stir up a little bit of controversy and we've now got a soap box and a letters page where people can let off steam.

An interviewee from a relatively small arthritis-related group said:

> We have a quarterly newsletter that goes out to our members and in it members are allowed to write in and we put members letters in. In that part...they say what they want, we won't edit it. It's up to them (gi15).

Newsletters were also used to consult on policy, to publicize development and business plans, and to generate support for campaigns. Typically, members were asked for their views or were presented with issues to prioritize as part of developing policy. Many groups had websites: some were developing chat rooms so that members could make contact through email. A few groups were exploring ways of using the internet or digital television interactively to develop a virtual network for support and provide help for those who lived in remote areas. In a recent paper, Powell (2003) discusses how the world-wide-web is changing the doctor–patient relationship.

Events and meetings
Most groups had annual conferences as well as more targeted events such as workshops, discussion groups, and gatherings for

fundraising. These serve a number of purposes. First, they reinforce togetherness, mutuality, and the development of a collective sense of identity. Second, they give an opportunity to provide information and to raise awareness. Third, they create opportunities for networking. Fourth, they reinforce the role of the leadership and, fifth, they help the leadership to develop a policy agenda.

Some events have a strong symbolic function in mediating the experience of pain and loss through providing an opportunity for a public acknowledgment. For example, one group fixes an annual consciousness-raising week around the time that a founder member's child died. To the participant observer, such gatherings can have a distinctly evangelistic flavour. Other groups organize special activities for members with caring responsibilities or disabling conditions, such as funding to attend a parliamentary gathering or an international meeting. These are part of a strategy for increasing the sense of inclusion.

Employment practices
Increasingly, longstanding groups formed in the altruistic tradition of providing services *for* users, now work *with* users. As the interviewee from Arthritis Care said:

> One of our most basic philosophies is the philosophy of user involvement...Right from the way in which the organization is governed, right down to the grassroots, we have people with arthritis very much at the centre of what we do, so that a majority of our trustees who are people with arthritis. We have a number of key posts that are designated for people with arthritis, like our help-line...All our trainers, all the people who run our self-management pro-grammes, they're all people who have arthritis. [The] people who work with young people are all young people with arthritis and nearly all our volunteers are people with arthritis...we will use our network to consult and discuss issues.

This philosophy also applied to a number of mental health groups. As one interviewee said:

> We do employ people with mental illness and...some of our jobs are particularly advertised. We stress the fact that applications are particularly welcome from people with a mental illness because of

the kind of job it is, and the skills and expertise that are required... We've carried out audits of our staff asking to find out what percentage have a mental illness... I'm sure... it's an under-representation... because even in our organization not everyone is happy to openly say that they have had, or have got, a mental illness... In our employment campaign and in our employment work we are encouraging employers to employ people with mental health problems so of course we couldn't do that if we weren't doing that here. (gi23)

A number of large population-based groups also stressed that they were driven from the bottom up. For example, the respondent from Help the Aged commented:

We are not in touch because we provide services to [them]. We are in touch because that is one of [our] objectives, to support them. Basically because they [the groups] reckon that real policy change is going to come from older people themselves and not from organizations like us. We have a role to play, but actually what really makes the difference is older people's own voices. Especially with all the government consultation going on now.

In summary, health consumer groups both large and small, across condition areas and types of organization, used broadly similar strategies to encourage social interaction and thus increase the level of engagement and activity. In so doing there was an emphasis on informal and personal modes of contact.

Social networks and health consumer groups

As well as providing help and support, health consumer groups could be said to constitute a network of expertise and intelligence-gathering that is used for political purposes. Networks of contacts were developed through working on projects over a period of time and also through both formal membership as well as informal links. For example, some health consumer groups drew on informal networks of specialist professionals, not only health professionals, but also lawyers and parliamentarians. Help and advice were also accessed through family and friends: a valuable resource for smaller groups, who could compensate to some extent for a low financial resource base with effective elite networking.

Such networks were particularly useful in accessing the political systems and identifying who to talk to in what organization. As the interviewee from one group said:

> [You have to ask the question] 'Who is behind what's happening?' 'Who is the driving force behind it?' 'Who are we going to go for?'...I mean, it isn't just going to be the Minister. You know it's the officials in the Department. It's the trust whose letter we've just got saying they're not going to provide this service. I think what we do is, when we are aware that there is something going on that we're not happy with, [we write a report] and we circulate it to quite a wide range of groups. And say, 'Look this is what's going on folks.' (gi3)

Networking activities are not sustained without the energy and commitment of an active membership. The motivation and experience of staff was also important. A number of the paid officers who were interviewed said they found working in the voluntary sector challenging and stimulating, with considerable opportunities for creative work. Many also had direct or indirect experience of a particular illness or condition themselves. There was also evidence of a transfer between the public and voluntary sector in both directions. For example Richard Gutch, at the time of writing a Director at the Community Fund, the body responsible for awarding National Lottery grants to the community and voluntary sector, was formerly the chief executive of Arthritis Care. Some groups in the interview sample had employed ex-civil servants in policy roles (see also McCurry, 2003). The exchange of expertise clearly aided networking and mutual understanding.

The political resources of health consumer groups

The values, knowledge base and ways of working helped health consumer groups to generate social resources to meet their own objectives and also, to contribute to the public interest. These same factors contributed to what groups saw as their political resources when putting pressure on government and influencing other health care stakeholders and public opinion. First, groups saw a major strength to be their 'expertise'. This consisted of a number of factors already mentioned: personal experiences of the disease or condition as patient, carer, or relative; acquired specialist knowledge of the disease or condition and its treatment; knowledge of user/carer priorities and needs; information on the realities of service delivery; their ability to come up with solutions and innovative ways of working; their social and political networks; and their knowledge of the workings of the policy process.

Examples from the data included the Stroke Association, whose respondent commented that they were listened to because they had

> knowledge and experience. We know what stroke is about; we know how it can affect people. We have funded, and know the research. We keep our finger on the pulse of what's going on world-wide. We can provide information...so it's our experience, our knowledge, our enthusiasm and our bloody-mindedness to improve the care of people affected by stroke.

The Mental Health Foundation, not a membership group, considered that they were considered part of the consumer movement and consulted because:

> [We draw on the experience of users] and it's a great strength. It serves to position us quite well with [the] service user movement and therefore we probably find it easier then to attract people to be involved in our other programmes of work. They see us as an organization, which has a commitment to working very strongly with, and employing, service users.

An interviewee from the Genetic Interest Group referred to their

> moral authority to talk about issues, if you're talking about changing the law to allow something like therapeutic cloning, clearly the fact that you're talking to a representative of [a patient group] gives [you this].

Others considered that they were consulted by government and other stakeholders for instrumental reasons. For example, the interviewee from the Maternity Alliance said they were consulted:

because we're useful. We tell them what's wrong with what they're doing. Well, we pointed out mistakes in legislation [to a Government Department] the other day, so they went away and rectified it. We tell them what women are saying to us about problems with legislation.

Another group commented that health consumer groups provided a training ground for the lay representatives that are now required for the new systems of governance introduced by post-1997 Labour governments. They said: 'You are entitled to have a consumer representative but there aren't enough knowledgeable people to go round. We are a precious resource, and a threatened resource' (gi3). Another interviewee also pointed out that there are now a number of controversial ethical issues on the health agenda, such as the need to prioritize and to ration access to certain services. There have also been technological changes that have enhanced the capability of medicine to prolong life. In her view, governments did not wish to take sole responsibility for these matters and looked to health consumer groups to help them deal with issues where there are ethical dilemmas.

Finally, interviewees also gave a range of examples of the strengths traditionally associated with voluntary organizations in the health and welfare sector: their ability to innovate and test out ideas. One group said they had pioneered the use of exercise regimes to delay the use of more invasive (and expensive) drug and surgical interventions for particular a form of arthritis. Pilot programmes had been developed for people and their carers with an early diagnosis of dementia. An interviewee from a mental health organization described the impact such programmes could have:

You know a minister goes to a good practice project in Wales, and thinks to himself 'mmm, that would work well', the next time he's in a meeting with someone from the [Department of Social Security] he makes a point of making sure that mental illness is covered under a certain section of one of the benefits. Things like that must happen because we win awards, we run good services, there's a lot of them, and influential people visit them and comment on them. (gi23)

Also, as pointed out in numerous National Council for Voluntary Organizations' reports, health consumer groups have raised significant financial resources and contribute to social welfare (Passey, Hems and Jas, 2000).

Barriers to using social and political resources

In the questionnaire, groups were asked to identify what they thought were the main barriers to influencing policy. Respondents said that these were the lack of resources in terms of staffing (83 per cent), finance (79 per cent), and political contacts (75 per cent) as well as the lack of prior consultation (71 per cent). The other barriers were seen as a lack of support within government (64 per cent) and lack of fit with the government's policy agenda (57 per cent) and their own lack of knowledge of the policy process (55 per cent). The interview data showed that some groups within the sector also faced particular problems in maintaining their social resources in the face of high levels of illness or disability among their members. A few organizations also gave examples of problems that may be typical for voluntary organizations in general, such as difficulties in maintaining group cohesion.

Illness or disability as a barrier

As Small and Rhodes (2000) have demonstrated in relation to people with serious and terminal illness, health consumer groups can face problems of maintaining an active membership due to the ill health of their members. Not all people with a condition wish to join groups and, even if they do, active participation can be precluded by an illness temporarily or permanently through degenerative illness or death. Many group leaders referred to specific barriers to participation and the special arrangements they had to make. As an interviewee from one arthritis group commented:

> Arthritis presents different types of obstacles. There is the obvious physical access issue, but a more subtle obstacle if you like is that arthritis is a fluctuating condition so that you can be kind of very bad in the morning and take a long time to get going or equally...you could go several months with being well under control and then have a flare-up which puts you out of action. You also obviously often have to have hospital treatment, joint replacement and things which can interrupt things...what we try and do is to make sure

that the way in which we plan our meetings and programmes takes account of all that...One of the best ways of course is having people with arthritis on the committee so they are there to point out [the difficulties]. (gi17)

Another interviewee said that 95 per cent of her group's members were wheelchair bound. So:

We can't get to meet each other. We're scattered all over the country. So we have what we call a pen pal register and they can contact people in their own area. And in London now they have a little group there of about twelve of them, who meet up once a month. That's the only way we can do it, we can't do it with a national body because we just can't get around. (gi14)

Maternity/childbirth organizations face a different kind of problem. Having a baby is a short-term issue. Many people join a group for a limited period and only a minority remain as active long-term members. An interviewee said:

The vast majority stay for about two years after they have given birth unless they're having another baby, which would prolong their membership. There's actually a huge turnover. (gi37)

In the case of cancer, members may become severely ill or die. As one interviewee commented:

[It's a] huge problem...in the wider user movement in cancer... you end up with them [those in leadership positions] dropping off the perch regularly. It's a big issue for cancer. (gi11)

However, another cancer organization said the length of survival was only a problem for some patients as: 'People can live with cancer for a long time or they will be recovered from cancer and [this] raises issues [about] whether they should still be considered patients or not' (gi31). However, this group also wished to involve patients who were terminally ill as they had a particular contribution to make in evaluating end-stage drug therapies and palliative care.

Maintaining group cohesion

Problems more typical of all forms of association were maintaining group cohesion and the 'market' position necessary for financial survival. In relation to the former, a few groups where there were issues that threatened consensus, followed a strategy of avoidance. Thus, a number of maternity/childbirth groups did not take a stance on abortion, and some mental health groups had no policy on electro-convulsant therapy as a form of treatment. An interviewee from the UK Federation of Smaller Mental Health Agencies said:

> We have within our organization one of the main groups in the country, which is campaigning against ECT, they would like it banned. Whereas, we have other people who find it a useful treatment... We will only be able to have a rather neutral policy ourselves.

Other groups commented on the difficulty of managing centre/periphery relations. As an interviewee commented:

> Most people join now really to support their branch. Because they've received something locally, they've decided to give something back to help, fundraising, functions, conferences and whatever else. And sometimes there are difficulties in that branches will suddenly wonder why headquarters is asking for money to be sent on to them, because they can use this money locally, thank you very much. They forget that if the central organization collapsed, they wouldn't have all the training back-up, the information leaflets and so on. (gi37)

Some interviewees referred to differences of opinion over strategy in relation to campaigning: about how confrontational a group should be; what kind of publicity should be sought; whether to collaborate with other organizations or professionals; and whether to accept drug company sponsorship (see Chapter 8). In a small minority of instances, these differences became public and led to a split. The interviews provided three examples from the recent past, for example, in one maternity/childbirth group, a conflict over the bottle-versus breast-feeding had led to the formation of a splinter group. For a time this threatened the stability, membership base and therefore income of the parent group (see also *The Independent*, 1997).

While most interviewees said their group had developed ways of maintaining a membership base, two groups (out of 39) referred to a slow decline. This was attributed by one to having achieved their objectives and by the other, a generalist group, to the rise of more specialist patient groups. A few other groups referred to the reverse problem – a rapid increase in the membership beyond the capability of the organization to respond. While not common, these examples are a reminder that health consumer groups are communities where a consensus must be constantly renegotiated. Membership is an act of choice and individuals seek to follow principles as well as needs. Furthermore, good managerial skills are necessary for group survival.

Are health consumer groups representative?

A criticism commonly made of voluntary organizations is that their very inclusiveness excludes others. A specific accusation is that those involved in voluntary organizations tend to be middle class and do not include ethnic minority groups. In relation to health consumer groups, it is true that only a minority of those with a particular condition join, although more people may seek help or information. Put another way, groups are accused of not representing a cross-section of people with a particular condition but only a white, middle-class, vocal minority. Health consumer groups may be low on linking social capital. To our knowledge, there are no systematic data on the social composition of health consumer groups in terms of gender, class, ethnicity, and age, let alone data that allows comparison over time, although some groups are likely to be composed mainly of women rather than men, or older as opposed to younger people, due to the nature of the condition.

Gender issues

Issues of gender and the membership, and leadership, of health consumer groups raise interesting issues. What little evidence there is on gender and civic engagement has recently been reviewed by Lowndes (2004). For example, the General Household Survey for 2000 shows that women were more likely to participate in formal volunteering, but only by a small margin (Coulthard, Walker and Morgan, 2002).[4] Earlier studies have shown that women are more active in terms of volunteering than men in the fields of health, education and social services. However, women are more likely to engage at a local or community level. This has been explained by women's patterns of sociability and their differential engagement in the public/private sphere. Community networks tend to be embedded in pre-existing networks of trust and mutuality among friends and neighbours. However, it has also been shown that women are less likely to occupy leadership positions at local and national level. This poses interesting questions about gender and health consumer group activity at both these levels. Many of the issues that concern health consumer groups are of major importance to women in the domestic sphere as carers and health workers (Lewin and Olesen, 1985; Doyal, 1998) Do they, however, occupy leadership positions within the sector?

The research did not cover local groups and the issue of gender did not arise except where it related to male medical dominance. It is not possible to tell whether the silence on the subject reflected its irrelevance in the work environment of health consumer groups. However, most of the interviewees from the 39 health consumer groups were women.[5] As subsequent chapters will show, they were often engaging in the policy process at the highest level. This appears to go against the trend in other spheres, where there is a 'tendency for the numbers of women and their potential for influence to decline inversely in relation to the most powerful positions' (Yule 2000, p. 33, quoted in Lowndes, 2004, p. 60).[6] It may be that the voluntary health sector has provided an area to which women have been drawn possibly because it is concerned with caring.[7] The topic certainly warrants more systematic study.

Class and ethnicity

In relation to class and ethnicity, interviewees perceived themselves to be open to criticism. A number of groups said they were perceived as 'middle-class'. For example, one cancer group said: '[the organization] does have an image that is I think slightly justified of catering for white middle-class, middle-aged people' (gi31). Some maternity/childbirth groups also described themselves as predominantly white and middle-class. Virtually all groups said they were concerned that they did not attract members from ethnic minorities. Only two groups in the interview sample were solely concerned with ethnic minorities and one of these had been established by a parent charity. It was suggested in interview that ethnic minorities are more strongly represented at a local, rather than national, level. The interviews indicated that some national groups had made considerable efforts to provide literature in a number of languages and had undertaken specific initiatives to attract members. For example, an interviewee from an arthritis group said: 'We have an advisory group on developing services to ethnic minorities because we don't have many members from ethnic minority communities' (gil7). Other groups had carried out research on the special needs of ethnic minorities and some mental health groups were active in protecting their rights.

Little is known about why people do, and do not, join groups and how this differs between sub-sets of the population. If culturally the UK is socially differentiated, health consumer groups are likely to reflect rather than counter these differences. Like other voluntary associations, health consumer groups may face a dilemma. A certain homogeneity of purpose may be necessary to encourage a sense of belonging, particularly at the small group level. Yet national groups with values related to inclusion will wish to attract a cross-section of those living with a particular condition. Moreover, for wider political reasons, they may wish to demonstrate that they can recruit, and therefore represent, people from diverse backgrounds.

Conclusion

In this chapter it has been demonstrated that health consumer groups, by and large, share particular values and have a knowledge base that draws on both experiential and biomedical knowledge relevant to their area. They also have particular ways of working that foster trust, sociability and participation. The relationship between leaders and members or clients is mutually supportive. Informal ways of working are more significant than formal rules and elections. From this base, health consumer groups derive the social resources to determine aims and activities and the financial and human resources necessary to provide support and to pursue policy objectives.

In pursuing these policy objectives, networks of social contacts, confidence about expertise and the claim to speak for clients and members provide the resources for the forums of political engagement discussed in later chapters. These social and political resources provide the social capital for continuing engagement both internally and externally. Relationships are maintained through shared values which relate to the ethics of caring. There were examples of a small number of groups where the drive towards purposeful activity for mutual benefit had failed. These provide a reminder that in voluntary associations, membership support is the vital ingredient and neither government support, nor media interest, can substitute for it.

6 Networks, and informal and formal alliances

The commonality of values between health consumer groups, and the small size of many, suggests considerable scope for the formation of alliances and networks. Although Wood (2000) was critical of the ability of patients' organizations to work together to challenge other interests, both he and others (Hogg, 1999) suggest that this might be changing, particularly through the creation of permanent alliances.

This chapter presents the findings of the De Montfort study on alliances and networks in this field. The questions the research set out to address included: What networks exist and what is their purpose? Are networks more evident in some condition areas than others? The answers to these questions raise broader issues. Evidence of extensive networking could indicate a broader health consumer movement and that the sector has the makings of a structured interest group and may be in a position to exercise influence in the wider health policy arena. The findings in this chapter could therefore provide further evidence about the actual or potential influence of health consumer groups in the national policy process.

The second issue is collaboration and competition. In one sense, the health consumer group sector is a market where a variety of groups compete for public attention and for funds. How do groups relate to each other? To answer this, one must examine theories of organizational behaviour.

Theoretical perspectives on alliance working

Networking is at the informal end of a spectrum of inter-relationships between organizations, while alliances are more permanent unions that are 'formed for mutual benefit' (OED, 1991). It has been argued in the policy studies literature that alliances are more likely to form in crowded policy environments where interests must compete for access, resources and status (Baumgartner and Jones, 1993). However, the nature and pattern of these alliances are likely to differ according to the issue at hand. The decision to join an alliance or work alone is viewed as a tactic in the policy process. Groups will join an alliance if they believe it will increase their chance of policy success (Gray and Lowery, 1998) or if they believe it will give them access to key decision-makers (Hojnacki, 1997). However, other organizations will seek to carve out 'issue niches' believing that it distinguishes them from similar organizations in the policy arena (Browne, 1990).

Leaders of interest groups must decide whether the potential benefits of joint working are sufficiently strong to warrant allying themselves with other groups. Gray and Lowery (1998) have argued that smaller, weaker groups are more likely to join alliances than stronger organizations because they are less able to 'hold their own' in the policy process. A strong and cohesive opposition may also encourage groups to co-operate. Others have argued groups are more likely to work together if they perceive the issue they are working on as controversial. An alliance helps them to spread risks (Heinz, 1993). By working together interest groups are able to share resources and lobby with a stronger voice (Lamb, 1997).

However, the decision to join an alliance must also include the costs to the organization (Riker, 1962). Salisbury (1987) argues that the downside to joint working is that any success must be shared between different players. Groups may have to compromise on their ideals and there is a danger of losing group identity. Other decision costs include: time costs, resource constraints, political costs (for example, of revealing one's stance on an issue). Although these decision costs are true for any organization in deciding whether to lobby together or to work alone (Hojnacki, 1997). In later work, Hojnacki (1998) suggested that not all groups who join alliances are willing or able to contribute to lobbying: they 'free-ride' on issues. Resources play a key factor in an organization's decision to contribute, and only well structured and managed coalitions ensure an input from all participants.

Links between health consumer groups

The data from the questionnaire indicated a high degree of networking, collaboration and joint working within the health consumer group sector, with 86 per cent of groups claiming to have links or alliances with other user/carer organizations. Of those groups who identified a specific organization, 41 named a group within their own condition area and 20 named one outside their area. Forty-two groups named a formal alliance organization with whom they were connected. Table 6.1 summarizes the frequency of contact health consumer groups reported with other user/carer organizations. From this it can be seen that groups are actively engaged with others on a regular basis. Population-based groups enjoyed more frequent contact with other health consumer groups than either formal alliance organizations or condition-based groups.

In the questionnaire, groups were asked whether they viewed alliances between groups as a facilitating factor in the policy process: three quarters of respondents said they were 'very important' or 'important'. However, despite the level of contact between groups, around half of the condition-based groups and population-based groups thought that a lack of cohesion in the sector was a barrier to influencing policy. Fewer formal alliance organizations (22 per cent) thought this was the case.

Table 6.1   Frequency of contact between health consumer groups, by type of group

	'At least monthly' (%)	'At least quarterly' (%)	'At least annually' (%)	'Not in past three years' (%)
All groups	46	77	90	10
Formal alliance organizations	56	100	none	none
Population-based groups	77	100	none	none
Condition-based groups	40	71	87	13

Source: Questionnaire data set 1999.

A number of alliances formed around a shared interest in a particular medical condition, or a shared interest in the experience of patients across a number of conditions. In terms of structure, these ranged from *ad hoc* collaborative networks to more permanent formal alliances. From the interview data, three different types of working arrangement were identified and are used in the analysis:

- *collaborative networks and ad hoc working*: intermittent activity involving various combinations of health consumer groups, such as joint projects convened by groups themselves. The development of a collaborative network tends to be based on a shared knowledge of an area;
- *informal alliances*: alliances where there were regular meetings over a number of years. Typically, administrative costs were shared between groups but they did not have a formal structure or staffing;
- *formal alliance organizations*: national organizations made up of other autonomous groups that could include both health consumer groups and other organizations. They tended to have paid administrative staff and their own office space.

Health consumer groups also worked with other health care stakeholders in broader coalitions, formed through third party arenas such as all-party groups, government taskforces and the patient and carer liaison committees created by professional organisations. These activities are dealt with in more detail in later chapters.

Differences between condition areas

The questionnaire and interview data revealed differences in the extent of collaboration within the condition areas. The questionnaire data showed that mental health groups were least likely to report links with other user/carer organizations, with only 75 per cent of groups reporting contact, compared to 100 per cent of maternity and childbirth groups; 89 per cent of cancer groups; 85 per cent of heart and circulatory disease groups and 81 per cent of arthritis groups. However, interview data indicated that joint working in the maternity/childbirth and mental health sectors was more deeply embedded than in the areas of arthritis, cancer or heart/circulatory disease. In the former, groups worked together on a wider range of issues and in a number of different fora. This may reflect both the structuring of the sectors and the policy environment. The Maternity Alliance acts as a broadly-based co-ordinated pressure group for maternity/childbirth as well as covering welfare and social security issues (Phillips, 2001). Moreover, there has been a long history of collaboration between health consumer groups in the sector. Despite a history of tension between groups in the mental health sector in recent times, a number of groups have begun collaborating over issues of joint concern, such as lobbying against proposed changes to legislation and supporting access to treatments. As one commentator said of the relationship: 'it has matured, it's not so much a problem as it used to be' (si28). The only formal alliance in the sector is the UK Federation of Smaller Mental Health Agencies (UKFSMHA) which brings together small local, regional and national organizations. At the time of interview this organisation was struggling to survive.

The configuration of groups has already been discussed in Chapter 3. In this context, the arthritis sector had a longstanding formal alliance organization, the British League Against Rheumatism (BLAR, now the Arthritis and Musculoskeletal Alliance), but had taken an interest in policy issues only recently. Arthritis groups also joined broader alliances. It should be noted that Arthritis Care was a founder member of the cross-condition Long-term Medical Conditions Alliance (LMCA). Cancer groups have tended to be more fragmented. This may be because they have specialized in particular areas and are of relatively recent origin. There was no formal alliance organization bringing together cancer sector groups, although one had formed around breast cancer. The heart/circulatory disease sector was served by two formal alliance organizations: the National Heart Forum, although this has only recently begun to incorporate health consumer groups which remain a minority in the membership, and the Children's Heart Federation, which includes only those health consumer groups dealing with heart conditions affecting children. A number of broad formal alliances served various condition areas, such as the LMCA, the Patients Forum and the Genetic Interest Group. These are discussed further below.

The development of links between health consumer groups

Collaborative networks and ad hoc working

At a basic level, the interview data indicated a number of networks, particularly within condition areas. At national level, groups generally knew of the particular specialism of other groups in their condition area. They also met in a variety of fora. Conferences, seminars and other meetings provided opportunities for networking with other groups. In the interests of helping members of the public who contacted them, a number of interviewees spoke of cross-referring members of the public to more appropriate source of support or information. For example, the respondent from the British Cardiac Patients Association (BCPA) said his organization passed on queries about children's heart conditions to the Children's Heart Federation: 'I have preferred to push people in their direction than deal with a small number [of children] badly.' The interviewee from the Zito Trust said: 'We don't just dismiss people, we actually refer them onto other organizations.' An interviewee from Association for Improvements in the Maternity Services (AIMS) said they received queries directed to them by the Stillbirth and Neonatal Death Society (SANDS) and: 'They refer their complaints cases to us because they're dealing with bereavement and people are not going to recover from bereavement if they think that the death was avoidable.'

Individual health consumer groups also worked together to share information, develop policy, pool resources, or simply to learn from each other. They also lobbied government or parliament. For example, one cancer group had developed links with other cancer groups to make joint representations to decision-makers about cancer screening. Another, CancerBACUP, was working with a number of breast cancer charities to produce information for patients on guidance on cancer treatment, published by the National Institute for Clinical Excellence (NICE), and had worked with other cancer charities on awareness campaigns for breast cancer and bowel cancer.

Two maternity/childbirth groups, AIMS and National Childbirth Trust, had collaborated to produce *A Charter for Ethical Research in Maternity Care* (AIMS and NCT, 1997). A number of maternity/childbirth groups established, with support from the Royal College of Midwives, a Maternity Care Working Party. This multidisciplinary group brought together health professionals and consumer organizations who shared a common concern that maternity services were losing out to other priorities in the NHS. In 2002 it produced *Modernising Maternity Care: A Commissioning Tool-Kit for Primary Care Trusts in England* (Maternity Care Working Party, 2002). In the mental health field, the National Schizophrenia Fellowship (now Rethink), MIND (the National Association for Mental Health) and the Manic Depressive Fellowship had surveyed their members to produce a research paper entitled *A Question of Choice* (National Schizophrenia Fellowship, 2000), which contributed to a NICE review of treatments for schizophrenia.

Joint working could also take place across condition areas. For example, the Arachnoiditis Trust had joined with other groups to campaign on informed consent for medical treatment. The campaign was being co-ordinated by the Action for the Victims of Medical Accidents so they 'could fight as a group'. Help the Aged had co-ordinated the input of various health consumer groups on the Older People's national service framework. Indeed, it was suggested by a small number of interviewees that coming together in third-party arenas such as government committees and taskforces, and particularly in discussions relating to government policies for patient and public involvement, had helped promote and build collaborative activity between health consumer groups.

Informal alliances

Another level of joint working was through informal alliances, which tended to be linked to specific conditions or around particular topics. For example, within the maternity/childbirth sector, Baby Network is a group of eight to ten organizations with similar interests. It meets periodically and shares the costs of meetings. Informal groupings can be a precursor of more formal working arrangements, an interviewee said attempts were being made to raise funding: 'to move this Baby Network forward because as you know, unless you've got a secretariat and a focal point, it's just a talking shop' (gi29).

CancerBACUP and Cancerlink have both contributed to the Cancer Information Charities Alliance which also shares good practice (Science and Technology Committee, 2000). Help the Aged was involved in the Social Policy Ageing Information Network, an alliance of policy, parliamentary or public affairs officers from about 20 different organizations. This was used to co-ordinate activity over a range of issues that had caused concern. Joint letters had been written to the press to raise awareness on particular issues, such as doctors who charged for visiting care homes. Other informal alliances had been established as a direct response to government policy. Patients Involved in NICE (PIN) helped health consumer groups share good practice in submitting evidence to NICE. The alliance had made representations to NICE based on its experiences of the appraisal process. The NICE annual report referred to its developing relationship with PIN as 'particularly important' (NICE, 2000).

In the late 1990s with the prospect of legislative changes to the 1983 Mental Health Act, a particularly influential informal alliance was formed of health consumer groups, professional organizations, research bodies and provider organizations, called the Mental Health Alliance. The alliance was concerned that the government was trying to expand the total number of people who could be treated compulsorily in the community or detained under treatment orders. Its administrative costs were met by a small number of groups. By 2003 it included over 50 organizations. Whilst the group had a standing committee and an agreed structure and agenda, it had no leadership structure. Its core members produced joint briefings on behalf of the wider network.

Formal alliance organizations

The questionnaire data showed that most formal alliance organizations, institutions whose memberships are made up of other national health consumer groups, were relatively recent phenomena, with a majority forming since 1981. The analysis of the interview data showed two common themes in the formation of these alliances. First, most had been set up when a need for greater co-ordination was identified through an informal organizational network. For example, before the LMCA was formally constituted and employed its own staff, administrative tasks were shared among a number of organizations associated with chronic illness. The Children's Heart Federation is a group of national and local support groups for families with a child with heart problems, their respondent describing its origins said:

> Most voluntary organizations start with a core of people who've seen something that needs doing and get together to do it and then they formalize things and they start looking for money to do what they want to do.

The Patients Forum developed from informal meetings at the Consumers' Association between the Patients Association and other statutory and voluntary health sector groups (see Chapter 2). In 1996, it adopted its own terms of reference and became a free-standing organization. The UKFSMHA (1996) was formed after the director of the Matthew Trust identified a need for an association which would represent smaller mental health groups.

Second, there is often a particular catalyst for the formation of formal alliances. The Genetic Interest Group was formed after various health consumer groups had jointly lobbied for changes to the 1990 Human Fertilization Embryology Act. Chapter 2 showed how the health service reforms of the late 1980s and early 1990s led indirectly to the formation of the Patients Forum and the LMCA. As one interviewee, describing the origins of the Patients Forum, said, there was a belief at the time that an alliance would have a 'stronger lobbying power' (gi25). Furthermore, as the pace of policy change gathered momentum and there was a flow of requests from government to provide a 'user perspective' to policy documents and consultative papers, there was a need for an organization or network that could minimize the workload by co-ordinating responses.

Not all formal alliances were established by patient/carer groups. In certain instances, organizations representing health professionals acted as initiators. Both BLAR, formed in 1972 and the National Heart Forum (1987), were started by professional organizations and societies that later broadened their remit to include health consumer groups. The structure and organization of group interaction also varied between formal alliances. Some focused on particular medical conditions; others addressed generic health issues across different conditions while others had a broader focus and dealt with social care and welfare issues as well. There were also differences in membership status. For example, the Patients Forum placed restrictions on the involvement of non-health consumer groups. Professional groups are associate members, pay higher fees and have no voting rights. There are also differences in the composition of memberships, the UK Breast Cancer Coalition (UKBCC) allowed local and regional groups to join alongside national health consumer groups, while the Maternity Alliance is primarily a lobby and campaigning group concerned with all aspects of maternity – income maintenance, employment, housing and health – and included trade unions as well as other interests.

The analysis of the interview data indicated considerable cross-group membership, For example, the Family Heart Association (now Heart UK) was a member of the National Heart Forum and the Genetic Interest Group. Arthritis Care was a member of the BLAR and the LMCA. In 1998/99, 18 health consumer groups were members of both the LMCA and Genetic Interest Group. It was also possible for different formal alliance organizations to be members of each other, for instance the Maternity Alliance and the LMCA were both members of the Patients Forum. Data indicated that formal alliances attracted both large and small groups into their membership, as well as groups that served population groups across all condition areas. However, population-based groups were more likely to join the Patients Forum and condition-based groups the LMCA. In recent years, the membership of three main cross-condition alliances has grown, in some instances, quite significantly. This is shown in Table 6.2.

Table 6.2   Growth in organizational membership of GIG, LMCA and Patients Forum 1998–2003

	1998/99	2003
Genetic Interest Group	116	120
Long-term Medical Conditions Alliance	87	112
Patients Forum[1]	33	81

[1] See note on p. 314.

Source: 1998/99 Annual Reports, 2003 websites.

The role of formal alliance organizations

Nine out of the eleven formal alliances identified in the questionnaire data set claimed that their primary purpose was to influence policy. This core aim was summarized in interview by a respondent from the UKFSMHA:

> [The main aim is] to lobby and engineer change specifically by influencing parliament...to give the smaller agencies a voice, organizations that weren't affiliated to anybody.

And the interviewee from the Genetic Interest Group said:

> [Our aims are] to promote a positive understanding in the public of the benefits of human genetics, and to improve the services, primarily in the health service, for people directly affected by genetic diseases within their families.

When consulted by government and other healthcare stakeholders, alliance leaders could speak on members' behalf; co-ordinate member responses or work alongside member organizations. An example of this process was described by the respondent from the National Heart Forum, who, in discussing a consultation on nutritional standards of school meals, said:

> It's not enough in terms of a public consultation for just one document to go in from the National Heart Forum. So then what we do is try and feed those ideas and get, for example, the British Diabetic Association, the Dietetic Association, to also send in submissions which reflect the policy recommendations and the values of the National Heart Forum.

Policy-related activity was not confined to responding to official consultations. Formal alliances produced position papers, reports and undertook research. Alliance members also attended party conferences and petitioned politicians. For example, BLAR had been involved in fringe meetings hosted by the LMCA. The Children's Heart Federation had presented a joint submission with the BCPA (not a member of the alliance) to Downing Street on heart services for children.

Formal alliances had a particular role to play in building the capacity of smaller groups and saw this as a way of attracting members. This could be achieved through sharing information on the policy process, setting up management training or using people from larger member organizations to act as mentors. A number of interviewees said that they particularly valued the Patients Forum briefing sessions. These provided an opportunity for networking and discussing the policy briefings produced by a member organization. In interview, a number of its members commented that it was a useful place to network. For example, one said: '[Its] a great opportunity to go and meet people face to face, have conversations, develop relationships, find out what we've got in common' (gi19). The LMCA had developed a Network of Smaller Organizations to encourage mutual support and information sharing and it also supported training for the groups on funding, planning and evaluation activities.

However, there was a possible downside. Expectations of what can be expected from membership of formal alliances may have been raised. For instance, the UKFSMHA established in 1996 to support smaller organizations, found that by 2000 members' demands were running beyond the funds available. In a consultation on the future of the organization, its leaders stated that the organization was a victim of its own success (UKFSMHA, 2000).

For larger organizations, membership of formal alliances could lead to joint campaigns. In 2000 a number of the interview groups were involved with the Peoples' Voice for Health Campaign, co-ordinated by the LMCA to promote a more patient-centred NHS. The LMCA did not take the lead on the campaign, but supported its member organizations in doing so, they said:

> Our role is to support the work of that group which will meet on a time-limited basis... If everything has to [be] channelled through me and through this little office... we will never achieve as much. Whereas if people feel that they can use the vehicle of an alliance to develop a thing that some people are interested in, I think we will achieve much more. [It's] the more risky tactic, but I think it will get us further in the end.

In summary, collaborative networks, informal alliances, and formal alliances between health consumer groups have both overlapping and specific purposes. This is shown in Figure 6.1.

	Mutual support		Influencing policy				Management structure
	Cross referral/sharing information/learning	Joint activities/resource pooling	Joint working	Lobbying	Campaigning	Developing capacity	
Networking	*	*					Loose/informal/*ad hoc*
Ad hoc working	*	*	*	*	*		Loose/informal/*ad hoc*
Informal alliances	*	*	*	*	*		Some management structure and continuity
Formal alliances	*	*	*	*	*	*	constitutional structure defining membership

Figure 6.1 Structure of joint working in the health consumer group sector

* potential outcome of collaborative working.

The benefits of working together

At the beginning of the chapter it was suggested the decision to work with other interest groups either on an *ad hoc* basis, or through alliances, was often made on rational grounds after weighing up the costs and benefits. In interview, the representatives from groups were asked what they saw as the benefits. These were seen to be sharing resources, drawing on each other's expertise and gaining access to other networks.

Joint activities and sharing resources

For groups with limited resources, funds for policy work were diverted from the direct support they were able to offer their members. Therefore, for smaller organizations, being part of an alliance may have been the only effective way of campaigning, as the interviewee from the Genetic Interest Group suggested:

> There're so many charities fighting in the field for funds – public awareness raising, medical professions awareness raising – its difficult for somebody who only has 12 people affected in the country...to have their voice heard.

This view was recognized by the interviewee from the LMCA, who, discussing why small groups joined the alliance, said: 'They wouldn't be big enough to have a policy officer or access to the media, so they're rather glad that we're getting on with that campaigning role.'

For larger organizations, joining an alliance provided an opportunity to add their voice to campaigns otherwise of peripheral interest. It was also a useful way of managing resources, as it enabled them to cover more issues than they would be able to alone. Thus, although the National Childbirth Trust was concerned with the socio-economic aspects of pregnancy and childbirth, its respondent believed that the Maternity Alliance could bring together necessary expertise and run more effective campaigns on these issues: 'They will take the lead on things like parental leave or child benefit or maternity pay and we would support them.' Members of the Mental Health Alliance had similar views. The respondent from MIND said:

'We do share the workload between groups – if others are focussed on an issue and it is not a central concern to us, we tend to leave it to them.'

Drawing on each other's expertise

A number of group representatives said that a benefit of working together was that their organization could learn from the experience of other groups. For example, the interviewee from BLAR, a formal alliance in the arthritis sector, described how her organization had joined the LMCA, because it was able to draw on the 'intellectual capital' of the organization.

In some instances groups had been formed with the assistance from other groups and links between them remained strong. Contact a Family and Cancerlink both played a role in supporting the development of other health consumer groups and in linking people with particular medical conditions or shared problems. For example, Cancer Black Care was established with the support of Cancerlink, which provided training for staff and referred the public as appropriate.

Given the difficulty that many groups have in attracting members from minority ethnic groups, Cancer Black Care was in demand. Its respondent said that his organization had been approached by a number of groups, including the National Cancer Alliance and Breast Cancer Care UK:

> Breast Cancer Care UK came here too to get some information. What happened is they have money from the Lottery, from the National Lottery Board, to provide information on the black woman and breast cancer. So they came in and worked with some of us here.

Irrespective of the setting, groups found that interaction with other groups brought practical support; a source of advice and information and the opportunity to learn from each other. Like condition-based and population-based groups, formal alliance organizations relied on their members for expertise and knowledge. For example, the Family Heart Association had provided evidence for a Genetic Interest Group report on patients' perceptions of care. The National Cancer Alliance had worked with the

LMCA to develop guidelines for working with the pharmaceutical industry. This work was mutually beneficial because the National Cancer Alliance was then able to adapt the guidelines to suit its own purpose. The expertise of member organizations often led to broader activities, for example, Arthritis Care had worked through the LMCA to promote interest in self-management techniques for patients with long-term medical conditions. The LMCA has since taken a leading role in the Department of Health's *Expert Patients Programme* (DoH, 2001a).

Access to networks of expertise

Interviewees said that working in alliances provided groups with access to a wider network of advice, support and expertise than would be available to them individually. In interview, respondents described the wealth of contacts that membership of formal and informal alliances brought. The Patients Forum has played a significant role in this respect. At the time of the research, the Forum met six times a year, although when responding to consultations or proposed legislation its leading members met more regularly. It also provided the opportunity to learn about different aspects of the health service by inviting speakers on key issues from health service organizations or academics with a particular expertise.

Groups could also use alliances as a gateway to expertise on how to influence policy. The interviewee from the UKBCC said that she had been approached by organizations who wished to learn from her experience in lobbying parliament:

> People will still phone to pick my brains about [how] to campaign... [They find the] relationship between central government and parliament [terribly confusing] and they don't get it right... Sometimes people just don't say the right things to the right person and it's wasted.

Accessing professional knowledge could also be a reason for joining an alliance. For example, the interviewee from BLAR believed groups joined because its member organizations included professional bodies such as the British Society of Rheumatology, a view which was shared by the interviewee from Arthritis Care:

We work closely with all the various societies like the British Society of Rheumatology, we are developing closer links with physiotherapists and primary care groups in Rheumatology and so on, and the BLAR umbrella is a good way of doing that.

The political advantages of working together

Analysis suggested that groups worked together to ensure policy success, confirming Hojnacki's (1997) argument that groups join alliances to gain tactical advantage. Interview data showed that health consumer groups would often join more than one alliance. In doing so, they were able to draw on different areas of expertise and position themselves strategically. Some larger organizations joined alliances because there was a perception that government preferred to work through them. This view was supported by the LMCA, whose respondent said:

I think they joined because we've got access to Ministers, senior civil servants, we get asked to nominate people to high-profile committees and so it gives them access through us if they [are] active members, they'll be in line for those sorts of roles.

Strength in numbers

For most interviewees, the desire to have a greater policy influence was the major reason for joining an alliance. This was the case for both the larger and better established groups as well as smaller organizations. An interviewee from BLAR, an alliance in its own right, said that her organization had 'hitched to the coat-tails' of the LMCA. Both the Arachnoiditis Trust and UKFSMHA said that by working in partnership with other organizations, their own public profile was raised rather than diminished.

There was strong evidence that smaller organizations saw particular benefits. There are large numbers of health consumer groups, supporting people with rare conditions, which have small memberships. However there were common concerns: access to specialist services; the implications for family members of a particular diagnosis and the issue of insurance cover for people with a genetically transmitted illness. An interviewee from the

Genetic Interest Group said groups joined the alliance because of 'strength in numbers' – an opinion that was confirmed by another interviewee who said of the Rare Conditions Alliance:

> There are 50 organizations in this country-wide. This has provided quite a powerful lobby because each condition is itself very small. There is power in numbers. (gi40)

The interviewee from the National Ankylosing Spondylitis Society also claimed that his organization was unlikely to succeed on its own. He said: 'Collectively we do it better than singlely [sic]'. A similar view was expressed by the Family Heart Association, who said that by working with the National Heart Forum their argument 'has more weight, significantly more weight to it'.

Collaboration between groups for tactical advantage

It was evident that health consumer groups developed tactics jointly so that they presented their issues to maximum advantage. In the maternity/childbirth sector, a number of interviewees informed us that whilst their objectives were similar, the larger and relatively well-funded National Childbirth Trust was more likely to adopt a conciliatory stance when lobbying government, whereas AIMS, a smaller and more vociferous pressure group had a more confrontational style. The National Childbirth Trust said: 'We both know that [we have different styles] and talk about that quite openly'. Indeed, these differences worked well as they could play 'good cop, bad cop' in order to achieve common goals.

However, compromises might have to be made in the interests of collaboration. For example, when discussing their work on the *Charter for Ethical Research in Maternity Services*, an interviewee from AIMS said:

> We persuaded the NCT [National Childbirth Trust] to come in and we knew that it was going to have much more clout if it came from a major group such as them. . . . we have a good relationship with the NCT but their structure and purposes are very different from ours. We have a lot of stuff in common but it took. . . much more time and effort than it would if we had produced it ourselves.

Groups believed that presenting a united front across a number of different organizations made it more difficult for other health care stakeholders to take advantage of differences between groups. Organizations working within the Mental Health Alliance laid particular stress on the importance of cohesion in relation to their campaign. One interviewee commented:

> I think there is a realization that if people work together and try and hold a common mind... that eventually it's going to be very difficult for the government to divide and rule. (gi13)

This was considered particularly important as differences between groups had previously been exploited by government. As one interviewee put it, unless groups work together: 'They [the government] talk to the ones that give them the answer they want' (gi38). In the case of MIND and Schizophrenia A National Emergency (SANE), past conflicts were used to underline the current consensus and to attract publicity to the alliance (Fazackerley and Parker, 2001). One interviewee commented:

> I hope that the differences will remain small and that we'll be able to keep together because if we do,... then we'll be able to get a much better Mental Health Act, and much better mental health services... there are some smaller organizations that aren't able to be involved in the Alliance because they have difficulty in letting go of particular issues and... seeing the benefits of compromise or working in a large group. (gi23)

Bringing together groups that might traditionally work independently of each other was a way of showing solidarity over core issues. The interviewee from the Mental Health Foundation said: 'There are a number of organizations in [the Mental Health Alliance], who you wouldn't expect to be there, to be there lobbying in parliament'. The need to show solidarity was echoed by a respondent from the National Heart Forum who commented that its strength 'derives from working... with influential but varied member organizations'.

Groups also aimed to simplify issues so that policy-makers such as MPs, civil servants or ministers would receive a clear and unambiguous message. One cancer organization had encouraged the use of standard statistics during Breast Cancer Awareness Week: 'so that people reading them don't get confused by one organization saying one thing and another, another' (gi36). The interviewee from the Maternity Alliance describing a regular meeting of groups with an interest in health issues said: 'We were treading on peoples toes, we realised that was stupid'. An interviewee from MIND, explaining why parliamentary officers from a number of mental health groups began to work together said:

> We thought the same way on many issues but the wording of briefing papers tended to be slightly different. We felt that this was confusing and weakening the impact of what we were trying to get across.

In some instances, not taking the lead could be advantageous as they could avoid publicity or being seen to be political. An interviewee from a mental health group said:

> In some ways it's quite good for us because we don't want to be a very sort of public profile and lobbying organization. It's not particularly appropriate...it's safer...to work with other organizations. (gi38)

Conflicts of interest and costs of collaboration

Strategies for managing difference and conflicts of interest

Wood (2000) contends that attempts to build permanent alliances may fail unless group leaders have the necessary political skills to forge links and develop trust between different interest groups. In order to reach agreement on policy issues and priorities, leaders of informal and formal alliances used similar mechanisms to those described in Chapter 5, such as newsletters, email and meetings. Their approach to decision-making was facilitative and consultative rather than directive. For instance, in preparing a report on the improvements required in both health and social care for people with long-term illnesses (LMCA, 1999b), the LMCA had used a variety of methods:

We used discussion groups, we used phone interviews and conventional questionnaires and so it meant that everybody, whatever their size and commitment, could take part.

However, for leaders of alliances, managing difference and avoiding conflict was a challenging task. Both informal and formal alliances had developed strategies for doing so. They chose to ignore issues known to be divisive. The UKFSMHA was policy neutral about electro-convulsant therapy, because its membership included organizations that supported its use and others that opposed it. Meanwhile, the National Heart Forum did not expect all its member organizations to respond to a government consultation on tobacco taxation.

We did not expect that Sport England would be able to sign up to that because... they are a government body and it was outside of their jurisdiction, if you like, to sign up to submission to the Chancellor.

Broadly-based coalitions such as the Patients Forum had to tread particularly carefully. There were broad 'value-based' issues where it was possible to get a consensus, but other matters where it was impractical. An interviewee commented:

Patient organizations will have different views... except for those very common [views], the kinds of views that are absolutely value-based, all the things about anti-discrimination and respect and dignity which are most often the things that patients and people using services say they want... at that level the Patients Forum can be a sort of a collective group. But going beyond that... with a huge forum and with hugely disparate organizations to speak for one voice... it's never attempted to do that.

Competition for funds from the public or government was a particularly difficult issue. A strategy to avoid conflicts when fundraising was to have tacit agreements about which funding sources should be approached by which group. As one interviewee commented: 'An umbrella body has to be very careful that it doesn't try and seek funding from the same sources [as] its members' (gi17).

In order to sustain collaboration and consensus, separate identities were respected. This is illustrated by a similar comments made by the spokespeople from a formal alliance organization and one of its larger member groups as they were concerned about the voice of smaller organizations being swamped. An interviewee from LMCA said:

> I think the downside [of the alliance] is that [in meeting] the specific needs of people with MS, Parkinson's, eczema it would be important that as well as speaking to us, that the people [civil servants] involved in those particular areas talk to the individual organizations and I would never claim that everything has to come through us.

This view was echoed by the interviewee from a member organization:

> You have to watch that you don't kind of dominate things and appear to be constantly ruling the show. Obviously it's easier for us to get people to meetings and things than it is for very small organizations. (gi17)

One of the rules of the game in managing difference was 'transparency and openness' and being prepared to 'talk things through'. The leaders of formal alliance organizations were very aware that their continuing existence depended upon being able to provide benefits. As one said of member organizations: 'They're just checking us out sometimes, that what we're saying is what they would approve of' (gi19). Indeed, a few groups said they had joined for negative reasons. They were concerned that if they did not do so, they might miss out on some crucial activity. Or their profile would be affected. A respondent from one mental health group commented:

> You know often you get ten people and nine of them are representing different kinds of physical health and you have one person representing mental health.... so very often in these bigger groups that's the role we're [playing]...The spin-off of being on those groups often is that mental health is included more than it was before. (gi23)

The costs of collaboration

Although more rarely mentioned, a few interviewees referred to the difficulties of collaboration. They said there was competition for funds and it was important to maintain a clear identity, with a high profile to attract public sponsorship and media support. Sharing a campaign meant sharing the spoils if they were successful (Salisbury, 1987). In the view of one mental health group, it was easier to work together on lobbying parliament than on media issues, because groups competed for media access. Indeed, one interviewee said that attempts to create permanent alliances in the mental health sector could not succeed because competition for resources and publicity.

Reference was also made to a few areas of conflict. A maternity/childbirth group had accepted funding from a commercial organization which made formula milk, which led to protests from other groups in the sector. There could be differences of opinion on tactics. For example, an organization concerned with the effect of steroids was accused of using scaremongering tactics by a group representing asthma patients. In another incident, one health consumer group refused to pass on the results of a survey to another because of the latter's criticism of a particular drug therapy.

One of the main lines of difference, if not conflict, was the degree to which health consumer groups should work with professional interests. Some groups criticized the Patients Forum for including organizations representing professionals as associate members because it was meant to be a consumer organization. The same issue was referred to in the arthritis area, where the BLAR's membership included both professionals and consumer groups:

> I think, for example, our partnership with LMCA, you have to be aware that some of the professional groups may not regard that as something of such high value for them, because LMCA is very much a patient groups' organization.

Another area of tension was how quickly a group could, or should respond to public policy issues. Generally, small groups with an executive committee could respond quickly. Larger groups with branches and consultative structures moved more slowly. One interviewee commented: 'Usually the bigger groups are more prepared to take it slowly. They don't want to upset the relationships they've established' (gi40). One interviewee claimed that her group was able to react on an issue after 'a few phone calls' whereas a larger organization would have to 'go through six committees and umpteen meetings' (gi3). These differences could make collaboration difficult.

The tensions were perhaps greatest in the cancer sector, where a number of interviewees said that collaboration was not a priority. It was acknowledged that there were a number of cancer charities with overlapping interests and competition for funding. However, the diversity was attributed by one interviewee to the complexity of cancer itself. She commented: 'A specialist in lung cancer wouldn't have the faintest clue about breast cancer and vice versa' (gi12). Others argued that groups fulfilled different roles as one respondent said:

> We all have slightly different ways that we emphasise things and in fact it in some cases is only going to strengthen things if different organizations are saying the same thing. (gi31)

Working alone

Collaboration was the norm for the majority of groups, although a few interviewees said their organization preferred to work alone. This could be due to limited resources or from choice. One respondent commented:

> We've been very adamant as a . . . board of trustees and patrons . . . in maintaining and retaining our independence and not actually working closely with other organizations. (gi28)

And another also expressed a reluctance to get involved in joint work:

> I really can't see the point of me joining, I know I'm not going to get any benefit from it at all. I plough my furrow. I do my patient education, I provide therapy . . . I don't need to do anything [else]. I can't learn anything from these people. I'm not a very good joiner, I hate locker rooms. (gi39)

Geography could also inhibit collaboration, and groups with headquarters in the provinces voiced concerns about the perceived advantages for London-based groups. As one interviewee commented:

> having wonderful 10 o'clock meetings with Lord somebody or other, or Lady somebody at eleven o'clock, with coffee and lunch from eleven till two, down in London. When it means [that] the only people who can get there are the 'lovies' who happen to work, already on salaries, around the area . . . Somebody in the voluntary sector in Sheffield or Newcastle or Manchester or whatever, they're talking about overnight accommodation for a start, as well as the train fare to get there for the day. (gi27)

Wider links

Links with other voluntary health organizations

The interviews showed that the health consumer groups had developed a network of contacts with other statutory or self-financing consumer organizations, as well as with similar organizations overseas. This section briefly describes these working arrangements and the benefits health consumer groups derived from them.

General consumer organizations such as the Consumers' Association played a significant role in getting groups together to discuss specific issues by providing a venue for meetings on neutral ground. Health consumer groups also had links with research charities (both medical and social policy) and social welfare organizations. Arthritis Care and the Arthritis Research Campaign met regularly to co-ordinate activity. Cancer Black Care and Cancerlink had received funding from Macmillan Cancer Relief and in 2001 Macmillan Cancer Relief and Cancerlink merged; the Children's Heart Federation received funding from the British Heart Foundation; the National Childbirth Trust had developed strong contacts with researchers at the Cochrane Collaboration and the Oxford-based National Perinatal Epidemiology Unit; the National Schizophrenia Fellowship had

links with the Sainsbury Centre for Mental Health whose interviewee said:

> If we want to make an impact on the carers' world, it's far better to
> do it through the NSF [National Schizophrenia Fellowship] and its
> constituency than try and do it ourselves.

Whilst relationships between medical research charities and health
consumer groups were in general co-operative at national level,
the De Montfort study found evidence of rivalry between
branches at local level. For example, there have been tensions
between branches of the BCPA and the support groups affiliated
to the British Heart Foundation and between branches of Arthritis
Care and the Arthritis Research Campaign. Whilst this could be
due to competition for members and resources, the respondent
from the Arthritis Research Campaign also suggested that it could
be due to the motivation people have for joining in the first
place, commenting:

> At the supporter level people are very clear about which way [they]
> want their money to go and they very rarely change their minds.
> Some people will think about the long term and want to invest for
> the future and others will think 'what about now, we need help now'.
> You very rarely get people crossing the floor.

International links and alliances

About half of the interview groups had international links. Four
groups had overseas members, for example the BCPA had a small
number of members in the USA, Canada, New Zealand and
Portugal. Groups had also developed relationships with parallel
or sister groups overseas, in particular groups in Western Europe,
North America, or New Zealand. These links typically involved
sharing information, newsletters, and offering advice or support
and learning from each other. Tyler (2002) comments on how
maternity user groups can benefit from each other's experience
despite social, political and cultural differences.

   While some groups maintained informal links with international
health consumer groups, nine groups in the interview sample had
joined international alliances. For the most part these alliances
were based in Europe. For example, the BLAR was a member of

the European League Against Rheumatism, an organization which sought to promote research, prevention and treatment of rheumatic conditions. The National Schizophrenia Fellowship was a founding member of the European Federation of Associations of Families of Mentally Ill People, an alliance of national and regional carers' organizations, established to provide support, share experience and campaign at European level. The National Ankylosing Spondylitis Society was a founding member of the Ankylosing Spondylitis International Federation, established in 1988 to share information and support the development of health consumer groups in countries where they did not exist.

Four groups in the interview sample had links to the International Alliance of Patients' Organizations, although only one, the LMCA, mentioned it in interview. The international alliance aims to place patients at the centre of health care through advocacy, partnership and capacity building. It was established in 1999 after the leaders of 40 patient groups recognized the need for a cross-disease, cross-national organization (Silver, 1999). Initial funding was provided by Pharmaceutical Partners for Better Health Care, a consortium of research companies (van der Zeijden, 2003).

Two of the arthritis organizations were members of the national taskforce for the World Health Organization's Bone and Joint Decade (2000–2010) which aimed to raise awareness, at national and international level, of the condition, improve prevention, diagnosis and treatment, promote research and empower patients. In 2000, Arthritis Care and the BLAR were also involved with the People with Arthritis/Rheumatism in Europe movement which launched a *Manifesto for the Third Millennium* as a basis for campaigning and lobbying on issues relating to arthritis and rheumatism (Jones, 2000). Three organizations were involved in lobbying at European level. For example, the Genetic Interest Group was pushing for an 'orphan' drugs act which would offer incentives to pharmaceutical companies to undertake research and develop treatments for rare conditions and a condition-based group had developed links with a Member of the European Parliament to gain support in a dispute with a pharmaceutical company over patient information leaflets.

For the most part interviewees were positive about their international links. Some used the links in order share ideas others, including the National Heart Forum and the Mental Health Foundation, talked about providing a model of good practice for colleagues overseas to follow. Others were members of international alliances because of the networking opportunities they provided for research. Whilst a number of groups talked about the growing potential for working in Europe, three respondents were concerned that differences in health systems meant that some activities could not be replicated between countries.

A confederation of health consumer groups?

At the time of the interviews, there was debate among the leaders of the health consumer group sector about the need for an over-arching alliance which would bring together the whole sector under one umbrella. Indeed, one interviewee criticized the Department of Health for not doing enough to strengthen the sector:

> I would like to see the government consider a more strategic approach to umbrellas in [the same] way that the Home Office funds the NCVO because they know they need that sort of organization to act as the filter and strengthener of the sector. The health sector hasn't got there yet, I'm not seeing any real demonstration that they want to. (gi19)

Such broad-based groupings exist in a few other countries, namely, the Australian Consumers' Health Forum (Bastian, 1998) and the Dutch Federation of Patient and Consumer Organizations (Dekkers, 1997). However, there was little consensus among the interviewees on the need for such an organization in the UK, or on its potential role. Respondents from five groups suggested that an over-arching organization already existed in some form or another naming, for example, the Patients Association or the Patients Forum. Groups were concerned that a new organization might ignore the voice of small organizations or people with rare conditions. Respondents were also concerned that a new organization could create more bureaucracy in the sector. These issues came to the surface during the debate about the creation of national patients' organization (see Chapter 2). In the event, however, the government decided to create a statutory body rather than a membership-based organization to which health consumer groups would be affiliated.

Conclusion

This chapter has shown that there is a high degree of networking and collaboration in the health consumer group sector, and that health consumer groups forge and join alliances as a means of influencing policy. This suggests that groups recognize the tactical advantages to be gained in working together. Chapter 9 discusses in more detail the influence of alliances in the policy process. It could be argued that the strategies developed to deal with difference, the sensitivity to smaller groups, and a concern to present a united front to decision-makers are illustrative of an underlying trust and a shared set of cultural assumptions. In this respect there has been a 'movement for patients'. Working together can strengthen groups' claim to represent the interests of all health care consumers. It is not necessarily a zero-sum game. Indeed, it can be argued that the capacity-building role adopted by some formal alliances has helped to structure and strengthen the sector by providing smaller organizations with the necessary skills to lobby and campaign.

However, it has also been shown that collaboration is contingent. Participation in alliances was dependent upon groups fulfilling their own particular goals and maintaining their particular identity. Group leaders made strategic decisions about joint working in the light of their particular position within the sector and the possible costs and some groups did not wish to join alliances. The extent of co-operation identified when this research was undertaken was high, yet this may change in the future. The fact that alliances often incorporate other interests in the health care arena must also be taken into account. Both government and professional associations have played a role in bringing health consumer groups together and may simply be attempting to control what they believe could be a powerful interest group in its own right. Finally, given that they are relatively new phenomena, it may simply be too early to judge the success of alliances in structuring the sector.

7

Collaboration with health professionals

It has already been shown that health consumer groups draw on the experience of their members or clients to provide support, services and to influence policy. Do health consumer groups also draw on professional knowledge and expertise and if so, in what ways? In the first section of this chapter, data from the questionnaire and interviews shows how, and for what reason, groups in different condition areas draw on professional knowledge. In the second section, interviews with the officers of a range of organizations representing professional interests in medicine and nursing provide an account of how, and why, professional associations have worked with health consumer groups, the importance they placed on involving the 'lay' interest and how this was done. This section also presents data on the views of professionals on the networks and alliances described in the previous chapter.

The relationship between professionals and groups representing health consumers is of particular interest in the contemporary context. From the establishment of the NHS, following the Second World War, until the 1990s commentators have described UK health policies as a state–professional alliance (Cawson, 1985; Moran, 1999; Klein, 2001). Among the health professions, organized medicine with its highly valued knowledge base and its dominance within the division of labour has enjoyed considerable clinical autonomy and an accepted social status (Elston 1991; Coburn and Willis 2000). Salter (1999) refers to an implicit bargain between the political forces of the state, the medical profession and the citizenry:

● Citizens receive health care from the state delivered to an appropriate standard by medical and other health professionals.

- The state gains politically from providing health care but relies on the medical profession and managers to allocate resources and manage demand and supply.
- By fulfilling the obligations to both, the profession is trusted by those who use services; enjoys a degree of autonomy to practice within a framework of resources; and has the advantage of financial security. Exposure to market forces is minimal as most private medicine is provided by doctors already employed within the state sector.

Over recent decades, this implicit bargain has failed either to meet the expectations of a more knowledgeable, critical and demanding public, or governments' concern to obtain greater value for money in health care. Therefore professional dominance, and particularly medical dominance, has come under challenge. In the 1960s and 1970s the women's movement, followed by the disability and HIV/AIDS movements, showed that professional clinical knowledge could be harnessed and used within support networks to give people greater control over their own body. These movements were often supported by individual health professionals sympathetic to this approach. Then, in the late 1980s, and 1990s, medical dominance came under challenge from the state. First, the health reforms strengthened the powers of managers both locally and centrally. Since 1997, the more recent regulatory reforms of Labour governments have created a raft of new regulatory bodies to monitor and oversee performance of health trusts and those who work within them. There has also been an enforced reform of professional self-regulation to increase the oversight of professional practice, through the revalidation of practising doctors, and the use of more accountable and transparent procedures for dealing with poor performance (Allsop and Saks, 2002).

While social attitude surveys show continuing high levels of trust in doctors and nurses (Johnson and Jowell, 2001), there has been concern among opinion-formers, such as parliament, national consumer organizations and members of professional bodies themselves, that systems for professional self-regulation are ineffective in dealing speedily with poor practice (Health Committee, 1999; National Consumer Council, 1999). These concerns have been exacerbated by wide media coverage of both individual, and systemic, failures. In these circumstances, have relationships between the groups that represent health consumer interests and those that represent the professions changed? Weberian theories of professional behaviour suggest that professionals seek to maintain control over their own practice and that a professional strategy might be to enter into new forms of alliance. It has been suggested that a new compact between the state, the professions and the citizenry is developing (Williamson, 1998; Ham and Alberti, 2002). Indeed, recent health reforms have increased networking between professional associations and health consumer groups. However, as shown in Chapter 3, the relations between health consumer groups and professionals in some condition areas is closer and more harmonious than in others. Furthermore, as subsequent chapters showed, groups differ in how they relate to professionals, some seeking to preserve a more independent stance, others perceiving greater advantages for their membership in having a close collaboration.

Health consumer groups and health professionals

The participation of professionals in health consumer groups

The questionnaire and interviews provided data on the extent to which individual health professionals participated in health consumer groups. Indicators of these inter-relationships included professionals' role in group formation and whether professionals actually joined groups. Among recently formed condition-based groups, doctors, generally hospital consultants, had played a significant role in the formation of some arthritis, cancer and heart/circulatory disease groups, either by initiating a groups' foundation or through encouraging patients and supporting them in their efforts. The objectives were to sustain a patient through a treatment regime; help them to maintain their health thereafter and by encouraging mutual support. Inter alia, this helped to raise the profile of a particular condition and to attract research funds (Clement-Jones, 1985; Williams, 1989).

In terms of membership, two-thirds of the questionnaire groups (68 per cent) had individual health care professionals as members. Doctors were the professionals most widely represented. Nearly half of the groups also said they had doctors on their main decision-making body (48 per cent), while a third had other health professionals. Medical professionals were most commonly members of condition-based groups (71 per cent) as compared to formal alliance organizations (64 per cent). Population-based groups were least likely (44 per cent) to have professionals as members, possibly reflecting their broader remit and larger size.

As well as these formal links, many groups in interview described close relationships with specialists – most commonly doctors but also nurses. Such relationships were seen to bring reciprocal benefits: access to up-to-date and accurate clinical information was important for group members and the wider public. Booklets and information sheets were commonly checked for accuracy by clinicians. As one heart/circulatory disease group said: 'You can't run a charity at the patient support end without having very highly qualified and a good range of professional advisers' (gi4). Networks of professional contacts were also used to set up study days, conferences and seminars. These could either be initiated by health consumer groups or professionals. In the view of one well-placed interviewee, the number of such events increased from the mid-1990s and were of critical importance in building mutual understanding and respect.

Close association with like-minded professionals has both practical and political advantages. The medical profession in particular was recognized by most groups as a powerful force because of its knowledge base, its ability to influence how a medical condition was perceived, and its influence over service delivery. Some groups supported and promoted research into particular conditions, particularly if these were rare. They sometimes helped recruit patients to research trials or test equipment. For example, CancerBACUP commissioned research on taxanes. The Stroke Association funded research on stroke and the availability of specialist stroke services. Other groups aimed to improve services for their members through developing networks with local providers. For example, some arthritis and heart/circulatory groups had funded additional facilities in local hospitals. Others had linked up with consultants, nurses or midwives in order to publicize their support services or to introduce enhanced service guidelines. Some health consumer groups saw their mission as informing generalists such as general practitioners, midwives, nurses, physiotherapists, or radiographers about rare conditions and promoting more patient-centred modes of care. As one questionnaire respondent said:

> As we develop as an organization, I feel it is important to create and maintain relationships with health professionals, so that they can become more aware of the needs of patients, carers, and their families, and as a result tailor their responses [in this way].

Health professionals and the policy process

In terms of external relations and influencing policy, groups saw political advantages in links with health professionals and particularly specialists who could provide a group with status and credibility. As the interviewee from one arthritis group said:

> It's a totally symbiotic relationship and I think that a patient organization involved in disease should have specialists on board, because I believe that gives them credibility . . . not just ordinary specialists but probably the best ones, the ones known to be associated with that disease. (gi39)

In the questionnaire, almost half the groups (49 per cent) believed that a lack of support from health professionals was a barrier to influencing policy. Nevertheless, there was a range of views about the terms of engagement. While some groups, like the one mentioned above, saw the relationship as mutually beneficial, a minority of groups said they were concerned to maintain their consumer identity and thus sought professional advice very selectively: they only consulted those who had similar values and either did not include them as members or, if they did, only as associates with no voting rights. A number of groups also had a suspicion of medical research charities. They were seen as vehicles for fundraising to support medical or pharmaceutical interests rather than representing patients and service users. As the interviewee from one cancer group said:

> They purport to represent patients and many of them are medical professionals, but they are there to raise money for the health care

professions who set them up, I don't have a problem with that, I have a problem with them pretending to be something they are not. (gi11)

For their part, medical research charities found they were sometimes the labelled as a 'consumer organization', which they were keen to reject. The British Heart Foundation's respondent believed it had been invited onto the Coronary Heart Disease Taskforce as a 'patient representative' organization, an assumption it had unsuccessfully tried to correct.

Variations between conditions

Overall, groups in the arthritis, heart/circulatory disease and cancer areas, were more likely to involve medical professionals over a range of activities. Groups in the maternity/childbirth and mental health area tended to be more selective about who they involved, and in what way. For example, only 12 per cent of maternity/childbirth groups had doctors on their decision-making body, compared to 63 per cent of arthritis groups, 62 per cent of heart and circulatory disease groups, 50 per cent of cancer groups and 43 per cent of mental health groups. However, some maternity/childbirth groups had a long history of collaboration with midwives at both local and national level. A common factor for both maternity/childbirth and mental health is a past history of struggle against a disease-based approach, in favour of a model of care that de-medicalizes treatments, offers choice, and values patient autonomy.

Networks with professional associations

The extent of contact

Health consumer groups had also established networks of contact with professional associations such as the Royal Colleges, the regulatory bodies and other specialist groups like the British Medical Association. These links were indicated formally through organizational affiliation. In the questionnaire a third (34 per cent) of all groups said they had professional associations as members.

This was higher for formal alliance organizations where over half (55 per cent) had a membership that included professional associations, a not unexpected finding given their policy remit. Table 7.1 shows the frequency of contact with professional organizations. One-fifth of groups said they were in contact with doctors' organizations at least once a month, compared to just over a third of groups being in touch with other professional organizations. Over three-quarters of groups had at least annual contact with doctors' organizations and nearly nine in ten groups, with other health professional organizations.

Table 7.1 Frequency of contact between health consumer groups and professional associations (all groups)

	'At least monthly' (%)	'At least quarterly' (%)	'At least annually' (%)	'Not in past three years' (%)
Doctors' organizations	21	48	78	22
Other professional organizations	36	71	87	13

Source: Questionnaire data set 1999.

Again, informal contacts were more frequent in the case of formal alliance organizations. Nearly three-quarters of these groups (73 per cent) said they were in at least quarterly contact with doctors' organizations compared to less that half of the condition-based groups (43 per cent). As Table 7.2 shows, the

Table 7.2 The issues health consumer groups discussed with professional associations (all groups)

	Health policy/ strategy (%)	Research issues (%)	Quality of care/ treatment (%)	User/ carer rights (%)	Other (%)
Doctors' organizations	51	38	65	42	18
Other professional organizations	44	28	51	44	34

Source: Questionnaire data set 1999.

issues discussed with professional associations were, shown in descending order of importance: the quality of care and treatment; health policy and strategy; user and carer rights; and research issues. The frequency of contact and the subject matter of that contact, indicate the shared interests and the possibility for building alliances, particularly through joint membership of formal alliance organizations.

The questionnaire data showed that a majority of groups were in regular contact with professional organizations and in interview, more than half of the groups had contact with the Royal Colleges representing specialist interests within medicine and nursing (54 per cent). This could be to share information or to work on particular projects; such as guideline development or in relation to more political campaigning activity. For example, a mental health group said:

> We build up, depending on the piece of work, a network of the organizations in the voluntary sector... professional organizations... [and] other mental health organizations where appropriate. (gi38)

For one maternity and childbirth group, there was regular and close contact with the Association of Radical Midwives (ARM) and for another, the Royal College of Midwives (RCM). As one interviewee commented in relation to the latter: 'We meet monthly, and I speak to my counterpart at the RCM, head of policy almost daily. We see ourselves having a lot of common goals' (gi35). In the cancer area, as well as strong links with cancer specialists supported by the Royal College of Physicians, groups had also developed links with nursing associations. One cancer group commented that contacts with the Royal College of Nursing had been particularly important for locally-based work but this had meant breaking down traditional boundaries. The interviewee said:

> I think we've reassured people that we're not after a 'them and us' scenario... we do a lot of work with the Royal College of Nursing and their Breast Care Nursing Association who are an incredibly powerful and useful contact for us in our local work... which is very exciting. We're increasingly asked to speak at the conferences of the various professional bodies, so we can get our perspective out

there and they're very useful information resources for us as well. (gi36)

Mental health groups referred to contact with a range of professionals, not only psychiatrists but clinical psychologists, mental health nurses and social workers.

As well as attending each other's conferences, representatives of professional associations and health consumer groups also met at a range of venues organized by formal alliance organizations, such as the British League Against Rheumatism (BLAR, now the Arthritis and Musculoskeletal Alliance) and the Patients Forum (see Chapter 6), and at events set up by third parties, such as general consumer organizations, pharmaceutical companies and all-party groups. Department of Health committees and new bodies set up since 1997 as part of the Labour government's health reforms also provided venues for interaction. The interview data showed areas of collaboration in lobbying to influence the decisions of the National Institute for Clinical Excellence (NICE) as well as opposition to new mental health legislation.

Closer relationships?

Health consumer groups described their relationships with health professionals as being more extensive and productive than in the past. This was attributed to a number of factors:

- Some health consumer groups were themselves large and influential, with considerable expertise in their area of specialization.
- A clear majority of groups interviewed believed that the general political environment was now more conducive to recognizing that service users and carers could bring a particular perspective to the policy table.
- It was felt that attitudes within the professions were changing as those with paternalistic views were being replaced by younger doctors who recognized the need for a greater partnership with patients.
- Both the professions and health consumer groups shared interests in research, and in developing an evidence-based approach to improving the quality of health care.

- It was increasingly recognized that professional and user groups needed to co-operate to improve NHS services.
- Evidence-based data had become more accessible to health consumer groups through the internet.
- Opportunities for health consumer groups and professional associations to engage had increased as governments now invited both parties to participate in policy developments.

As a consequence of these changes, there was a better basis for dialogue. As one large group concerned with the elderly said: 'It's all about trust and understanding about where each [of us] is coming from' (gi22).

However, despite the acknowledgement that there was considerably more interaction with professional groups and greater commonality of interest, trust was contingent and the medical profession in particular was perceived as both powerful and seeking to protect its own interests. As one seasoned campaigner within the maternity/childbirth area commented:

We try to work with them now as far as possible as equal partners. We are clearly not equal partners because we do not have the clout that they have. (gi35)

Another interviewee said that the now influential position of her organization within the cancer movement depended on support from powerful clinicians:

There are individual oncologists who have championed the cause and they have been important to people like [us]. We don't have a health background, we actually rely on the clinicians to help us get into positions of power and influence... cancer is such a traditional world it's almost impossible to have any influence unless you ally yourself with the powerful people and in cancer, it actually happens to be the oncologists. [This has allowed me access] to lots of the key research meetings where you can start to influence the agenda. (gi2)

The cognitive dominance of the methodologies and the knowledge base of clinical science were identified as sources of strength for medical interests which could act as a barrier to health consumer groups. For example, interviewees referred to the difficulties of contributing to discussions about which drugs and medicines were effective. In the context of decisions made by NICE, the only source of information considered valid was evidence based on findings from random controlled trials. Some mental health groups also argued that evidence from psychiatrists was given more weight than the views of consumer groups during discussions on the Mental Health national service framework (see also Hogg, 2002).

It is possible that where issues of medical autonomy or medical leadership in the division of labour were at stake, as in some national service framework deliberations, medical professionals attempted to guard their territory. However, leading professionals could also give public support to causes about which they felt strongly, even if this was not in line with current clinical practice. For example, in one interview a support group for people suffering from the effects of steroid use commented that their position on over-prescribing had been supported by an eminent specialist in a television documentary. Also, within the maternity/childbirth field for example, some obstetricians and midwives have been supported by health consumer groups for the stance they have taken following criticism from professional colleagues (Savage, 1986).

Working with the 'consumer interest': the perspective of medical and nursing associations

The policy context

Professional associations such as the Royal Colleges and other professional societies exist at least in part to promote and defend the interests of their membership. Moreover, these bodies are extensively networked in government and have considerable influence (Davies and Beach, 2000; Klein, 2001). In addition, government employs health professionals as civil servants, while professional associations are consulted on policy changes and contribute to policy development. Interviews with ministers and civil servants, showed that in 1997 the in-coming Labour government continued to draw extensively on professional expertise. However, as subsequent chapters will show, increasingly, the consumer interest has also been strongly represented. Interviews with medical and nursing professionals undertaken for the De Montfort study showed that the professions, too, have established stronger links with the consumer interest in the last decade.[1]

Structures for involvement

At the time of the research the Royal College of Physicians had a Patients' Representative Liaison Committee; the Royal College of Obstetricians and Gynaecologists (RCOG) had a Consumers' Forum; and the Royal College of Psychiatrists, a Patients' and Carers' Liaison Committee.[2] These bodies met three to four times a year and in addition, lay people were represented on a range of working groups and participated in professional conferences and seminars. The laity or consumer interest was perceived in different ways by the Colleges.[3] The RCOG chose the term Consumers' Forum deliberately and their approach has been developed carefully. Their respondent said:

> Other Colleges talk about patients – but we wanted to move away from this terminology and consult with consumer opinion.

In this College, the consumer members were all representatives from voluntary health sector organizations with an interest and expertise in women and/or maternity and childbirth – the Family Planning Association, National Childbirth Trust, the National Council of Women, Maternity Alliance, Women's Health, Association for Improvement in the Maternity Services (AIMS) and Maternity and Health Links are permanent members. In addition, the consumer interest is represented on all the College committees through Forum members. The interviewee explained:

> To begin with it was experimental ... [for example], we organized a meeting on the menopause so that we could give information that way. Now we work in a different way. If we are drawing up guidelines [on various areas of practice], these are shared. First, we nominate someone from the Consumers' Forum to sit on the working party which is drawing up the guidelines. Second, when the guidelines

are nearing completion we get feedback from the Forum. We also
use the web to get wider feedback.

The Consumers' Forum has helped to promote a shared agenda.
For example, two recent issues of concern to doctors, womens'
and maternity/childbirth groups have been the high rates for
hysterectomy and caesareans in the UK. In relation to the latter,
it was agreed that the reasons for this were not understood and
a joint audit and research project was undertaken with support
from various organizations (RCOG, Royal College of Midwives
and National Childbirth Trust, 1999, 2000).

Other colleges approached particular individuals, 'lay notables',
service users and carers as well as well as representatives from
health consumer groups. The Royal College of Physicians said
the aims of its Patients' Representative Liaison Committee were:
to act as a forum for the lay public to voice its concerns about
health and health care; to review policy documents for the College
and to advise on issues from the consumers perspective. They
have appointed lay notables as well as representatives from larger
and more 'successful' consumer organizations. As an interviewee
commented:

> We wanted people who had social care, social work backgrounds,
> and those who had experience of representing the views of
> patients...[people with passion and/or consumer groups where]
> we could benefit from their knowledge.

The College is planning to restructure and strengthen its patients'
committee to include carers and may in future have consumer
members on its governing council.

The Royal College of Psychiatrists said it had representatives
from most of the main national mental health and learning disability
organizations. It asks the organization for a representative so may
include people who have used mental health services, their carers,
and paid officials.

> I suppose that in a way we've invited those [organizations] that
> have been the most politically engaged and are national. We've got
> MINDlink, which is the user organization from MIND, Hearing
> Voices which is the user organization from the National Schizophrenia

Fellowship, NSF, Alzheimer's Disease Society, Eating Disorders Association, Northern Ireland Association of Mental Health, Patients Association, Mencap, Rescare, Carers National Association, Age Concern, Depression Alliance and Manic Depression Fellowship.

Recently, the Royal College of Psychiatrists has involved their consumer members in training initiatives; on working parties related to policies and guidelines for community care and in the development of an advocacy service provided by 'expert patients'. The working process has been iterative and consultative, aiming to establish a consensus between different interests.

All the Royal Colleges referred to the importance of the 'expertise' of their consumer or patient members and all had drawn on their expertise to assist in developing clinical guidelines for practice standards. The latter are now seen as a product to be shared (Williamson, 2000).

The British Medical Association

In contrast to the Colleges, the British Medical Association does not have a standing committee, rather it supports what it calls the Doctor–Patient Partnership through which patients/carers, specialist lay people or representatives of voluntary groups specializing in particular issues are asked to serve on committees and working parties on an ad hoc basis. They have also called upon the expertise of health groups in area where there are ethical dilemmas which have implications for the doctor–patient relationship. For example, it has worked with a number of health consumer groups, including the Patients Association and the British Kidney Patients Association in developing a position paper on the changes required to legislation on organ donation.

The British Medical Association is an associate member of the Patients Forum and has also worked with other health consumer groups on policy issues. For example, with the Impotence Association in relation to the initial guidelines on the use of Viagra; with the Multiple Sclerosis Society over prescribing beta-interferon within the NHS; and with the Carers National Association (now Carers UK), the Alzheimer's Disease Society (now Alzheimer's Society) and Help the Aged in relation to the Taking Care of the Carers initiative.

Nursing and midwifery

The professions of nursing and midwifery have a longer history of representing the lay interest. For example, the professions' regulatory body, the UK Central Council for Nursing, Midwifery and Health Visiting (now the Nursing and Midwifery Council, NMC) has appointed increasing numbers of lay members to its Council and committees. It was one of the first regulatory Councils to develop a public involvement strategy (Davies and Beach, 2000; UKCC, 2000). The NMC now has the one of the highest ratios of lay to professional members, 48 per cent (Allsop *et al.*, 2004). Within the Royal College of Nursing, the lay interest is represented not through a formal committee structure, but through representation on thirteen special fields of interest such as cancer, mental health, and so on. Each has a programme director, a steering group and an advisory panel that includes patient/carer representatives. How members are selected appears to depend on the programme director and may include actual service users as well as health consumer groups. For example, representatives from larger groups, such as the National Consumer Council and the LMCA, all serve on Royal College of Nursing committees.

In interview, the Royal College of Midwives said that midwives had worked in partnership with women's groups long before the issue of user involvement became fashionable. The main advantage of working with groups, rather than individual lay people, was that it provided a 'critical but considered perspective' and they believed that the long history of collaboration had built a high level of trust so that collaboration, both formal and informal, took place automatically in relation to a wide range of policy issues. Currently, the main committee for user involvement is the Maternity Services Committee which has representatives of the main maternity/childbirth groups with others co-opted as necessary.

Trends in representation

Looking at professional associations as a whole, a number of trends were discernible. Representatives from health consumer groups have tended to replace lay 'notables'. Involvement has deepened (ie: there is more frequent and more structured contact). It has broadened (contact occurs in more arenas within the association), become more embedded (there are longer-term relationships) and been strengthened (instead of one lay or consumer group member there are at least two and often more). Nevertheless, structures differ and the objectives of the professional associations in drawing on the consumer interest are more, or less, clearly worked out.

What are the benefits of working with health consumer groups?

The practical benefits

The reasons that professional associations gave for working with health consumer groups were both practical and political. For the medical associations, a major area of activity was drawing on the knowledge and expertise of groups to develop guidelines for practice, develop information booklets, and submit joint press releases (see also Williamson, 2000). As one respondent said:

> I think we get a better product in guidelines, on the advice we give, statements to the press and so on. It isn't just political correctness bolted on – it's getting something more robust which can stand up to scrutiny. So it's a genuine quality issue. (si13)

There was an acknowledgement that health consumer groups could draw on the experience of users and that this was different from professional knowledge and could be of benefit in communicating better with patients. One interviewee commented:

> [We need to] hear, because there is a difference between listening and hearing... you have to put away your technical baggage and just listen to what people say. (si18)

Another association said that patients and carers were changing and one way of keeping up was through listening to user representatives:

> Assumptions are changing continually and the groups are in touch with a well-informed clientele. People are getting more information

and they always understand more than you think they do.... It's only when you're made to confront people who think differently through a formal structure that you begin to understand the point of view of others . ... So I don't think we can ever say we haven't got more to learn, particularly in relation to language. [For example, some technical terms] can carry a message of blame. (si13)

Groups could also bring an experienced-based knowledge of how the NHS was working for patients and a network of contacts that could aid the dissemination of information. One interviewee echoed others when he said:

They bring such things as a network of contacts and a network of communications – simple things like receiving things from their membership and sending things back....Having groups...round the table is a great advantage. They bring the expertise they have gained to our members. They can say: 'However much you think things work like this is your hospital, we know that there are other hospitals where it doesn't.' (si13)

For medical associations, the experience of working with health consumers was relatively new. For nursing associations and particularly for midwives, the practice was more deeply embedded in their structures and processes.

Political influence

All the professional associations saw health consumer groups as being very influential on bodies set up by recent governments. The cancer groups in particular were perceived to have been very powerful. According to one respondent, the influence of breast cancer groups in helping to draw up clinical and service guidelines was described as 'mega' (si1). Interestingly, cancer groups also recognized the medical profession as a powerful interest group so there was mutual recognition of sources of power that could be complementary. There were seen to be political advantages in working with the lay interest as this brought greater credibility and acceptance of the work of the professional organisations. As one respondent said: '[to show] we're not in an ivory tower with minimal action...it's a demonstration that the College is listening' (si13). There was also an acknowledgement that the professions were under pressure and it was important to have allies. An interviewee commented in relation to mental health:

> The mental health user movement is very, very political and can be exceedingly adversarial and it's extremely important that if you are representing a medical professional group [to] be seen to be listening, be seen to be taking on board patients/carers needs. I know that the BMA is very concerned about the adversarial nature of the media coverage of the medical profession..... You have to move with the times....Working with groups is much more powerful than just the voice of the profession.

The difficulties and dilemmas of increased interaction

It was also acknowledged by interviewees from professional organisations that there were risks, difficulties and dilemmas in working with consumer groups. For example, one said: 'There are confrontational groups, but there are those who wish to engage in constructive politics' (si32). He went on to comment that there was sometimes a need to reach a compromise and gave an example:

> The [name withheld] has worked with us on considering a therapy....There were said to be benefits but the research is not sound. It is not without risk – we have discussed this with them and we have been able to reach agreement on a set of recommendations on which we both agree. (si32)

Some professional interviewees referred to problems of dealing with consumer representatives who tried to highjack the agenda with their own particular 'horror story' or 'hobby horse'. They also commented on the difficulties in establishing clear rules of engagement, a matter also of concern to health consumer groups. A few interviewees from the latter constituency felt that their contribution had been 'edited-out'. From their perspective, they wanted recognition of the fact that they represented others to whom they felt accountable. On some issues, it was necessary to consult with their own membership.

How consumer representatives were selected and paid was an issue that caused difficulty, particularly for the medical professional associations. As one interviewee said:

> You have people representing themselves or other organizations. How do you select people? Do you advertise for them? Do you have contracts, do you pay them? There is a danger of incorporation – there is a distinct possibility that you can loose the grassroots element – what we don't want is it to be stuffed with suits. (si18)

Problems of accountability were reduced by drawing on the officials of health consumer groups to represent their membership. Such people not only had organizational backing and a constituency, but also managerial and political experience. Nevertheless, informal and 'gossip' networks could still be a channel for recruitment. There was a belief among nursing organizations that officials often end up by recruiting people they know and that they can work with. There is currently no national database of health consumer groups, or of people interested in acting as a lay representative, so it is not surprising that professional associations seek out well-known groups or people they know. The Royal College of Midwives with long experience of working with health consumer groups, simply asked groups to nominate the most appropriate person to act as a representative.

As with health consumer groups themselves, there was general concern among professional associations about the lack of representation of ethnic minority groups. The Royal College of Psychiatrists was particularly worried about this deficit as certain mental health policies have a marked impact on ethnic minorities. They acknowledged that while progress had been made at the local level, more remained to be done nationally. The Royal College of Midwives has made a particular effort to work with such communities and has a comprehensive database for seeking comment on relevant consultation documents. It has considerable experience in working with black and ethnic minority groups at a local and national level, a constituency that is well represented in the College itself. The College has set up working parties on many sensitive issues related to pregnancy and childbirth where the representation of different communities is necessary for effective policies. Furthermore, when responding to consultation documents, it seeks comments from a wide constituency who are listed on a comprehensive database kept at the College.

From their perspective, people appointed as general health user 'representatives', said they were often uncomfortable about being asked to give an opinion on issues of which they had no direct experience or knowledge. Some also referred to feeling that they had been 'captured' and could not openly criticize a professional group when they were a member of one of its committees – particularly if lay representation was small. Others said they did not know how to report back and there were anxieties about payment. While medical committee members and officers of health consumer groups were normally covered for the time spent on committee work through salaries or remuneration, patients, carers, or volunteer officers of consumer associations were not. As one interviewee said:

> There was nobody else in that room who was doing anything on a voluntary basis and there are days when you miss the train home and it all gets protracted and you think, 'why the heck am I doing this?' However... that's one's own decision at the end of the day. (gi37)

There were also opportunity costs for people with a regular working or caring commitment which ruled out certain people from engaging in this sort of activity.

Political campaigning

Health consumer groups were sensitive about the costs of collaboration in terms of a possible loss of identity and capture by a professional interest. Examples of where health consumer groups had campaigned actively alongside professional associations were found in the maternity/childbirth and mental health fields. Maternity/childbirth groups had gained political experience in campaigning for a more woman-sensitive service. However, at the time of the interviews, these services were no longer a priority for government – a matter of concern for consultant obstetricians, midwives, and health consumer groups. The Maternity Care Working Party described in Chapter 6, was a precursor to the creation of an All-party Group on Maternity. The aim of the group was to campaign and stimulate parliamentary concern about the high rates for caesarean section in the UK and what is seen as the low level of provision for neonatal care. As a professional interviewee said:

> We now have a potentially very important alliance. Half the electorate have been through the process of bearing children and it should have a strong voice. The alliance of midwives, obstetricians, and public can have shared aims. (si13)

In the case of mental health, the Royal College of Psychiatrists has provided administrative support for the All-party Group on Mental Health for some years. It originally decided not to join the Mental Health Alliance established to co-ordinate a campaign against the government's proposed revision of the 1983 Mental Health Act and which included the Royal College of General Practitioners and the Royal College of Nursing (see Chapters 10). However, by July 2002 it had changed its mind and joined the campaign (Boseley, 2002).

Conclusion

Despite the difficulties, there is strong evidence that health consumer groups and professional associations perceive a mutual interest in collaboration. Each constituency recognises that the other possesses expertise and knowledge that complements their own. In addition, each constituency can benefit from access to the social and political networks of the other. The politics of collaboration differs according the type of group and the particular sector. Formal alliance and larger population-based groups represent the wider constituency of health consumer interests. They often have extensive contacts within the Whitehall policy arena and can speak for a range of groups. For professional associations, such groups offer access to a broad constituency of health care users through newsletters and conferences. Equally, for groups, access to clinical knowledge and professional networks can help them keep up to date with innovations and policy changes. These forms of collaboration are now extremely important developments.

For groups in particular condition areas such as arthritis, heart and circulatory disease and cancer, access to clinical specialists is an important part of providing a service to their membership. There is close collaboration with professional specialists in the production of leaflets giving information on clinical conditions. Equally, professional bodies benefit from a consumer input on guidelines for protocols and practice. Maternity and childbirth and mental health groups too see advantages in having access to professional knowledge, although these groups have tended to be selective in deciding on the particular professionals with whom they wish to work.

The politics of health care has changed over the past decade as professionals have come under pressure to work more closely to government agendas. Service frameworks have been developed for many condition areas. They are based on evidence of what is considered as best practice and will shape patterns of service delivery and the division of labour in health care for the future. Governments have urged doctors and professional associations to develop greater partnership with patients; to move away from paternalistic modes of practice and to recognise that those who use health care wish to be well informed about their condition, and be in a position to make choices about their own care.

In this new environment, professional bodies and associations can maintain legitimacy and credibility from being seen to collaborate with health consumers, and in many cases the involvement of health consumer groups is actively welcomed, as shown in Irvine's (2003) account of the role of consumer organizations in consultations on the reform of the General Medical Council. From the interviews it was clear that the professional associations believed that jointly produced documents on practice guidelines or ethical issues carried greater credibility than those drawn up by the profession acting alone. The data also suggest that many professionals and their associations believed that a partnership with health care users and health consumer groups had two benefits. First, it led to better health care outcomes and, second, resources for health could be increased as a result of combined pressure from both constituencies.

It is worth noting that both professional associations and health consumer groups saw each other as 'influential' and 'powerful' on the national level committees set up to develop service frameworks and their associated working parties. Some health consumer groups believed that professionals continued to dominate, but others were prepared to engage in a struggle to represent their perception of the consumer interest. There was also a willingness on the part of both interests to collaborate in political action, to modify government policy, or to get issues on the policy agenda which currently had a low priority. To some extent, the landscape of health politics has shifted. For both practical and political reasons there are mutual advantages in collaboration. Both professional associations and government see themselves as gaining an advantage by incorporating the health consumer interest.

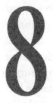

8 The pharmaceutical industry

There are several reasons why it is important to look at the links between health consumer groups and the pharmaceutical industry. First, the two sectors have a mutual interest in ensuring that patients have access to treatments, although their motivations differ. Second, little is known about how health consumer groups view relationships with the pharmaceutical industry and how they work with them. Third, links between the two sectors have been viewed with suspicion by many commentators due to the profit motive of pharmaceutical companies and their massive resources compared to health consumer groups. Drawing on data from the De Montfort study, this chapter will address how and why groups choose to work with drugs companies and explore how the industry might benefit from working with them. It will also assess how the relationship between health consumer groups and the pharmaceutical sector is handled in practice.[1]

The pharmaceutical industry, health consumers and the policy context

The industry

Pharmaceutical companies are driven by a profit motive. As Moran (1999, 2002) has pointed out, in modern economies they are at the frontier of innovation, production, and marketing through the creation of 'world brands' that have deeply penetrated health care systems. Moreover, culturally, the pharmaceutical industry corresponds to science-based medicine, which has historically driven developments in health care. These factors place the pharmaceutical sector in a powerful position in relation to governments, professionals and consumers. For governments in countries such as the UK, pharmaceutical companies contribute to exports, provide employment and through research and development, contribute to economic growth. In the UK, the pharmaceutical trade association, the Association of the British Pharmaceutical Industry (ABPI), claims that annually the sector creates almost £3 billion in trade surplus. It also spends around £2 billion each year on research and development (ABPI, 2002). Indeed 15 out of the top 75 prescribed drugs in the world today were developed in the UK (ABPI, 2002).

The industry is regulated to ensure the safety, efficacy, quality, manufacture, sale and promotion of drugs. The ABPI also enforces a code of practice, particularly in relation to the promotion and advertisement of drugs. The sector is bound by relevant European regulations and legislation. As the NHS is tax-funded, the government is a major consumer of health and medical technology. Its monoponist position has enabled successive governments to control prices of branded drugs through the Pharmaceutical Price Regulatory Scheme (PPRS). A different mechanism is in place for generic drugs.[2] Nonetheless, the NHS drugs budget is huge and in 1999/2000, accounted for 14 per cent of total expenditure (Kay, 2001).

Although public safety considerations have led to a high degree of regulation over the sector, there have been concerns that globalization and the concentration of business among a few large companies has made regulation more difficult in practice. Critics argue that problems remain including 'brand' name marketing of very similar products, assertive marketing and poor quality information about the efficacy of products (Medewar, 2002).

Health consumers

Health consumers demand pharmaceutical products that are effective and accessible. But they also want drugs that are safe and reliable. Health consumer groups have an important role here. They can facilitate access to accurate information about products. As bodies representing or promoting the interests of patients, users and carers, they have variously supported the licensing of products of proven effectiveness and have led campaigns against products where unacceptable risks have been identified. Indeed, some groups have been formed in direct response to adverse effects of drugs and other medical technologies, for example, the Vaccine Victims Support Group UK (1985), Group Action into Steroid Prescribing (1994) and the Radiotherapy Action Group Exposure (1991).

In analysing the research data, the underlying assumption was that the relationship between health consumer groups and the pharmaceutical companies was likely to vary. The willingness of health consumer groups to engage with the industry was likely to depend on the nature of the condition affecting their members; the formation and history of the group; and whether or not there were drug therapies available or for future development. It was also considered likely that the pharmaceutical companies would aim to build relationships with groups where there was a profitable market related to current or future products.

The current policy context

The pharmaceutical sector is a key stakeholder in the health care arena. Collier (1989, p. 29) argues that the industry is now the 'single most dominant influence' in medicine, with interests in medical research, education and practice. In recent years however, it has been claimed that companies are now struggling to develop new treatments which can sustain and promote levels of growth previously achieved. As a consequence, the past decade has seen an increase in mergers, acquisitions and the creation of large multinational corporations within the sector (Medewar, 2002; Busfield, 2003). Busfield (2003) argues that profit levels depend on the innovation of new drugs and the protection of patents. Furthermore, industry analysts believe that the push to increase profits has meant that the pharmaceutical sector is spending more on marketing their products (Medewar, 2002; Moynihan, Heath and Henry, 2002).

Currently it is illegal in the UK and the European Union to advertise directly to consumers. In 2003, proposals to allow a limited amount of direct-to-consumer advertising in three condition areas – AIDS/HIV, diabetes and asthma – were rejected by the European Commission. Yet even with a ban on direct advertising, health service users are becoming more aware of different treatment options. The internet has enabled patients to identify treatment protocols and to advocate for their introduction within the NHS (Kendall, 2001; Judd, 2003). Health consumer groups play a role in channelling information about drugs and the pharmaceutical industry. Within the wider voluntary sector, the Consumers' Association as a broadly-based subscription association has been particularly active as a watchdog on the pharmaceutical industry (see for example, Consumers' Association, 2001a). Medical research charities have also played a role in disseminating information about, and promoting access to, new treatments and particularly where they have been involved in their research and development.

As referred to above, in the UK the main buyer in the pharmaceutical sector is the NHS, which purchases two classes of medicine: branded drugs, which are produced under patent, and generic drugs, produced once the patent runs out. The health consumer groups in the research were mainly concerned about access to newer branded treatments. The price of drugs under the PPRS were revised in October 1999, with current agreements running until 2004. The scheme aims to ensure that the NHS gets access to effective medicines at prices that are not excessive but which are high enough to fund the research necessary for UK-based companies to remain competitive both nationally and internationally (Lawton, 1999). Concerned with a growing drugs bill, successive governments have also introduced mechanisms to improve the cost-effectiveness of prescribing by general practitioners and within the hospital sector.

Governments have also aimed to identify cost-effective treatments and in April 1999 the National Institute for Clinical Excellence (NICE) was established to appraise the cost-effectiveness of new technologies including drug therapies and to determine whether they should be made available within the health service. According to Kay (2001), the establishment of NICE, and the revision of the pharmaceutical prices under PPRS, caused some friction in industry–government relationships, with the former raising concerns that cost-containment would affect competitiveness and profitability. The pharmaceutical industry has an interest in ensuring its products are utilized as soon as possible and delays in acceptance, or an outright rejection of particular treatments, can affect profitability. It has been critical of delays in the assessment process and in the implementation of NICE recommendations.

In response, the government established the Pharmaceutical Industry Competitiveness Taskforce. This body was matched at a European level, with the European Commission establishing the G10 working group to identify ways of increasing both innovation and competitiveness in the pharmaceutical industry. In 2002 it recommended a continuation of restrictions on direct to consumer advertising and declared that legislation relating to drug information leaflets should be reviewed to take account of user views. The review also considered the industry's links with health consumer groups and whether industry funding compromised the independence of patients' groups. The report stated:

> The Commission should consider providing core funding for European patient groups to enable them to participate independently in the debates and decision-making on health matters in the EU. (High Level Group on Innovation and Provision of Medicines, 2002, p. 23)

For some years, the pharmaceutical sector has been aware of the potential benefits of working with patients' groups. For example, UK cancer groups, in relation to Taxol, and AIDS/HIV groups, on AZT, have campaigned successfully to make these medicines available through the health service. Whitehead (2000) has suggested that this activity made drug companies take notice of the health consumer group sector. In recent years, the drugs trade association, the ABPI has sponsored publications which examine the role of patients and their support groups in the health sector, in, for example, *Putting Patients First* (Kirkness, 1996) and *Expert Patient* (Illman, 2000). The industry has also established the Informed Patient Initiative which promotes health awareness campaigns that encourage the public to consult their doctor if they think they have symptoms of a particular condition (Illman, 2000).

Relationships with the pharmaceutical sector

Contact between groups and the drugs industry

The relevant questionnaire findings from the De Montfort study are shown in Table 8.1 below. Nearly two-thirds of groups in our

Table 8.1 Level of contact with pharmaceutical industry, by type of group

	'At least monthly' (%)	'At least quarterly' (%)	'At least annually' (%)	'Not in past three years' (%)
Formal alliance organizations	27	46	55	46
Population-based groups	9	73	82	18
Condition-based groups	23	41	61	39
All groups	22	45	63	38

Source: Questionnaire data 1999. Due to rounding up some totals exceed 100.

data set had some contact with pharmaceutical industry. The majority of these had at least quarterly contact (45 per cent). However, nearly 40 per cent of groups reported they had no recent contact with industry. When broken down by category, formal alliance organizations and condition-based groups had a similar pattern, with over 40 per cent reporting quarterly contact and over 20 per cent monthly contact. Population-based groups had less regular contact with industry, but a significant proportion (73 per cent) had at least quarterly contact.

The questionnaire data also showed that smaller groups (with an income of £100 000 or less per annum) were less likely to have contact with the pharmaceutical industry than medium-sized (with an income of between £100 001 and £1 million per annum), or larger groups (with an income of over £1 million): 28 per cent of smaller groups had 'at least quarterly' contact with industry compared to 59 per cent of medium-sized groups and 69 per cent of large groups. One explanation could be that medium-sized and large groups have the resources and infrastructure to engage with industry. Indeed, the questionnaire showed that only 8 per cent of the large groups had no contact with industry within the previous three years, compared to 30 per cent of medium-sized groups and half of the smaller groups. Another explanation could be that the smaller groups were not big enough for the pharmaceutical sector to engage with, either because they did not represent a large enough constituency or because many smaller groups cover rare conditions for which few treatments are available and where there is little economic incentive to develop new products.

The main reason for contact between pharmaceutical companies and health consumer groups related to funding, either through sponsorship or grants. It was shown in Figure 4.2 above that 34 per cent of groups accepted private sector sponsorship a category which included drugs companies. In interview, a number of groups said that funding from this source had been used to update publications, run seminars and conferences, and that contact tended to be initiated by the pharmaceutical companies. In one instance, a group had been approached by a public relations company on behalf of a manufacturer of an over-the-counter medication who wished to work with a health charity. Such sponsoring activity could be interpreted as an indication of goodwill, or as a way of influencing the group and thereby public policy.

A recurring theme across the interviews with groups was uncertainty about the benefits and costs of accepting support from, and working with, drugs companies. The benefits included additional support for projects and being informed about new medicines or products – useful to the membership and the public in contact. However, such sponsorship could be seen as compromising the independence and integrity of a group. Indeed, in 1994 the Insulin Dependent Diabetes Trust (IDDT) was formed in part due to concerns that the British Diabetic Association (now Diabetes UK) had not adequately publicised the adverse effects of synthetic human insulin. The latter had accepted funding from two manufacturers of the drug, and whilst there was no question of undue influence or impropriety, the founders of the IDDT were uneasy about the link and formed their own group (*Which?* 2003, p. 25). In interview, there was widespread mistrust about the motivation of pharmaceutical companies and the strings that could be attached to funding. The relationship was seen as unequal with the pharmaceutical companies seen as having a substantial wealth, power and status. Writing about patients' groups, both Hogg (1999) and Wood (2000) commented that those who work with the sector risk 'capture', that is, the profit motive of drug companies will ultimately dictate the terms of any relationship that develops. The sensitivities of the sector were reflected in a comment made by the president of the American Alzheimer's Association who argued that the pharmaceutical industry must: 'Appreciate and accept the unique role of patient-based organizations, and help them maintain the only real capital they can control: their integrity, credibility and independence' (quoted in Buttle and Boldrini, 2001, p. 206). In a submission to the G10 working group, the Consumers' Association argued that in relation to pharmaceutical industry funding: 'some organizations are much better than others at managing these relationships and at ensuring they do not compromise their position' (Consumers' Association, 2001, p. 4.).

Arguably, it is the symbolic position of the industry as much as its actual power, status and resources that underpins these fears. In the UK there has been no systematic analysis of consumer/industry relations. Within the health consumer group sector, however, there are three positions:

● There are groups who have no contact with the pharmaceutical sector on principle. This may be because they prefer to seek funding from other sources or because they are against technological interventions, as in the case of certain maternity/childbirth groups, or because there has been a history of adverse reactions, as is the case with some mental health groups.
● There are groups that have no contact because the area that they represent does not require drug treatments. For example, some health consumer groups promote patient participation and do not deal with illnesses or particular conditions.
● There are groups that represent condition areas which rely heavily on medicines for treating and alleviating illness. Such groups have varying degrees of sponsorship and were the most likely to have a relationship with the industry.

Sponsorship and funding

Most groups in the interview sample were pragmatic about accepting sponsorship. For three of the five condition areas, advances in treatment meant that contact with the pharmaceutical industry was almost inevitable. One arthritis group was lobbying for access to anti-TNF drugs for rheumatoid arthritis (see Chapter 3). Cancer groups had lobbied for access to taxanes for breast and ovarian cancer while mental health groups were concerned about the availability of a new generation of anti-psychotic drugs for schizophrenia. Some groups argued that without the drugs industry there would be little effective treatment for their members. They also recognized that decisions within the drugs industry would ultimately affect future treatment options. New medicines could be more acceptable because they had fewer side effects – an issue raised by some mental health groups, although other groups in this condition area were strongly opposed to any drug treatment and indeed half the mental health groups in the questionnaire data set stated they had no recent contact with the pharmaceutical industry. Arthritis groups and cancer groups were concerned both about side effects and access to drugs that might prevent a recurrence of the disease.

A minority of groups would not accept sponsorship at all or, in very limited circumstances, when, for example, they were a member of a formal alliance. Most alliance groups had well-established relationships with the pharmaceutical industry, or were considering them, although some did not accept funding. Links with the pharmaceutical industry could also occur at European level through membership of international alliances (see Chapter 6). A number of pan-European alliances received support from the pharmaceutical sector including People with Arthritis/Rheumatism in Europe and the International Alliance of Patients' Organizations. It is possible that sponsorship through a larger organization provided some protection in an unbalanced power relationship, a point discussed further below.

Perhaps because of the sensitivity of the issue, the annual reports of health consumer groups do not always give detailed information about sources of funding. Some merely identified drug companies as 'supporters' or 'sponsors' and gave no data on the amount of funding received. Others gave brief information about funding, for example the National Schizophrenia Fellowship (1999b) stated that in 1998/99 it had received over £2000, from five separate pharmaceutical companies. In the same period the Genetic Interest Group received over £1000 from five pharmaceutical companies (Genetic Interest Group, 1999). Other groups gave more detail on the level of funding received. In 1999 the LMCA declared that it received a fifth of its income from the pharmaceutical sector (LMCA, 2000a).

Just under half of the 39 interview groups had received industry sponsorship although many were highly selective in the purposes for which the funds were used. Funding was most widely used to support publications, subsidise meetings and to increase the amount of information available for consumers. For example, the *Guidebook for Patients* produced by the National Ankylosing Spondylitis Society was sponsored by a pharmaceutical company, as was the British League Against Rheumatism's (BLAR, now the Arthritis and Musculoskeletal Alliance) report *Standards of Care for Osteoarthritis and Rheumatoid Arthritis*. Other groups used drug industry funding to produce research reports or position papers, for example Bristol Myers Squibb sponsored CancerBACUPs' *Living with Cancer in the 21st Century*. A pharmaceutical company sponsored the publication of a training pack for the Family Heart Association (now Heart UK) and their interviewee said 'They had no influence on the contents at all, but they actually helped provide financial support to get it published.' The newsletter of a cancer group was sponsored by the pharmaceutical industry. The Long-term Medical Condition Alliance's (LMCA) *Living Well* video, which helped to develop the concept of self-management of medical conditions, was sponsored through an educational grant from GlaxoWellcome (now GlaxoSmithKline). Eli Lilley had sponsored the National Schizophrenia Fellowships' national conference programme since 1997 and in 2000 named the organization as its 'charity of the year' (Rethink, 2003). In recent years pharmaceutical companies have sponsored websites, including one for Arthritis Care. It should be noted, however, that not all requests for assistance were supported. For example, one cancer group reported that it had approached a number of companies to sponsor their magazine but had been unsuccessful.

Some companies sponsored services which groups provided for members. For example, a drugs company sponsored the telephone help-line of one population-based group. Funding could also been used to develop good practice. Arthritis Care had worked with Pharmacia (now Pfizer), the Department of Health and Coventry University, to develop a self-management programme *Challenging Arthritis* for use in primary care. This was a precursor to the *Expert Patients Programme* (see Chapter 3). Other groups have worked with the pharmaceutical industry to publicize information about clinical developments, such as new drug treatments and protocols. The ABPI drew on the expertise of health consumer groups when producing its 'Target...' series. This series provided information about current research on medical conditions such as diabetes, arthritis and schizophrenia.

A shared agenda?

The interview data showed that in some areas there was a shared agenda between health consumer groups and the pharmaceutical industry. For example, Arthritis Care argued that both the industry and arthritis groups wished to raise public awareness and move arthritis up the political agenda. In November 2000 Arthritis Care had used company sponsorship for an advertisement in *The Guardian* newspaper, as part of a campaign for enhanced access to newer and potentially more effective treatments (*The Guardian*, 2000a). A heart/circulatory disease group was funded to undertake research on the availability and take-up of particular treatments across the country. An interviewee from the organization said:

> On a number of issues recently we've inserted questionnaires into the magazine... It's tended to be on specific drug-related issues to help inform, very often, the drug companies themselves. We did a survey on Warfarin users that was funded by... the lead [drug company] on that front. (gi1)

Campaigning activity was also supported. For example, Merck Sharp & Dohme funded the LMCA's fringe meetings at party conferences (LMCA, 2001b) and Roche sponsored the UK Breast Cancer Coalition's (UKBCC) advocacy online campaign (Covington, 2001).

Working with the pharmaceutical companies: rationale and strategy

Health consumer groups that worked with the pharmaceutical industry justified this in terms of the interests of patients. For example, a respondent from one group stated:

> Yes, we do get criticized because it could be seen that there's a conflict of interest there, but [the company] provides a resource

for patients that wouldn't otherwise have that information . . . if we've got our information across to patients and it's benefited patients, I don't care who's paid for it. (gi33)

For most groups the decision to accept funding from the pharmaceutical industry was not taken lightly. One interviewee said: 'When times are hard you might have to sleep with the devil' (gi4). Another stated: 'it is an incredibly sensitive issue . . . once you stop being aware of how sensitive and difficult it is, you're probably doing the wrong thing' (gi36). When considering accepting sponsorship, prior consultation with the membership was seen as important. A formal alliance organization commented: 'We've done an extensive search on their range of products and their future products . . . it took us six months, and about six board meetings to actually agree to work with one of the companies' (gi36).

Guidelines and written agreements were used by some groups to avoid being compromised. As one interviewee said: 'If you can get money out of people with no strings attached, and you watch yourself very carefully, and it's all very clear and written down in abundance then it doesn't really matter' (gi11). However, this could restrict access, another group commented: 'We don't particularly have a lot of contacts with the pharmaceutical industry, probably as a result of that policy [of strict ethical guidelines]' (gi38). One larger organization had also laid down guidelines for staff:

We have a very specific commercial working policy and there are certain things that staff members can and cannot do. I think the drug companies are also a bit wary to be getting to a bad PR situation, so they're a little bit wary of going too far. (gi10)

Formal alliance organizations such as the LMCA, have played an important role in developing guidelines for use by their member organizations. In 1998, LMCA produced policy guidelines stating that any relationship should be based on four principles: integrity and openness; the maintenance of independence; maintaining equality in the partnership; and mutual benefits for both parties. LMCA argued that health consumer groups should set boundaries, particularly in relation to the endorsement of products and the acknowledgement of funding, and pay attention to procedures and contractual matters. Groups were also advised to safeguard their independence with a 'get-out' clause (Wilson, 1998). An updated version of their guidelines said: 'Ideally, every VHO [voluntary health organization] would have a clear, uncompromising policy to show to pharmaceutical companies at the outset of any relationship' (LMCA, 2000b, p. 2). For the industry, the ABPI (2001) *Code of Practice for the Pharmaceutical Industry* covered relationships with the general public but did not explicitly mention health consumer groups. However, since the research was undertaken, the ABPI has published a new briefing paper clarifying the industry's relationships with patient organizations.[3]

The available evidence suggests that few health consumer groups that accept support from the pharmaceutical industry have codes of good practice. In 2003 a Consumers' Association survey found that only 32 out of 125 patient organizations listed donor information on their website and just two groups provided information about their funding policy (*Which?* 2003, p. 25). It was suggested that lack of guidelines may be a particular problem in continental Europe. As one interviewee commented, European patients groups were '"in hock" to the pharmaceutical industry' (si12).

Dilemmas: product endorsement

For those groups representing members whose illness required drug treatment, there were particular dilemmas. This arose in relation to accepting funding and lobbying for a particular drug or product. As the interviewee from CancerBACUP, commented in relation to the cancer drug, Taxol:

> It is a difficult line to tread really because Taxol obviously is made by one company, and what are we supposed to do? Say that because we don't want to look like we're supporting the drugs industry, we shouldn't support patients having the drug?

While the UKBCC, said:

> Sometimes you have to be realistic and actually say the point is, some drugs are best and if we're campaigning for equality of

access to the best then there's going to be times when we're campaigning for equality of access to a specific drug.

One strategy adopted to maintain independence was not to use funding from a company to sponsor a particular campaign. An interviewee from one group said:

> If we're doing something like . . . . research where we're asking people about medicine, we can't have that funded by the pharmaceutical industry. When we try and influence the government, NICE or journalists with our findings, they will if they're any good, say 'Who funded this . . . the drug companies? Aha, well that's a bias' (gi23)

Another strategy was to be well informed about research findings from drug trials and use this external source of knowledge. One arthritis group said:

> There have been cases where some of the claims that drug companies have made for their new product have been questioned in research articles and we would usually want to publicize that in our magazine and it's possible that in the same issue . . . the magazine might be carrying a section on exercise or something sponsored by that pharmaceutical company. . . . It might seem in a sense odd that we are carrying articles critical of that company while we are also taking their money. But I mean that is understood or we certainly try to make it clear that we would always want to preserve our independence. (gi17)

It should be noted that these dilemmas also apply to links with other commercial organizations whose activities have a health dimension. For example, there has been recent media criticism of charities that support manufactured food products (Food Commission, 2002). Although this kind of endorsement is more prevalent in research charities, a few groups in the interview sample had done this. For instance, one of the heart/circulatory disease group studied had endorsed a breakfast cereal. For some years there has been a direct link between one maternity/childbirth group and a company manufacturing breast-feeding aids, with the management of the company and profits being shared by the group (gi37).

Why the pharmaceutical sector works with health consumer groups

The analysis of the interviews with health consumer groups and the ABPI, and of the pharmaceutical marketing literature, indicate the reasons why a drugs company may wish to work with health consumer groups. First, the alliance offers the opportunity to promote awareness of products that may help to market a particular brand and their corporate image. Second, groups are an invaluable and unique source of information about consumers' views and needs. Third, they are a potential ally in the debates on direct-to-consumer advertising. Fourth, they may support funding for particular treatments. Fifth, they make the company appear generous rather than exclusively concerned with profit. Finally, contact with groups carries legitimacy in a drug company's dealings with other healthcare stakeholders.

A changing relationship?

Buttle and Boldrini (2001) argue that in recent years the ways in which pharmaceutical companies work with health consumer groups has changed. As the visibility, influence and capacity of groups has increased, so companies have become more aware of the potential for alliances. As a consequence, funding has tended to become more closely targeted to focus on particular projects with particular groups rather than on generalized charitable giving. Government policies to include patients and their representatives in decision-making, and the recruitment of patients to research trials may also have persuaded companies of the value of working with health consumer groups. One commentator on pharmaceutical marketing said: 'The industry needs to think more creatively about building alliances between it and patient groups in all disease areas like never before' (Rowden, 2002, p. 3).

The closer involvement with groups appears to have brought recognition of the diversity of the sector and respect for their activities. For example, the interviewee from the ABPI saw health consumer groups as 'anything but dependent' and as 'quite strong bodies', with 'an in-depth understanding of the nature of illness and its impact on people's lives, the research going on, the range of treatment options, state and other support available'. The respondent commented on the political values of groups:

> They are socially responsible. They are not demanding just for themselves. And they certainly don't want the health service to spend in their area at the expense of other people with other debilitating health problems. They are a vital part of the broader health service and expect to be properly valued for the job they do. They make a major contribution to the nation by helping people affected by illness to lead full lives.

As a trade association, the ABPI saw its role as facilitating dialogue and promoting networks between health consumer groups and industry. It therefore sponsored and hosted meetings and workshops on important topics where different healthcare sectors could meet. As its respondent commented:

> It provides a backdrop for co-operation. We can all work constructively together partly because we do see each other often. There are a variety of events over the year where challenging issues are tackled and differing voices heard. People from different stakeholder groups meet with time to talk. Inevitably ideas for useful projects arise that might not otherwise have come up.

For the ABPI, encouraging contact between the sectors provided a useful way of encouraging mutual respect and understanding:

> When groups have issues they'd like to discuss, they know they can set up those discussions at the level they need to in a company, they are familiar with how the pharmaceutical industry works and industry has a better understanding of the voluntary sector. So it's much easier to get things done or changed.

The importance of health consumer groups remaining independent of the industry is accepted. As one Pfizer media relations manager said: 'It is vital to avoid any risk of voluntary organizations appearing simply to be the mouthpiece for industry. That perception doesn't do anybody any good' (quoted in Gander, 2000, p. 3).

The political resources of health consumer groups

From the research findings, it is apparent that closer relationships have developed between some health consumer groups and the pharmaceutical industry. These ties are particularly important in relation to two policy issues already referred to – the approval of new treatments and the question of direct advertising of medicines. Health consumer groups are concerned to increase access to effective treatments and Boseley (2000, p. 9) has argued that: 'Drugs companies anticipating that some of their new expensive medicines will be rationed, are looking to patient power', and indeed, the industry has provided funding for the Campaign for Effective and Rational Treatment which acts as a conduit between industry, charities, professions and government (CERT, 2002).

The interviews showed that several health consumer groups had, or were in the process of, submitting evidence to NICE (see also Chapter 9). This arena has given health consumer groups an important new mechanism to promote access to treatments. However, there are also temptations for pharmaceutical companies to demonstrate consumer support by setting up a patients' group. In 2000, the Medicines Control Agency took action against two pharmaceutical companies for their tactics in demonstrating patient support for access to beta interferon, a drug used in the treatment of multiple sclerosis (Dillon and Gould, 2000). According to the then director of the Multiple Sclerosis Society (MS Society), this approach: 'Destroyed in a matter of weeks the trust that had been painfully built up between the MS Society and the companies over the previous five years' (Peter Cardy, quoted in Gander, 2000, p.1).

Despite a common interest in the outcome of NICE deliberations, there was little evidence from the De Montfort study to suggest that health consumer groups and the pharmaceutical sector openly worked together on either appraisals or in the appeal process. However, there were cases where interest coincided, such as the Taxol case (see Chapter 9). Research by Rangnekar and Duckenfield (2002) found that between 2000 and 2002, in the five cases where both industry and patients' groups appealed against NICE decisions, four were referred back for re-evaluation and for the fifth (beta-interferon) a risk-sharing venture between the Department of Health and the pharmaceutical industry was devised which made the drug available to certain patients. This suggests that, as with other health policy decisions, a common position between different interests can be very effective. Whilst government can accuse the pharmaceutical sector of having a vested commercial interest, independent support from patients may be more difficult to ignore.

Another key issue is direct advertising to the public of 'prescription only' medicines. Currently European legislation places restrictions on contact between companies and individual members of the general public and on direct advertising. In the event of requests for information, a company may only recommend that individuals contact their doctor. Companies are allowed however, to contact and work with health consumer groups. The pharmaceutical sector is keen to engage with health consumer groups on a relaxation of this law and to seek their support if possible. Opinion in the voluntary health sector is divided on the issue. In June 2002 the Patients Association hosted a conference, sponsored by the ABPI, which included discussions on direct advertising (*Which?* 2002). The Consumers' Association has lobbied against direct advertising as it could lead to an increase in the NHS drugs bill and the exploitation of patients. Accordingly, it has been opposed to consumer groups accepting funding from industry in the absence of guidelines to manage the relationship (*Which?* 2002).

During the De Montfort study, two new health consumer groups were formed with support from the pharmaceutical industry, although no information was available about the extent of support received. Both Bristol-Myers Squibb and Pfizer were founding corporate sponsors of the Blood Pressure Association, launched in October 2000, which seeks inform and education the public about the dangers of high blood pressure. In 2001 Aventis, Pharmacia and Schering-Plough were among the pharmaceutical companies that supported the launch and the subsequent work by the National Rheumatoid Arthritis Society (NRAS). A specific objective of the NRAS is to: 'provide objective and easily available information on the treatments available...especially with the recent introduction of the radically improved and effective drugs'

(NRAS, 2002). In the short space of time since their launch both groups have been active in the policy process. The Blood Pressure Association is represented on a number of government committees (Blood Pressure Association, 2003). The NRAS has set up the All-party Group on Rheumatoid Arthritis and successfully appealed with other organizations against a NICE decision to reject anti-TNF drugs and has initiated a further group, the Inflammatory Arthritis Alliance (NRAS, 2002). In both these cases, the role of the industry in establishing and sponsoring these groups has been openly acknowledged.

Conclusion

In this chapter it has been shown that as representatives of the interests of their members and the public, health consumer groups have been drawn into relationships with pharmaceutical companies and their trade association, the ABPI. Within the sector, groups have had different relationships depending on the condition area and type of group. Those in condition areas where drug therapies are heavily used in treatment – arthritis, cancer, heart/circulatory disease and mental health – have had more contact. However, a number of groups on principle did not seek support at all. Indeed, one group was considering legal action on the basis that a drugs company did not give out sufficient information regarding adverse drug reactions.

Health consumer groups see the industry is a possible funder for projects and a key source of information about new treatments. The reasons why pharmaceutical companies have developed closer links with groups were similar to those advanced by health professionals. The groups were considered knowledgeable about the needs of patients and were an important source of information about patient experiences. Relationships had developed through these mutual interests on an ad hoc basis. In addition there were political motives on both sides. Both saw each other as potential allies in building support for decisions relating to a particular drug.

Even so, pharmaceutical companies have greater financial resources than health consumer groups and can dominate the relationship. For some, the profit motive that drives the industry is paramount. One interviewee with long experience of the health consumer group sector was critical of the relationship that some groups were building with industry. In his view, any health consumer group that printed pharmaceutical brand names or company logos on their publications was acting as a sales representative for the industry. He considered it would be naïve to assume that industry would act in any way other than to maximize profit. Similarly, Hogg (1999, p. 133) warned that 'by supporting voluntary organizations, pharmaceutical companies can help create consumer demand for their drugs and exert pressure to fast track a drug through licensing procedures'. Although there are occasions when health consumer groups can benefit substantially from support from the industry, as has been shown, the industry is likely to be the biggest beneficiary from what is a highly unequal relationship.

9 Working with government

In the UK, central government dominates the policy process. In order to shape the direction and detail of most policies, groups must participate in the institutions, policy processes and networks of central government, seeking to persuade ministers, civil servants, and their advisors. It has been assumed that groups that build a close relationship with government become insiders (Grant, 1995), as members of closely knit policy communities, and thereby increase their chances of influencing policy (Marsh and Rhodes, 1992). For this to happen, government must accept the group's legitimacy, acknowledge its expertise and be assured that it will play by the rules. Above all, the admittance of a group into various decision-making, consultative and advisory fora will depend on the extent to which it can contribute to the political and administrative objectives of the government. This presents a dilemma for groups whose desire to exert influence may be tempered by a fear of manipulation by government and a loss of independence.

In this chapter, the interaction of health consumer groups with central government is discussed, drawing on data from the De Montfort study. The nature and extent of engagement is examined alongside the reasons for participation from the perspective of both groups and government. The chapter also explores variations in activity between different types of group and some of the key barriers to involvement. There then follows a discussion of how access to government relates to influence over policy, focusing on issues where groups have claimed to influence outcomes.

Engagement with central government

Frequency of contact

The De Montfort study found that health consumer groups had little difficulty gaining access to central government to discuss policy matters. The questionnaire survey showed that three-quarters of groups had had at least some contact with central government in the previous three years. Not surprisingly, groups were more frequently in contact with Department of Health ministers and civil servants than other departments (see Table 9.1), although some groups established contact with other central government departments. For example, the Carers National Association (now Carers UK) reported contact with the Department for Education and Skills and the Department of Social Security (now the Department for Work and Pensions); mental health groups with the Home Office; and the Maternity Alliance with Department of Trade and Industry and the Department of Social Security. In interview, groups elaborated on the reasons why they did not rely solely on links with the Department of Health. The interviewee from Carers National Association argued that links with the Treasury were essential to press for further financial assistance for carers. A further impetus was the need to 'join-up' the activities of government departments. Indeed, there were instances where groups facilitated collaboration across government. For instance, the Mental Health Foundation promoted an interdepartmental conference on children's mental health that brought together civil servants from eight different government departments.

Table 9.1   Percentage of groups reporting 'at least quarterly' contact with ministers and civil servants (all groups)

	(%)
Department of Health civil servants	48
Department of Health ministers	30
Other Departmental civil servants	22
Other Departmental ministers	16
Prime Minister's Office	8

Source: Questionnaire data set 1999.

Compared with links to government departments, contact with the core executive of central government was reported less frequently in the questionnaire survey (see Table 9.1) and in interview. Examples mainly took the form of a letter to the prime minister or a petition to Number Ten, rather than direct contact, though there were a few instances where groups had been able to put their case directly to the prime minister or his advisors. Nonetheless, the perceived importance of high level contact was widely held. One respondent, from a mental health group, said it was important to have contact with Number Ten, but that the core executive discouraged such lobbying: 'If they open themselves to every sort of lobby group on every subject they would have difficulties. So they've built up some pretty good barriers' (gi38). Other groups identified Number Ten as being very influential over health policy and noted that policy documents were extensively rewritten at this level, notably in relation to national service frameworks, discussed below. The important role of the prime minister's health policy advisor was specifically mentioned and has been reflected in the observations of others.[1]

Increased opportunities

Aside from problems of contacting the higher echelons of government, the De Montfort study found that government departments were relatively accessible and that contact was becoming more frequent. The majority of groups responding to the questionnaire (62 per cent) stated that in the previous three years, opportunities for involvement in central government had increased. Only 9 per cent reported decreased opportunities, the remainder perceiving no change. Increased opportunities were confirmed by interviews with groups and other stakeholders. Most interviewees noted that health consumer groups were now frequently invited to comment on proposals and meet with ministers and civil servants. Most reported an environment of inclusiveness that was conducive to involvement, illustrated by the following observations. An interviewee from one cancer organization said: 'The climate of the Department of Health and health policy-making is becoming more inclusive' (gi31), another from a mental health group commented: 'I know personally the guy who's in charge of mental health policy. . . . A few years ago I would have never seen this person, never heard of this person' (gi23).

It is difficult to pinpoint a specific point in time when central government became more accessible, although, as shown in Chapter 2, some respondents suggested that efforts to incorporate the patient perspective began in earnest during the mid-1990s. Under the Labour government, groups were apparently drawn closer into the process of policy formation and implementation. The Department of Health civil servants interviewed saw changes since 1997 as being particularly significant, given the emphasis on the patient and consumer experience. One stated that the change in group involvement was 'massive ... compared with a couple of years ago' (si4). This was confirmed in interviews with former ministers.

Relationships with Department of Health ministers and civil servants

As noted, questionnaire and interview data suggested that most contact between groups and the Department of Health was through civil servants. These relationships were described mostly in positive terms, with groups commenting on the professionalism, integrity and energy of the civil servants. Most respondents viewed civil servants as accessible and reported little difficulty gaining access even to senior personnel. Groups described relationships with officials as 'crucial' in view of their role in advising and briefing ministers. They also recognized that civil servants developed specific expertise in a particular area and were able to grasp the fine detail of policy. The length of time civil servants stayed in a post was viewed as giving the process some stability. By the same token, when civil servants moved on to other posts this often caused disruption, as an interviewee from the Patients Forum noted: 'It's very vulnerable to changes in personnel.... every time someone comes and goes you have to re-educate them'.

Many groups had learned how to deal with civil servants and the importance of identifying and targeting the most appropriate person. Existing contacts were used to pinpoint the relevant officials inside the Department. This insider knowledge was enhanced where groups employed civil servants who had formerly worked for the Department. These people were regarded as useful because of their knowledge of government structures. Of particular importance here was knowing the appropriate language, as an interviewee from one group commented:

> You need to use the appropriate language because many civil servants either can't understand, or won't understand, the emotional bit. They're trained that way. (gi5)

However, not all groups had this insider knowledge. Groups also recognized that at times civil servants could be obstructive. They could restrict the supply of information to groups and could attempt to block or delay policy developments through the advice they gave to more senior colleagues and ministers. In this situation, relationships with ministers took on greater significance. This was neatly expressed by the interviewee from one of the maternity and childbirth groups:

> If policy is going to be changed, it's the civil servants who draft it, so you need to influence civil servants and all the time. Civil servants are both your obstacle and the means to an end because they often get in the way. One feels that the minister understands our problem better then the civil servants and the civil servants hold them back and you want to kind of leap frog over the civil servants and get to the ministers. (gi35)

Although contact between groups and health ministers was less frequent than with civil servants, and in some respect access to them was more problematic, groups realized that there were occasions when an approach to ministers was essential. Ministers were seen as powerful drivers of policy. They were regarded as more in tune with public opinion on health issues than civil servants and more willing to consider policy developments likely to be judged as popular or arousing public sympathy. They were seen by groups as valuable allies in 'breaking the logjam' when policies were being impeded by civil servants. A number of examples were given by interviewees. For instance, maternity/childbirth groups believed that their arguments for 'women-centred' maternity services had been strengthened because the junior minister chairing the Department of Health's Expert

Maternity Group back in the early 1990s (Baroness Cumberlege) shared their vision (see also Chapter 3).

Former ministers stated that, despite the limited time available, they were generally accessible to groups. One minister, who had held office under the Major government, said she had insisted that civil servants refer all requests by groups for a meeting to her (after discovering that they had been 'filtered' by the Department). Another, who had served in the first Blair government, stated that she could not ever recall turning down a request for such a meeting during her time in office. Nonetheless, the pressure on ministers' time meant that meetings had to be prioritized. From a group's perspective, a meeting scheduled three months ahead was of little use if an issue was being decided tomorrow. Groups mentioned that they had to use informal links with ministers, what one interviewee called the 'magic card' (gi43) in order to secure access quickly when needed.

Formal and informal contact

Informal networks cover a range of activity including friendships, common educational or occupational backgrounds and long-standing political allegiances. These operate across a range of settings, including social and recreational venues such as dinner parties, restaurants and clubs. Some of our interviewees provided a glimpse of these networks. In one case a senior officer of a health consumer group had previously worked alongside a current health minister in a voluntary organization and was able to secure a meeting between his new organization and his former colleague. Informal networks were also believed to be important in influencing the composition of official committees, with ministers and civil servants preferring to select individuals that were known to them. This is one reason why there was a tendency for the same people to be appointed to these bodies, an issue discussed later in this chapter.

Groups did not lack informal contacts, as illustrated by the number of health ministers with a voluntary sector background (see Chapter 2). Even so, it was generally acknowledged by several interviewees that, compared with other interests, notably the medical profession and the drugs industry, health consumer groups lacked the 'heavyweight' informal contacts that were most effective, especially at the higher echelons of government.

Building relationships with government: the rationale

Relationships between groups and government emerged out of mutual interests and the perception of mutual benefits. As noted in Chapter 2, there was a pull by government to involve groups and a push by the groups to get involved. However, there were also tensions arising from the interplay of these interests, recognized by both sides.

Why did groups form a closer relationship with government?

In seeking to explain why groups and government began to work more closely, the motivating factors on both sides should be understood. From the perspective of most groups, engagement with central government was essential as a means of influencing policy and developing services. They believed, rightly, that central government had a key role of setting priorities and allocating resources to the health care system and that this role was becoming even more important in the light of national service frameworks and clinical governance introduced by the 1997 Labour government.

When seeking to influence government, most groups tried to build a mutually beneficial and trusting relationship. One group interviewee noted how the longer-term nature of the relationship encouraged trust on both sides:

We aren't trying to trick them or get them to do something they don't want to, and they are not trying to manipulate us or get something out of us, then sort of chuck us away. (gi23)

While another emphasized reciprocal benefits:

It's a matter of being able to do something for them and then expecting a pay back. (gi40)

However, groups mentioned the dangers of becoming 'too close' to government, fearing that their independence might be compromised. Particular concerns were expressed about seeking government funding, and maintaining autonomy and independence. A minority of groups clearly believed that the Department of Health disliked their confrontational style and preferred to meet with those who were less adversarial. Some even believed they were regarded as beyond the pale; that government simply did not like what they did, or disagreed with their views, so there was little point in having a dialogue.

Nonetheless, even groups that worked closely with government recognized that there were occasions when they had to be assertive, even if this invoked the displeasure of ministers and officials. A respondent from National Childbirth Trust likened this to 'walking a tightrope'. She went on: '[We] want to be on good terms with them and yet our purpose is to make life difficult for them.'

Similarly, an Age Concern respondent referred to the need to put pressure on government, even if this meant putting a strain on their relationship. Referring to age discrimination in the NHS, she said:

> We've told them that we will continue to bring forward evidence, and essentially embarrass the government until we're more convinced than we currently are that there is a sea-change and that something will happen.

If they felt strongly enough about an issue, groups claimed they would not hesitate to adopt tactics that might irritate those in government, such as lobbying parliament and raising concerns in the media. But their tactics were pragmatic. Most groups acknowledged that in order to influence policy and service development they needed a good working relationship with government. They accepted that this might place some constraints on them, but this was the price to be paid for access to decision-makers.

Why did government involve groups?

As noted in Chapter 2, during the 1990s two key policy streams were relevant to the closer relationship between government and groups, namely initiatives to promote patient and public involvement, and, indirectly, policies that acknowledged the role of the voluntary sector in policy and service provision. In the late 1990s, reform processes created further opportunities for health consumer groups to engage in arenas that shaped policy and NHS guidance, including the NHS Modernisation Action Teams, national service framework external reference groups and National Institute for Clinical Excellence (NICE) committees and appraisals.

In addition, the broader social and political context was conducive to extending user and carer participation. Respondents, from groups and government, referred to a decline in deference to doctors; the growth of health information available to the public; the rise of consumerism in health care; the demands of patients/users and carers for more responsive services; the recognition of the importance of self-help and self-management and an acknowledgement that the quality of health care could be improved by greater patient involvement. Links were made between the wider user/carer participation agenda and the specific role of health consumer groups. According to one group interviewee, the strength of the case for greater participation made it difficult to deny a role for groups: 'I think there is just a momentum, perhaps beyond any government to make a decision on whether they want to involve ... patient groups' (gi31).

Other groups were more cynical and saw government attempts to include groups as a means by which it could control the agenda. As a result, policy options could be restricted or even foreclosed. The interviewee from one group said:

In so far as the government has a fairly set idea of what it wants to do, and what it wants to achieve, then that will tend to mean that they are not going to be so open to anything that doesn't fit with their agenda. But I suppose that's true of any government. You've got to find a way of presenting what you want to happen in ways that will be attractive or convincing to them. You have obviously got to work with their agenda and their political philosophy. (gi17)

From the perspective of ministers and civil servants, engagement with health consumer groups was part of an effort to respond to demands for greater user and carer involvement. One civil servant acknowledged that 'patients have shifted to centre stage' (si4) and this was why the Department was now more proactive in dealing with groups. Civil servants also noted other advantages such as gaining support for policies and, by the same token, limiting dissent. The need for a 'shared realism' (si4) between service providers and users was referred to, that is, a mutual acceptance of what could be achieved, as well as shared ownership of policy. As another civil servant frankly acknowledged: 'Let's face it, presentation is also an advantage because we can say we've consulted users...so the ministers can say, well we've got users in there' (si17).

By contrast, the more confrontational groups were regarded as troublesome. As one civil servant put it: 'When we try and consult, it's not much use at all if all we get back are destructive comments' (si17). Another said that in one particular case, they excluded a group because it was 'very vociferous and cause[d] a lot of trouble' (si36). However, ministers denied that confrontational or troublesome groups would automatically be refused access. One former minister claimed that she wanted to encourage debate, and had been prepared to grant access, and even financial support, to such groups. However, she did concede that ministers tended to work more closely with those groups that shared their overall policy aims. In short, government could tolerate criticism, providing that these aims were not challenged or undermined. Yet both ministers and civil servants were wary that open opposition by groups to a particular policy might cause political embarrassment, and acknowledged this could be a problem when coupled with adverse media coverage and parliamentary pressures.

Ministers and civil servants also identified other, 'technical' reasons for engaging with groups. Groups were seen as repositories of expertise, particularly with regard to patient/carer experiences. Their involvement was justified because, as one civil servant bluntly put it: 'You get better policy out of it' (si36). More specifically, the involvement of groups was justified in terms of attuning policy more closely to the needs of users, and thereby improving policy outcomes, as the following comments indicated:

I don't think any policy can be developed without their involvement because...they bring a sharper perspective and focus. They ensure that we are actually producing policy that's going hopefully to make a difference and improve patient care. (si8)

The policy is more robust, we get better interaction of ideas, an understanding of what will work. (si23)

A number of possible disadvantages were also identified. It was noted that greater involvement could raise expectations. If these were not met, disillusionment with government policy could follow. According to one civil servant: 'Patients' groups do help to raise the profile, but you do have to be very careful, if you raise the profile and nothing happens, then all you get is angry letters' (si36).

Those in government were aware that efforts to involve groups could rebound, fuelling opposition and criticism, particularly if groups were unrealistic in their aims. A further disadvantage was that policy initiatives could be delayed by extensive consultation. Finally, some of the civil servants interviewed expressed fears that the involvement of health consumer groups could make it more difficult to protect confidentiality within the policy process. On balance, ministers and civil servants appreciated that involving health consumer groups added to the complexity of the policy process, but saw their contribution as a means of improving the quality of policy-making.

The contribution of groups to the policy process

What did groups bring to the policy process? Essentially this came down to two distinct but related elements. On the one hand, the groups' ability to *represent* patients, users and carers; on the other, their *expertise* – about the patient experience of conditions and services, as well as wider issues relating to patient and carer involvement.

Representation

Government saw groups as being able to represent patients, users and carers. However, they were careful to distinguish between the representation of these interests and the wider public interest. Ministers and civil servants stated that they did not believe that groups could represent the latter, because their interests were by their very nature, sectional. As one civil servant put it: 'They represent views which are strongly held and genuine, and have to be listened to. The idea that they might represent all patients is not tenable. They don't' (si36).

Nonetheless, it was acknowledged that some formal alliances – those which covered a range of conditions – could encapsulate a broader perspective. For other groups, if they could satisfy government that they could speak authoritatively on behalf of their constituency, then their position was strengthened considerably. However, groups with weaker representational claims would not necessarily be excluded, providing they had relevant expertise or knowledge to offer.

The task of evaluating these claims fell mainly to civil servants, though ministers were able to challenge their judgements. There was no clear formula for determining 'representativeness'. Nor was there an explicit threshold which groups had to achieve to be so regarded. Rather there were several criteria used to justify inclusion. The most significant was the group's ability to engage with its members and its wider 'client-base', such as people who used a group's services – for example, help-lines – but who were not formal members. One former minister stated that she liked to see evidence of a 'governance structure'. This could include mechanisms for electing leaders, a clear organizational framework, and forums to encourage dialogue between service users and group leaders or officers. However, it would be wrong to see credibility being judged solely in terms of formal constitutions. Those in government were keen to work with groups that facilitated engagement with members and clients and who could speak with authority on their behalf. This relates to the notion of social resources, discussed in Chapter 5. Much depended on how groups could demonstrate active engagement with their constituency. This was illustrated by comments from the civil servants. As one said:

> It's not really important that they are democratically representative, it's important that they represent a series of views which are credible. (si36)

And another:

> It is important that we know those attending carry the confidence of their constituents . (si23)

Large membership groups could claim to represent more people, but they were not necessarily seen as more representative than smaller organizations. Civil servants appeared less impressed with the size of membership than ministers – the latter perhaps had an eye to the numbers of voters involved. For both, the quality of a group's interaction with its membership appeared to be more important than sheer membership size. However, size was inevitably linked to income and resources, which favoured the larger groups in ways that will be discussed later.

A further criteria was the ability of a group to mobilize the wider public behind an issue. Ministers and civil servants were aware that some groups were more adept than others in building public support, largely through sympathetic media coverage. If a group could demonstrate wider public support it could strengthen its position considerably. By the same token, a group could be seriously disadvantaged if its view was at odds with the government's perception of public opinion. In interview a number of civil servants expressed concern about the difficulties of ensuring the voice of excluded populations, including ethnic minorities, was heard. Indeed, a particular problem identified was that few groups representing ethnic minorities existed at national level.

In their contact with government, many groups sought to strengthen their representative claims by involving actual service users or carers from the ranks of members or staff. In some cases groups acted as a means of access to a wider network of current users and carers, who could advise government on policy or services. However, both groups and government recognized that policy skills were also necessary, which actual service users and carers sometimes lacked. Another problem was that the condition itself could provide a significant barrier to involvement: people with dementia, communication difficulties, severe degenerative conditions and psychotic illnesses faced considerable obstacles in participating in conventional settings, such as committees (see also Chapter 4).

Some respondents, both from groups and from government, argued that it was difficult for some individual patients and carers to be objective. The condition could dominate their outlook. As one civil servant noted, some patients could be 'hopelessly introspective' (si17). Similarly, a former minister observed that what she had wanted was patients who could encapsulate a broader base of experience and not just talk about the impact the condition had had on them personally.

Groups reported that the selection of people to act as representatives on official committees and working groups was geared towards people who were not currently experiencing a particular condition. People were chosen because they were experienced representatives, or were regarded by government as trustworthy. Some group respondents were not comfortable about this and saw it as promoting a rather tokenistic form of involvement. However, ministers and officials, along with most of the groups, accepted that there had to be some 'experienced' representatives largely because of the problems already referred to and the shortage of policy skills and knowledge across the sector.

The broader question of who should represent patients, users and carers was reflected in committee appointments. In the questionnaire, nearly two-thirds of groups replied that someone from their organization had acted as a user or carer representative on an official Department of Health or NHS advisory committee. Interviews suggested that the civil servants used their previous knowledge of groups and individuals to recommend appointment. Individuals were often 'sounded out' about their willingness to participate, but ministers would make the ultimate decision. In the view of ministers, civil servants were clearly reluctant to include vociferous or difficult people. However, civil servants denied that the intention was to select, in the words of one respondent, 'a bunch of "yes men"' (si33). Another view expressed was that 'difficult people' were sometimes brought into the fold in an effort to restrain their public criticism of policy.

The number of individuals involved in official committees was relatively small. Some group respondents, civil servants and some other stakeholder respondents, referred to this phenomenon as the 'usual suspects', or 'familiar faces'. One civil servant said that in a review of committee membership one health consumer group representative's name: 'turned up on...six or eight committees' (si16). While some civil servants agreed that the same people tended be chosen, they argued in most cases that this was inevitable, given the small number of people capable, in their view, of performing this role. Some civil servants however expressed a desire for change, one declaring: 'It is a mould that I would love us to be able to break' (si8). The term 'usual suspects' is often used pejoratively. But there was little doubt that those who served on these committees, including some of our interviewees, worked tirelessly on behalf of users and carers (see also Anderson *et al.*, 2002). Nevertheless, the narrow base of eligible representatives caused problems of overload for what was a scarce resource. These people were highly valued by government as one former minister testified: 'sometimes you absolutely needed the usual suspects' (si2).

Expertise

As noted in Chapter 5, the expertise of health consumer groups is one of their key resources. In particular, their experiential knowledge is highly regarded by other policy actors. Research findings demonstrated that a group's ability to accumulate and communicate the experiential knowledge of its constituency was an important factor in determining its credibility with ministers and civil servants. The importance of experiential knowledge as a resource has also been noted by others (Wilson, 1999; Tyler, 2002; Prior, 2003). As one former minister noted: 'People with experience of illness can teach the doctor something. If they can do this, they can also teach the policy-makers' (si2), and according to one civil servant:

> We can draw on their expertise and their experience, and also just understand what are the things that are worrying them, what is the impact of government policies on the people who are meant to be delivering them or who have a particular interest in the way they are delivered. (si33)

Policy-makers acknowledged that experiential knowledge constituted an important resource for the groups, enabling them to secure access to the policy process and exert influence. However, it was important that groups were able to communicate this to policy-makers in a coherent way. Those in government identified three key factors which could strengthen a group's case. First, it was important that experiential knowledge was based on properly conducted research. Groups that collected and analysed data from members of the public could build a stronger case than those relying wholly on individual anecdote and case studies. Individual cases were useful in illustrating particular problems or issues, but these had to be set in the context of wider research findings. Secondly, groups had to present their findings in a way that was meaningful to policy-makers: that is, in a concise manner with clear recommendations. Thirdly, groups had to demonstrate awareness of the policy context and in particular the political and practical constraints which ministers and civil servants worked under. In short, the experiential knowledge had to be targeted, tailored and timely to meet the specific needs of policy-makers. As one former minister put it, the most effective groups not only highlighted problems but provided possible solutions.

Organizations that met these criteria were highly regarded. This was summarized neatly in the following comment from one civil servant speaking about a maternity/childbirth group she believed was highly effective:

> They do the research and are able to validate what they say, they back it up with evidence and offer solutions. They have to show it will work and show it to be effective. (si23)

In summary, groups that could demonstrate their representativeness, interaction with their members or clients and their specialized knowledge; and who sought a constructive relationship, abiding by the 'rules of the game', had few problems in accessing government and having their say. However, the analysis highlighted other structural factors, which gave some health consumer groups an added advantage.

Organizational size and financial resources

A voluntary organization's size, and in particular the financial resources at its disposal, has been acknowledged as an important factor in securing access to government (Vincent, 2002). With regard to health consumer groups, larger and better-resourced organizations had greater capacity for engagement. They could send delegations to meetings and respond to consultations, often at short notice. They could employ officials with valuable policy skills and knowledge and were in a better position to fund, or undertake research, and present findings in an acceptable form. Groups with a large membership could claim to represent a large number of voters, and thereby attract ministerial attention. Table 9.2, summarizing questionnaire data, shows that organizational size had an impact on the frequency of contact with government:

Table 9.2 Percentage of groups having 'at least quarterly' contact with Department of Health ministers and civil servants, by income band

Income band	Department of Health ministers (%)	Department of Health civil servants (%)
£100 000 or less	12	33
£ 100 001–£1 000 000	38	55
£ 1 000 001 and over	79	86

Source: Questionnaire data set 1999.

Alliances

Whilst the questionnaire data showed that formal alliance organizations tended to have slightly less frequent contact with Department of Health civil servants and health ministers than population-based groups, it also showed that they both had much more frequent contact than condition-based groups. Chapter 6 described how health consumer groups believed that working together, and joining alliances, was a source of strength in the policy process as it enabled them to make the most of scarce resources and present a united front on substantive issues. Indeed, a significant number of groups in the questionnaire data set had links with other user/carer organizations. Interviews with civil servants and ministers showed that they valued the contribution that formal alliance organizations (which they labelled 'umbrella groups') could make. Bodies such as the Long-term Medical Conditions Alliance (LMCA) and the Patients Forum were mentioned as examples of effective alliances, knowledgeable, and skilled in the policy process. Working through alliances enabled civil servants to avoid duplication of effort. As one said: 'They are a good way into a huge range of disparate conditions... if you get in through there you can do a huge amount with not very much money' (si36) and another suggested that alliance groups were 'useful' because: 'If they respond to [a] consultation we know we've talked to a large number of people' (si23). However, it was also acknowledged by some that not all alliances were easy to deal with. One alliance was referred to by a civil servant as 'a horrendous talking shop' (si17).

Government priorities

Most group respondents believed that current health priorities had a strong bearing on their relationship with government. The consensus was that heart disease and cancer groups had a closer relationship with government than mental health, arthritis, and maternity/childbirth groups (notwithstanding the fact that mental health is a stated government priority – see Chapter 3). Ministers and civil servants acknowledged that this was inevitable. Indeed one civil servant noted that cancer and heart/circulatory disease groups had been 'knocking at an open door' (si4). Others described how groups had been drawn in by policy development in the priority areas, such as the *Cancer Plan* and the *National Service Framework for Coronary Heart Disease*. Civil servants observed that relations with arthritis groups were not close because of the relatively low priority given to the condition and the lack of a condition-specific service framework. Indeed, arthritis groups seemed the least satisfied with access to government.

Surprisingly, questionnaire data indicated that priority status did not appear to have a clear impact on the extent of contact between groups and government. As Table 9.3 shows, although a much higher proportion of cancer and heart/circulatory disease groups reported contact with government in the previous three years compared with arthritis groups (83 per cent and 69 percent respectively, compared with 53 per cent), the *frequency* of reported contact with the Department of Health did not vary significantly. This suggests that priority status has more impact on the quality, rather than the frequency, of interaction between government and groups.

Table 9.3   Frequency of contact with Department of Health ministers and civil servants, by condition area

	'At least quarterly' contact with Department of Health ministers (%)	'At least quarterly' contact with Department of Health civil servants (%)
Arthritis and related conditions	23	33
Cancer	18	38
Heart and circulatory disease	23	42
Maternity and childbirth	9	27
Mental health	36	52

Source: Questionnaire data set 1999.

Barriers to effective consultation

The burden of consultation

Despite the closer relationship between groups and government, significant barriers to participation were also identified. One set of problems noted by the groups concerned the consultation process: 71 per cent of those responding to the questionnaire believed that lack of consultation was a 'very important' or 'important' barrier. In interview, groups complained about the problems of responding to a torrent of consultation documents. A common criticism was that there was insufficient time given for consultation. Groups claimed that deadlines were unrealistically short and prohibited dialogue with members, users, and carers. This led some groups to question the value of participation. According to one questionnaire respondent: 'Sometimes I think consultation is token. Deadlines are often short, particularly if we want to involve our network in response'.

Another concern was lack of feedback from government to the evidence submitted. As one mental health group observed:

There's streams of this stuff we respond too, then silence. A document appears which may or may not take into account our views. It doesn't say whether they have taken our arguments on board or why they haven't taken on board 'x' which we suggested. (gi6)

A second set of problems related to the costs of involvement and the constraints placed on groups. Groups identified the opportunity costs of participation in policy consultations, discussions, and attendance at meetings. Other activities, such as providing services and working with members suffered (see Chapter 4). Many interviewees believed that government should reimburse the costs of involvement, noting that professionals usually received payment for attending meetings whereas user/carer representatives were regarded as volunteers. Several respondents felt that government should make a greater financial contribution for this advisory role, and wanted more stable funding arrangements (see also McCurry, 2001).

Confidentiality

Groups also felt constrained by government rules on confidentiality, noting instances where individuals serving on committees had been prevented from sharing official papers with their colleagues. There was clearly a tension between the government's desire to be inclusive and their need for secrecy. However, there seems to have been considerable variation in practice. For example, the circulation of papers relating to the development of some national service frameworks was wider than in others.

Government structures

Another set of issues related to problems faced by groups when dealing with government structures. There was considerable cynicism among groups about 'joined-up government', both within the Department of Health and between departments. Examples were given of related activities, of which civil servants were apparently unaware, being undertaken by different sections of the same department, resulting in a duplication of effort. Consultation processes could also vary and this could add to the burden on groups. Despite the existence of a database of groups held by the Department of Health, some groups said they were overlooked when they had relevant expertise. In practice, each departmental section tended to develop its own network of contacts. A related problem was lack of knowledge about government and the 'rules of the game' among some groups. Some respondents appeared to have a good knowledge of inter and intra-department structures. As one former minister observed of these groups, 'they know how to work the patch' (si15). Other groups admitted that their knowledge and understanding of policy structures and processes was limited. A large number felt that the Department of Health could do more to clarify its structure and provide more information about the responsibilities of various sections and of the individuals within it.

The civil servants' view

The civil servants interviewed largely agreed with these short-comings and to some extent sympathized with them. Despite attempts to increase consistency, they acknowledged that different sections of the Department of Health adopted different approaches to consultation[2] and that some sections were more active than others in consulting with groups. However, one civil servant maintained that the introduction of national service frameworks was helping to address this problem by bringing together different sections of the Department and their various user and carer networks. The role of national clinical directors (or 'czars') in promoting cross-departmental co-ordination was also mentioned as a positive development.

Confidentiality was seen as an important requirement by civil servants, who maintained that rules must be clear and groups should be made aware of the consequences of leaking information to the press. They appreciated that group representatives on official committees might need to share ideas with colleagues in order to make an effective contribution. In this situation, civil servants stated that they had no objections to ideas and general principles being discussed by a wider constituency, but not the actual draft policy documents.

On the question of resources, civil servants stated that limited funding was available for attendance at meetings and training, however, there seemed to be variations in practice. Most sections of the Department of Health paid expenses, while others compensated for loss of income as well. One respondent stated that in exceptional circumstances, groups could be recompensed for sending a representative to a meeting. Section 64 funding was available to organizations, though increasingly this was for specific projects rather than for core funding (see Chapter 4). One civil servant, echoed the views of some groups that there were dangers of relying overly on state funding. He gave an example of how one group which had received significant levels of funding from government had been admonished for issuing a negative press release:

> One organization...got itself into real trouble with a minister because they issued this very negative press release, the day before they saw him, which was a bad move, and he swore at them and said 'We're bloody well giving you half your income, you can't then act as a campaigning organization against your main funder, you can't have your cake and eat it.' It rather rocked them back on their chair. (si17)

The civil servants sympathized with the problems caused by timescales for consultation but argued that this was inevitable given the political pressures on policy-makers. They were aware too that some groups faced problems with the workload brought by consultation. One way forward was to develop more effective forms of consultation, through seminars for example, where user and carer views could be channelled more quickly and efficiently.

Access and influence

While it has been demonstrated that groups now have access to government, and participation has increased, what impact has this had? Access does not equal influence and participation does not guarantee that groups will secure their objectives. Moreover, policy influence is a product of complex forces that include not only government, but other interests and policy actors, such as the professions, the drugs industry, research charities, other voluntary organizations, MPs and peers, and the media.

The perceived influence of groups

In interview, two-thirds of groups identified at least one instance where they believed they had influenced policy. The examples given covered all stages of the policy cycle from agenda setting, to formulation and implementation. The issues that groups believed they had brought to the agenda included: carers' needs; the woman's perspective in childbirth; the problems of mixed-sex wards; the discrimination against, and the neglect of, elderly people in hospital and shortcomings in community care for mentally ill people. More generally, groups believed they had focused government attention on issues that tended to be neglected within the health policy process, including quality of life issues, psycho-social aspects of health, and the need for providers to better inform and communicate with patients, users, and carers. They believed that they had influenced the development of national service frameworks and NICE guidelines by introducing this perspective. Groups also claimed to have strongly influenced the development of certain key initiatives, such as *Changing Childbirth* (Expert Maternity Group, 1993), the *Carers' Strategy* (HM Government, 1999) and the *Expert Patients Programme* (DoH, 2001a). Some gave instances of how they had successfully tabled amendments to legislation, usually with ministerial backing. These are discussed in more detail in the next chapter. Often the interviewees described their influence in quite narrow and detailed terms. As one cancer group noted, for example: 'Patient organizations can be better at influencing the detail rather than the overall direction' (gi31). In contrast, ministers and civil servants were reluctant to discuss specific instances where groups had been influential, preferring to talk in general terms. Nonetheless, they accepted that groups had brought a fresh perspective to the policy process and that their influence was reflected in policy outputs, notably the national service frameworks.

Groups also believed they had influenced the implementation of policy. This view was supported by a civil servant who said that while groups in some cases may not be able to stop the 'direction of travel' of policy, it was in 'the implementation guidance where you can smooth the rough edges so it will work in practice' (si17). However, the implementation phase of policy-making could also be frustrating for groups. For example, the maternity/childbirth groups had been pleased with the proposals from the 1993 Expert Maternity Group, but were very disappointed with the implementation of *Changing Childbirth*.

Variations in influence between groups

Although examples of policy influence were identified by a majority of groups, it appeared that they enjoyed varying levels of success. Groups that had insider status were more likely than outsiders to report an instance of influence. Other characteristics such as group strategy, structure, acceptance by government and focus also had an effect on group influence (Whiteley and Winyard, 1987 – see Chapter 1). Groups that pursued an open strategy, targeting the media, parliament and government, were more likely to report at least one example of their influence than those that focused their attention on government alone. The choice of an open strategy meant they could bring additional pressure to bear on government. Ministers and civil servants also acknowledged that the groups that could mobilize support in the media and parliament, as well as having good contacts with government, were most likely to be influential.

The overall size of groups, in terms of the resources at their disposal, was linked to self-reported influence over government policy. The larger groups (annual income over £1 million) were more likely than other groups to report an example of influence. Similarly, the medium-sized groups (income £100 001–£ 1 million) were more likely than the smaller groups (income £ 100 000 or less) to report an example of influence. This did not square with the comments of ministers and civil servants, however, who, as noted earlier, argued that the size and resources of groups did not make a crucial difference and smaller groups could be influential, particularly when they produced a well researched case.

Among health consumer groups, there was a strong belief that influence varied according to condition area. Groups in the arthritis and maternity/childbirth sectors for example claimed that their influence was limited because these conditions were not currently government priorities. Yet groups in mental health (a stated priority) also believed that they lacked the influence of cancer and heart/circulatory disease groups:

> If you are cancer, or heart disease, or children then I think it is much easier to drive the political agenda in those areas, but when you are in mental illness, it is harder to drive, you're often on the back foot. (gi23)

A similar point was made by the interviewee from the Stroke Association, who said:

> Heart disease and cancer have such a high profile, that's an automatic: stroke we've got to work at it.

Even so, cancer and heart/circulatory disease groups, while recognizing that they were pushing at an open door, did not accept that influence automatically followed. Nor did other policy actors believe that health consumer groups in these priority areas were always more influential, although they had more opportunities to influence policies. Whether their suggestions were taken up depended on the quality of input, the practicality of proposals and their political acceptability. Data on self-reported influence showed that although arthritis groups were less likely to report an instance of influence than others, as might be expected given the low priority of this condition, mental health and maternity/childbirth groups were more likely than heart/circulatory and cancer groups to report an example of influence, suggesting that the relationship between priority status and influence remains uncertain.

Indeed, groups realized that success in influencing policy depended heavily on their fit with the current government agenda rather than simply the priority status of their condition. For example, a respondent from one mental health group said that their efforts to influence policy had foundered because government's main concern lay in protecting the public rather in than protecting the rights of mentally ill people, a message clearly communicated to them by ministers. Compatibility not only opened doors, but enabled groups to have opportunities to raise issues and influence important policy details.

Influence of health consumer groups relative to other policy actors

Any assessment of the influence of health consumer groups must account for the position of professional and commercial interests. The De Montfort study did not find any examples of where health consumer groups had achieved influence in the face of opposition from these interests. In practice, influence was more subtle, with other interests conceding ground voluntarily on some issues and occasionally joining forces with health consumer groups or others to fight a common cause, as in the cases of both caesarean section and mental health legislation (discussed further in Chapter 10).

For the most part, health consumer groups acknowledged and were realistic about the power of these established interests. A number of interviewees believed that professionals, particularly the medical profession, continued to have preferential access or status in the policy process:

> I think the big problem is that it's really the power of the medical profession...they have mechanisms whereby they can get in to see people of influence in ways that we simply can't. (gi3)

> At the moment you're grateful to be included in things, but you recognize that you are behind the medical profession and commercial organizations. (gi31)

Health consumer groups also realized that the agenda tended to be set by these interests, and the traditional link between doctors and civil servants remained well-embedded, as the following comments from an interviewee from a cancer group illustrate:

> We...and other people who participated in it [the Cancer Information Strategy] felt that we wouldn't have started from where [it did] and that it had all been decided in advance. (gi31)

These views were echoed by those in government. According to the civil servants, health professionals had more power and a better knowledge of the political system. Their contacts were generally stronger, especially informal contacts with decision-makers. The medical profession were seen by civil servants as dominating the agenda. They also recognized the ability of the professions, particularly the medical profession, to affect the implementation of policies. As one civil servant observed:

> At the end of the day, with the NSFs [national service frameworks] for example, we've got to carry the professionals with us, they may not like everything but we have got to carry them with us. They've got to implement them and they can be really destructive if they want to be. (si17)

Interestingly, some ministers departed from this line and argued that the inclusion of health consumer groups represented a major challenge to the traditional ways of making policy. Ministers noted that health consumer groups were more influential over some issues than others. Nonetheless, they accepted that the power bases of professional and commercial interests were substantial and that they had very good political contacts, knowledge and skills. Ministers and civil servants also pointed out that health consumer groups often worked collaboratively with each other and with other interests and these broader alliances could be very influential, particularly in relation to some national service frameworks and NICE decisions. When health consumer interests were allied with those of the drugs industry, as on issues of drug licensing and availability, they could be formidable.

National service frameworks

In the period covered by the De Montfort project, national service frameworks were introduced for mental health, coronary heart disease and older people. In addition, the *National Cancer Plan* was developed, which set out standards and implementation plans in this priority area. Each evolved in a slightly different way, although the general features of the process were similar (see Chapter 3). Many respondents from the groups referred to their own or their organization's experiences of national service frameworks and in particular the role of the external reference groups that helped to formulate them. They applauded the government's efforts to engage with users and carers and believed that the outcomes would have been different had they not been involved. Emphasis on health promotion in the Older People's national service framework and the standards for carers in the Mental Health national service framework were two examples cited by respondents as fruits of their involvement.

Some health consumer group respondents commented positively on the national service framework process, noting that the external reference groups worked well and that, at this stage at least, consultation was genuine. However, experiences varied. Mental health groups were highly critical of the process and there were resignations among members on an external reference group working party (Hogg, 2002). Most group representatives commented adversely on delays and alterations made to the national service framework by health ministers, Number Ten and the Treasury, apparently without explanation. Some expressed disappointment and felt that their views had been ignored. There was a suspicion that the agenda had already been decided by professionals and civil servants before the external reference groups began their work. Reiterating an earlier point, confidentiality was a problem, with user and carer representatives expressing frustration at not being able to share relevant documents with colleagues in their organization.

These findings supported Hogg's (2002) study, which reported that agendas were set by medical and government interests, expressed reservations about the use of confidentiality as a control mechanism, and was critical of a drafting process that slowed momentum as government considered political and resource issues. Despite these observations, Hogg concluded that the involvement of groups had made a difference and helped to develop comprehensive service standards.

The National Institute for Clinical Excellence

The National Institute for Clinical Excellence (NICE), established in 1999, has an important role in appraising and producing guidance on the cost-effectiveness of new and existing technologies (see Chapters 3 and 8). Health consumer groups submit evidence for appraisals and may appeal against draft guidance. Representatives of health consumer groups sit on various NICE committees, such as the appraisal committee and appeals panel. In addition, members of the Partner's Council, a consultative body, are drawn from health consumer groups, as well as clinicians and representatives from the health technologies industry, health service managers, researchers and other experts, and trade unions. Finally, there is an informal alliance called Patients Involved in NICE (PIN) which meets with senior personnel at NICE on issues of concern (see also Chapter 6 and Quennell, 2001).

In the De Montfort study, several respondents spoke of their relationship with NICE. They noted that patients, users and carer representatives were in a minority on committees and on the Partners' Council. They believed the agenda was dominated by professional and political agendas. Some talked of 'tokenism'. There were also comments that groups had been denied important background information that would have enabled them to make a fuller contribution to debates. Nonetheless, most acknowledged that there was some scope to influence decisions, through the submission of evidence, based on the qualitative analysis of patients' views and experiences.[3]

Although the study did not attempt to analyse the impact of groups on NICE decisions in a systematic way, it found examples where groups had been successful in shaping guidance. In one example, cancer groups, notably CancerBACUP, opposed an initial decision by NICE to recommend the anti-cancer drug, Taxotere, for breast cancer patients, and not to recommend a second drug, Taxol. The manufacturer of the latter drug also appealed against the ruling. Following the appeal, NICE ruled that both drugs should be recommended.

Some of the points made by respondents to the De Montfort study have been raised in other reports. The Consumers' Association (2001b) criticized NICE for the lack of transparency of its procedures. It found that patients' groups incurred high costs in making submissions, but received insufficient feedback on how their efforts had affected the final decision. It also reported that groups believed NICE placed much greater emphasis on clinical trial data than on the quality-of-life data they provided. A House of Commons inquiry (Health Committee, 2002) made similar comments, notably about the lack of transparency of NICE decisions. Quennell's (2001) study showed that groups are now heavily engaged with NICE and its processes and that this engagement is evolving in ways that might strengthen patients' representative bodies in the longer term. However, she also criticized the lack of transparency, poor feedback and the fundamental tension between evidence-based medicine and evidence from patients that challenges the dominant scientific-bureaucratic paradigm.

Conclusion

The barriers that limit the contribution of groups in the policy process should not obscure the advances they have made. The political and policy context has been favourable to the inclusion of consumer interests. Groups have had more access to government and greater opportunities to influence policy than before. Government sought their views on policy and their expertise, in particular their experiential knowledge, was valued. They are regarded as the legitimate representatives of specific constituencies. Alliance groups in particular were valued for the broader perspective they brought to the policy process. In short, groups can be regarded as new members of an expanded health policy network, though one that is strongly shaped by government and traditionally powerful interests such as the medical profession and the drugs industry.

In terms of Grant's (1995) typology, most groups had little difficulty in securing insider status. Moreover, as the interviews indicated, the majority of groups wanted to play such a role and wished to engage in government consultations and to serve on official committees. This suggests, as Maloney, Jordan and McLaughlin (1994) have argued, that whether a group has insider status or not may be less important than variations in the standing and influence of groups that have already secured such status. In other words, it is their status as core insiders that is crucial. The findings of this chapter suggest that few groups were regarded as core insiders, the exception perhaps being Carers National Association (now Carers UK), and possibly the Patients Forum and the LMCA. Some groups do however appear to have achieved specialist insider status on issues such as public involvement (College of Health),[4] on condition-specific issues British Cardiac Patients Association,[5] MIND (the National Association for Mental Health) and the National Childbirth Trust, and on issues affecting population groups (Age Concern, Help the Aged and Action for Sick Children).

One possible explanation is that, in line with Saward's (1990) model discussed in Chapter 1, health consumer group resources have increased. They are no longer simply representing a small minority that can easily be brushed aside, they represent a 'significant minority', which gives them greater leverage. Second, they have expertise which government accepts as important for improved services. Health consumer groups therefore have more scope for influence. They emphasize issues that have traditionally been neglected in the policy process. The established interests in health policy remain powerful. This is partly because of their wider informal contacts, their greater knowledge of the rules of the game, their resources, and the sanctions they can bring to bear. Nonetheless, health consumer groups are not without influence, particularly when they combine with other interests.

An important theme of this chapter has been the variation between groups, in terms of access and influence. A variety of factors have been examined as possible explanations. With regard to access, the status of the condition seems to be an important factor, certainly as far as the quality of contact with decision-makers is concerned. Much more seems to depend on how a group approaches government. A group that is well organized; that can claim with some justification that it speaks for a particular constituency; is knowledgeable and skilled in the policy process; has a network of informal contacts; has experiential knowledge that is backed by evidence and can offer potential solutions, will tend to be included in the policy process. If it understands and complies with the rules of the game, particularly with regard to confidentiality, and does not engage in destructive criticism of policy, its chances of inclusion are further increased.

Although access does not equate with influence, those groups that are 'at the table' have greater opportunities to put their case. Insiders tend to be regarded as more influential than outsiders. However, the scope for government to control and manipulate the groups should not be underestimated. Small concessions may be offered in return for overall compliance. Indeed the entire process of involving groups may be regarded as an attempt at control within an authoritarian system of governance. If so, the ability of the groups to mobilize not only their 'constituency' but broader public sentiment, through media support as well as parliamentary lobbying, becomes important to their independence as advocates. The open strategy may well be the best approach, and will be examined further in the next two chapters.

10 Working with parliament

As the previous chapter suggested, it is not enough for groups to form good working relationships with government. Other institutions, notably parliament and the media can be used to exert influence over policy agendas and decisions. These institutions can articulate and mobilize specific interests and broader public opinion. They act as alternative arenas, where problems and policy options are floated. In undertaking these functions, parliament and the media do not operate in isolation. Each affects the other, enabling issues to move between different policy arenas, including the government's own agenda. This dynamic process can neither be ignored, nor controlled by the executive, though it seeks to manipulate both parliament and the media – through party discipline, in the case of the former, and media/public relations with regard to the latter. This chapter focuses on the relationships between health consumer groups and parliament. It begins by looking at the relevance of parliament to policy formation and then moves on to discuss the links between health consumer groups and parliament, the nature and extent of parliamentary activities, and the implications for policy.

Parliament and policy influence

The UK parliament is regarded as a policy-influencing rather than a policy-making body. According to Norton (1993, p. 88), it is: 'At best, a proximate – at worst, a marginal – actor in determining the content of measures of public policy.' Several factors combine to leave parliament in a relatively weak position vis-à-vis the executive: the government's control of the parliamentary agenda; the systems of party discipline, including the whips who seek to ensure that MPs vote according to the party line; patronage (many MPs and peers actually serve the government as ministers or as private secretaries) and the limited powers of the House of Lords. When government enjoys a large working majority, as most recent governments have, the ability of parliament to challenge government is further weakened.

For these reasons, many observers believe that parliament is increasingly bypassed and that the real debate and decision-making takes place elsewhere (Adonis, 1990; Riddell, 1998). If this is true, how can the apparent increase in parliamentary lobbying be explained (Baggott, 1995)? According to Rush (1990), there are three possible explanations. Those seeking to lobby may not fully comprehend the weakness of parliament against central government. This may be true for those who lobby rarely or infrequently. Alternatively, parliamentary lobbying may be the only opportunity for some groups to put their case, as government may be unwilling to discuss policy matters directly with them. Engagement with parliament may therefore be a last resort. Another explanation is that parliament may actually have some influence over policy, particularly with regard to residual legislation, and therefore even groups that have good relationships with the government are wise not to neglect it.

There are several ways in which parliament can be used by groups to influence policy. First, it is an indirect of way of lobbying government. Ministers and civil servants monitor parliamentary opinion and are aware of issues being raised there (Adonis, 1990). This may supplement direct lobbying of government departments and agencies (Norton, 1993). Parliament can also shape a broader climate of opinion, which encourages or discourages government intervention in a particular policy area (Jordan and Richardson, 1987). Many parliamentary activities shed light on government in a way that attracts wider public attention (Silk and Walters, 1995). These include select committee inquiries, parliamentary debates and questions, as well as scrutiny of legislation, all of which can be used to raise issues, criticize government policy and promote alternatives. Ministers, and in some cases their civil servants, have to explain and defend their policies in these various settings and this creates opportunities for parliament to probe their thinking and to influence both the policy agenda and specific policy initiatives.

Parliament therefore can be a useful target for voluntary organizations, including health consumer groups, seeking to influence policy. By working with MPs and peers, groups can build political support, acquire political intelligence and raise policy issues which may then be taken up with government. The De Montfort study found that groups had considerable involvement with parliament. Nearly three-quarters of the groups had contact with parliament in the previous three years, over a fifth had at least monthly contact, while almost half had at least quarterly contact. In interview, almost all the groups referred to some parliamentary contact or activity.

Why lobby parliament?

Health consumer groups believed that establishing and maintaining contact with parliament was an important part of their strategy. MPs and peers were seen as well-connected and able to use their networks to influence policy. Although only a small minority (6 per cent) of groups had MPs or peers on their main decision-making body, when asked to identify the most important non-financial resources at the organization's disposal, almost two-thirds of the groups stated that links with the Commons and the Lords were either 'very important' or 'important'. However, this was lower than the proportion rating links with central government and the media as 'very important' or 'important'. In addition, MPs and peers were regarded as a useful source of intelligence about political processes and the specific measures currently under consideration.

Making and establishing contacts

The accessibility of parliament was confirmed by interviews with MPs and peers. One of the MPs acknowledged that members were highly dependent on briefings provided by outside organizations, especially where this helped them to acquire knowledge on issues of interest to their constituents. This supports a more general point made by Norton (1993) that MPs (and peers) are often dependent on outside organizations for information because their resources for independent research are limited. MPs welcomed health consumer groups as they were well-informed about a range of health issues. Likewise, many groups referred to their role in briefing MPs and believed this was useful in establishing their credibility.

Some health consumer groups worked with small groups of MPs and peers who had already endorsed the views of the group or had campaigned previously on their behalf. For example, the National Childbirth Trust's main contacts included Nicholas Winterton, who had chaired a Health Committee inquiry into childbirth in the early 1990s (see Chapter 3). The late Audrey Wise had also been an important parliamentary ally of the maternity and childbirth groups over the years. The Stroke Association said it had a cluster of 40 to 50 MPs and peers whom it briefed regularly. Similarly the Mental After Care Association targeted 30 active MPs and 20 peers who, in the view of the Association, were 'really interested' in mental health. In many of the groups' accounts a distinction was made between a 'hard core' of MPs and peers with a strong interest in key issues, or who had actively supported the group in the past, and the wider network of interested parliamentarians. Some groups explicitly identified the latter by monitoring parliamentary proceedings to assess whether individual MPs and peers had an interest in the health issues relevant to their group. These members were sent regular written briefings and, when a particular issue arose, were invited to briefing events. Some groups undertook surveys of parliamentary opinion, including the Mental After Care Association (Lawton-Smith, 1999). Several groups mentioned that they had held meetings in the Commons to brief MPs. For example, Arthritis Care, along with other arthritis groups, held a reception at the House of Commons in December 1999 with an estimated attendance of 170 members. Groups claimed that such meetings had several purposes: to inform MPs and peers about specific health issues; to raise awareness about conditions and to challenge common misconceptions and stereotypes.

Political parties

In seeking contact with MPs and peers, groups avoided partisanship. All were seen as potentially useful, irrespective of party allegiance.

Groups did not wish to alienate those without affiliation in the House of Lords, either. In the case of groups that were charities, any suggestion of party political bias could compromise their charitable status. Some did seek to inform MPs and party members by having a presence at party conferences, but were usually careful to engage with more than one party during the conference season.

In parliament too, groups were keen to avoid being too closely linked to a single political party. However, when opportunities arose they did operate through informal political networks, some of which were based on party political allegiances. Groups were also happy to work with opposition party spokespersons when the need arose, mainly to raise issues of concern and put pressure on government to act. In this regard, links with 'shadow ministers' in the House of Lords appear to have been particularly useful.

Targeting individual MPs

Wherever possible, groups targeted the particular interests and needs of MPs and peers. Some provided background information relating directly to the MP's constituency. For example, both the British League Against Rheumatism (BLAR, now the Arthritis and Musculoskeletal Alliance) and Arthritis Care supplied MPs with constituency statistics on arthritis, while the UK Breast Cancer Coalition (UKBCC) provided them with a constituency resource pack on breast cancer. As another cancer group noted:

> We very much recognize that the way to get an MP's attention on something is to draw a constituency link and we try to do that. For example...we had MPs writing to their local Health Authorities asking them what their policy was on funding...and we got quite a good response on that. (gi31)

The MPs and peers interviewed valued constituency-relevant material and welcomed the briefings supplied by groups. They and their colleagues who had a longstanding interest in health issues sought closer relationships with health consumer groups. Some members had a health background, including medical research and medical practice. Others had a background in the voluntary sector. For example, Virginia Bottomley (a former Secretary of

State for Health), Malcolm Wicks and Sylvia Heal, were all connected with the Carers National Association (now Carers UK): Bottomley was a patron; Wicks a vice-president and Heal had previously worked for the organization. All had been active in parliament on carers' issues. Personal factors were also important. There were cases of members, or their relatives and close friends, having suffered from a particular illness or disability, which led them to take a greater interest in specific conditions and relevant health consumer groups. For example, one of the MPs interviewed for the De Montfort study mentioned that a case of severe mental illness in the family had prompted an interest in mental health issues. Examination of parliamentary debates revealed other examples of MPs drawing on personal and family experiences when contributing to debates on health and social care issues.[1]

Direct lobbying of MPs

Some groups encouraged their members to contact their MPs directly. Several, including the British Cardiac Patients Association (BCPA), the UKBCC and the Arachnoiditis Trust, mentioned that they had given information to their members showing how they could lobby their MP on an individual basis. Arthritis Care had produced a campaigning pack to help inform members about how to contact their MP. The National Childbirth Trust also encouraged members to approach their MPs, and with regard to concern about the rising caesarean rate, provided a standard letter which could be used for this purpose.

Some groups encouraged members to go to Westminster '*en masse*' to directly lobby their MPs. Mass lobbying can be a useful tactic because unlike individual letters and meetings with MPs, it attracts publicity. Several groups initiated mass lobbies, including the National Childbirth Trust, the Stroke Association and the Arachnoiditis Trust. The mental health groups also used this tactic to express concerns about proposed legislation. From the point of view of the groups, all these examples attracted good publicity. However, the downside of mass lobbies is that they can be difficult to organize (Dubs, 1989). Also, it is possible that MPs and peers may feel intimidated by mass lobbies, and this can be counter-productive when trying to win added support from parliament (Baggott, 1995).

Parliamentary organization

In relation to parliamentary lobbying, MPs and peers believed that some groups were better organized, more skilled and knowledgeable than others. Some groups, in the words of a former minister, were 'very astute' (si15). Others, in contrast, lacked political organization, skills and knowledge. In addition, some groups were viewed as having limited ambitions, such as getting a mention in *Hansard*, the record of parliamentary proceedings. However, most groups were aware of the importance of good parliamentary organization. Some had appointed a parliamentary officer, which could be a full-time post or part of the wider remit of a policy or public relations officer. The groups with larger incomes had the resources to make such appointments and indeed had more paid staff working on policy than other groups (see Table 10.1).

In interview, groups acknowledged the value of having paid staff to work on policy and parliamentary matters. The less well-resourced groups admitted that they felt disadvantaged and that they lacked skills and knowledge about political processes generally, and parliament in particular (see also Chapter 4).

Joint working between groups

Another problem mentioned by MPs interviewed was that groups could do more to overcome fragmentation and the associated problems of duplication. Joint working was acknowledged in the arthritis, mental health and maternity/childbirth field, but in contrast, the cancer lobby was seen as highly fragmented and

Table 10.1 Groups having paid staff working on policy, by income

Income per annum	Groups having paid staff working on policy	
	(%)	(n)
Less than £100 000	57	26
£100 001–£1 000 000	85	28
£1 000 001 and over	93	13

Source: Questionnaire data set 1999.

MPs would have preferred greater collaboration between groups and a more coherently organized parliamentary presence.

In the mental health field a Mental Health Parliamentary Officers' Group was formed by the National Schizophrenia Fellowship (now Rethink), MIND (the National Association for Mental Health), the Royal College of Psychiatrists, Mental After Care Association, Manic Depression Fellowship, Mental Health Foundation and the UK Federation of Smaller Mental Health Agencies (UKFSMHA). This group organized meetings in the Commons about twice a year to keep mental health issues on the agenda and to provide a forum for discussion when relevant parliamentary matters arose. The group services meetings, decides who to invite, sets the agenda and provides any necessary follow-up. It also issues press releases and briefs MPs on mental health matters. One of the health consumer groups involved described the advantages of this joint operation as follows:

> We've been able to do joint briefings to parliament which everyone prefers. It's easier for us, it's less work. It's easier for the parliamentarians because they're getting a clear message from the mental health lobby. (gi23)

The MPs also noted that joint working had improved in the mental health field and that briefings had become more effective and coherent as a result.

Variations in parliamentary activity

There was considerable variation between different types of group in their parliamentary activity. The questionnaire revealed that population-based groups were particularly active: a majority in the survey (69 per cent) had at least quarterly contact with MPs and peers (compared with 40 per cent of condition-based groups and 60 per cent of formal alliance organizations). There was also considerable variation by income. Only 29 per cent of groups with annual incomes of £100 000 or less a year reported contact with MPs and peers at least quarterly, compared with 44 per cent of groups with incomes between £100 001 and £1 million. The wealthiest groups, those with incomes over £1 million per annum were most frequently in contact with parliament, with 93 per cent of these groups having at least quarterly contact. Of the different conditions, cancer and mental health groups appeared to be the most active: 32 per cent of mental health groups had at least monthly contact; while 53 per cent of cancer groups (and 50 per cent of mental health groups) had at least quarterly contact. Out of all the health consumer groups, heart and circulatory groups had the lowest frequency of contact with parliament. This was also evident from the interviews, with few of the heart/circulatory disease groups referring to contact with parliament. It should also be noted that parliamentary links were rated as 'very important' or 'important' by more groups in cancer (67 per cent), maternity/childbirth (67 per cent) and mental health (60 per cent), than groups in arthritis (55 per cent) or heart/circulatory disease (50 per cent).

Parliamentary activities

MPs and peers can raise issues on behalf of outside organizations in a number of different ways: through parliamentary questions; contributions to debates; or proposing amendments to legislation. They can also raise issues in committees of the House, such as select committees and all-party groups.

Parliamentary questions, debates and motions

Parliamentary questions (PQs) are tabled by MPs and peers to elicit information, press for action or to advance a case or argument (Silk and Walters, 1995). They receive a response from ministers (based on drafts by civil servants) and therefore can attract Whitehall's attention to particular matters. They are also a means of getting ministers to clarify or restate their policy. If picked up by the media, PQs and answers can attract publicity, although, prime minister's questions apart, their profile is believed to have declined in recent years.

In interview, a number of examples were given by groups on the use of PQs. One mental health group, unable to obtain details of homicide inquiry reports that involved mentally ill people, persuaded an MP with an interest in the field to table a question on their behalf. This was undertaken to elicit information not publicly available, and also highlighted the lack of a standardized system for homicide inquiries involving mentally ill people. Many of the groups interviewed were aware that PQs attracted the attention of government and were not simply a means of getting information. They used them to highlight particular issues or to follow through a particular course of action. PQs were also used as part of a broader lobbying campaign in Parliament – to secure amendments to legislation for example. Groups appeared to have little problem in getting MPs to ask questions on their behalf and usually contacted them through the networks mentioned earlier in this chapter.

Parliamentary debates on the other hand have been described as 'blunderbusses' (Silk and Walters, 1995, p. 207). They cannot probe the government's policy in detail, but can force a public statement on an issue. As with other parliamentary devices, the impact of debates depends greatly on publicity and other campaigning activities. Health consumer groups were active in promoting and encouraging debates in both the Commons and the Lords. Examples included Commons adjournment debates on arthritis on the 13 December 1999, backed by several arthritis groups, including BLAR and Arthritis Care, and on chronic illness on 29 March 2000, prompted by the LMCA. In addition, groups were active in briefing MPs when a debate was tabled by government or the opposition, For example, this occurred when an opposition debate on mental health took place on 25 June 2002. Groups interviewed demonstrated that they were prepared to invest time and effort urging MPs to introduce debates and briefing them when these took place. Despite their limitations – few attract media coverage and most (particularly the adjournment debates held at the end of each parliamentary day) are poorly attended – debates were seen as useful in highlighting concerns, especially in conjunction with other parliamentary activities.

While debates and PQs can indicate backbench opinion on a particular matter, they do not indicate levels of support or opposition to a policy. For this reason MPs often table early day motions (EDMs), which are in effect, statements that attract support for a particular viewpoint. MPs can endorse them by adding their names to the motion. Alternatively, they may indicate a different view by proposing an amendment, which may subsequently be endorsed by others. By these means, the government, MPs and those seeking to lobby parliament can gauge the support for, or opposition to, a particular cause. When the numbers of MPs involved are small, EDMs are of minor significance. But when they attract larger numbers, particularly from across the different parties at Westminster, they provide a useful barometer of opinion. In combination with other parliamentary activities, such as PQs and debates, EDMs can attract wider attention.

In recent years EDMs have been tabled on a range of health issues. For example, in the 1999/2000 session of Parliament an EDM on the availability of the anti-cancer drug, Taxol, tabled by Joan Ruddock (at the time the chair of the All-party Group on Breast Cancer) attracted over 150 signatures. Other EDMs in the following session referred to stroke care, mentioning the work of the Stroke Association (146 signatures); osteoporosis, referring to the National Osteoporosis Society (131 signatures) and Parkinson's Disease, mentioning the Parkinson's Disease Society (128 signatures).

Select committees

Select committees are official committees of parliament that examine the conduct and policies of government. In the House of Commons, select committees include backbench MPs from different parties. Select committees inquire into areas of policy and administration, with the Commons' departmental select committees focusing on the work of specific Whitehall departments. The House of Lords also has select committees, but unlike those of the Commons they do not 'shadow' particular departments.

Select committees have been credited with improving the scrutiny of government (Silk and Walters, 1995) and it is acknowledged that through their inquiries and reports they can have an impact on policy agendas and debates. For example, they may add further weight to pressure on government to adopt or change a particular policy (Judge, 1992). The media, as in other areas of parliamentary activity, can play a crucial role in highlighting concerns raised by select committees. According to Silk and Walters (1995, p. 220): 'Journalists have become aware that select committees are an alternative focus for news about political issues and can expose matters which otherwise might escape scrutiny.'

Health consumer groups were aware of the importance of select committees. They believed that they could help them to advance their aims and objectives. For example, the Health Committee was credited with getting the issue of choice in childbirth on the agenda during the early 1990s, by both the National Childbirth Trust and the Association for Improvements in the Maternity Services (AIMS) (see also Chapter 3). The Health Committee's inquiry into complaints and adverse clinical incidents (Health Committee, 1999) highlighted issues that had been neglected in the past and recommended that the NHS take organizational responsibility for improving complaints procedures and reporting adverse incidents. Alongside other developments, notably the Bristol Royal Infirmary Inquiry (Bristol Inquiry, 2001), it added further momentum to pressures for reform in this area, which culminated in changes to complaint systems and a new system for reporting errors and 'near misses'.

Health consumer groups believed that committees contributed to their particular policy objectives in two ways. First, they considered that committee recommendations could give added legitimacy to their arguments in discussions with government. Second, government might have to consider a particular matter as a result of any media attention given to a committee's proceedings or following its final report.

Select committees operate on the basis of *persons, papers* and *records.* Individuals, acting independently or as representatives of an organization, can be called in as witnesses and examined. Individuals and organizations may also submit written evidence. About half the health consumer groups in the interview sample mentioned giving evidence to select committees. However, not all had been invited to give oral evidence and indeed some of the smaller and lower-profile groups felt that they had less chance of being chosen to do so.

An examination of the Health Committee inquiries between 2000 and 2002 showed that health consumer groups submitted a substantial body of evidence. In 2002 an inquiry into the National Institute for Clinical Excellence (NICE) received evidence from the Multiple Sclerosis Society, the BCPA and Pituitary Foundation, among others (Health Committee, 2002). Other inquiries receiving evidence from health consumer groups included: 'Head Injury: Rehabilitation' (Health Committee, 2001a), where Headway – the National Brian Injury Association gave evidence; 'Procedures Related to Adverse Clinical Incidents and Outcomes in

Medical Care' (Health Committee, 1999), where evidence was provided by, among others, Action for the Victims of Medical Accidents, Haemophilia Society, Victims of Tranquillisers and the [Rodney] Ledward Victims' Group. In the inquiry into 'The Provision of Information by Government Relating to the Safety of Breast Implants' (Health Committee, 2001b), evidence was submitted by Action Against Silicon Gel UK and Sufferers of Iatrogenic Neglect; and in the inquiry into 'The Provision of Mental Health Services' (Health Committee, 2000) MIND, the Manic Depression Fellowship, Schizophrenia A National Emergency (SANE) and the National Schizophrenia Fellowship gave evidence.

A majority of groups involved with select committees mentioned only the Health Committee. However, other select committees explored policy areas relevant to some health consumer groups – including Work and Pensions, Home Affairs and the Environment, Food and Rural Affairs – all of which in recent years have touched on health-related issues. Non-departmental select committees, such as the Committee of Public Accounts, also examines health-related issues in the course of its inquiries into public expenditure.

Select committees' choice of topics for inquiry can have a major impact on the ability of groups to make their views known on policy. Some groups were clearly aware of this and pressed members of select committees to choose a particular topic. In one case, an MP successfully pushed for the House of Commons' Science and Technology Committee to enquire into cancer research – where three health consumer groups were subsequently invited to give oral evidence. It appeared that MPs sitting on select committees attempted to influence the terms of reference and the scope of inquiries so as to increase the opportunities for health consumer groups and other organizations to contribute.

All-party groups

As mentioned earlier, health consumer groups were careful not to be seen as partisan. When lobbying parliament they preferred to seek cross-party support for their particular cause. One way of building this was to work with all-party subject groups, which focus on particular topics of interest to MPs. Parliament has a number of all-party groups which MPs and peers may join.

These have no official standing or powers, and there are contrasting views about their effectiveness. Some observers dismiss them as poorly attended and under-resourced (Norton, 1993), while others acknowledge their utility in building cross-party support (Jones, 1990). They may also be seen as conducive to a two-way process of communication between backbench MPs and ministers (Administration Committee, 1995). Ministers occasionally attend meetings and explain their policies in an informal setting, which allows MPs and Peers to raise matters. The effectiveness of all-party groups depends on how well they are organized. The most effective groups work closely with outside organizations, and derive important resources from them, such as secretarial support, information and expertise (Dubs, 1989; Jones, 1990).

In 2000, over 200 all-party groups were approved and listed by the House of Commons: 38 were health-related and 16 focused on specific conditions.[2] In several cases, these all-party groups were supported by health consumer groups, including asthma (National Asthma Campaign), cancer (CancerBACUP), diabetes (Diabetes UK), acquired brain injury (Headway – the National Brain Injury Association), multiple sclerosis (Multiple Sclerosis Society), osteoporosis (National Osteoporosis Society) and ageing and older people (Age Concern). In all, ten health consumer groups interviewed in the De Montfort study mentioned involvement with all-party groups. Those that were involved pointed out several advantages. For example, one cancer group said:

> It's informing parliamentarians about developments in research and treatment, it's raising the profile of cancer in parliament, you know, reminding them of the issues, and it's also a way of campaigning. (gi31)

All-party groups were seen as a useful platform for raising issues and building political support within parliament. The Mental Health Foundation respondent commented on the usefulness of all-party groups in engaging MPs and building links:

> I think they can be an extremely good way of engaging usually quite a small group of MPs who are particularly interested in a particular subject area and...is a useful process. It means that when legislation comes up or you want parliamentary questions asked there is a way in.

But the same group also acknowledged that while 'some of them are brilliant' others 'are a complete waste of time'. A few groups were similarly dismissive of all-party groups. For example, a respondent from Carers National Association did not believe that the absence of an all-party group for carers was a problem:

> On the whole, I don't think all-party groups are particularly useful .... We have tremendous contacts in parliament, we don't need an all-party group.

In the cancer field, several all-party groups co-existed and some health consumer groups maintained links with more than one. In some cases this worked well. For example, UKBCC had worked closely with three all-party groups (breast cancer, cancer and ageing/older people) on the issue of extending automatic breast screening to those aged 65–69. Generally though, respondents felt that the number of cancer all-party groups was confusing and symptomatic of the lack of coherence among cancer groups in parliament. At the time of writing attempts were being made to bring together the work of these separate groups.

Although at the time of the De Montfort study there was no all-party group for maternity services, the maternity/childbirth groups were in the process of establishing one. A maternity all-party group was subsequently set up in 2000, serviced by the National Childbirth Trust. Similarly, two arthritis groups (Arthritis Care and BLAR) were considering setting up an all-party group. In 2002 a rheumatoid arthritis all-party group was established with support from the National Rheumatoid Arthritis Society (see Chapter 8).

From the perspective of MPs and peers, all-party groups were regarded as informative and enabled co-ordination of briefings. However, their strategic use was seen as limited and less important than other forms of contact with health consumer groups. Former ministers, on the other hand, commented that all-party groups were useful. They were seen by one as giving groups 'a foot in the door' (si22) in the parliamentary process. Another stated that they formed a channel of communication with MPs, enabling ministers to explain their policies, as well as providing an opportunity for members to put points across to ministers. Although the civil servants interviewed were reluctant to discuss parliamentary matters, one did observe that all-party groups provided a means by which interested MPs could get together and communicate with ministers on policy issues.

The Lords

This chapter so far has focused mainly on the House of Commons. However, the House of Lords should not be ignored. Although its powers are weaker than the Commons, the upper house scrutinizes and revises legislation and can be useful to outside organizations seeking to influence policy. Although the Lords can defeat government on legislation, the Commons usually reverses amendments made in the Lords with which the government disagrees. Even so, the upper house can force government to think again about legislation and can secure important concessions (see Baldwin, 1990; Shell, 1993).

While most of the contact reported by health consumer groups related to the Commons, several groups mentioned the Lords. Peers were approached to table amendments, ask questions and raise debates. For example, in January 2000 Baroness Cumberlege, a former health minister and patron of the National Childbirth Trust, introduced a debate on maternity services. Peers were generally regarded by groups as very accessible, open to argument and willing to act on behalf of groups. Contacts with peers were also established through informal networks and through all-party groups. It was also noted that the Lords had a tradition of campaigning on behalf of elderly and disabled people and that consequently they were receptive to groups representing these particular constituencies.

In some cases, peers were associated with a specific health consumer group. For example, Lord Skelmersdale has served as chairperson of the Stroke Association; Lord Clement-Jones was a trustee director of CancerBACUP and patron of the National Childbirth Trust as well as a health spokesman for the Liberal Democrats from 1998 onwards; Baroness Greengross was previously director of Age Concern, England, and Baroness Pitkeathley a former director of the Carers National Association. These peers were regarded by groups as well-connected, both within the voluntary sector and in wider political networks. It was believed that they exercised influence beyond their role as peers and had good political contacts, which could be useful. Some peers had also previously served as ministers and were approached by health consumer groups because of their knowledge of the policy process, as well as their wider political contacts and networks.

Influencing legislation

The legislative process provides a major opportunity to influence policy, and in recent years there have been several examples where health consumer groups have played an active role. In general, groups realized the importance of getting ministers and officials 'on-side' before legislation was introduced. This was reflected in their efforts to build a constructive relationship with Whitehall, discussed in the previous chapter. Once positions became entrenched, it was more difficult to change things. As the respondent from MIND observed with regard to mental health legislation: 'You have to do work early in order to influence. The government has a huge majority and there would have to be a massive back bench revolt to overturn it.'

In the following cases, groups secured amendments to legislation or other concessions through parliamentary lobbying, coupled with discussions with ministers and civil servants as legislation progressed through its various stages.

The Health Bill 1998/99

The first example related to the Health Bill of 1998/99, which became the Health Act, 1999. This was the first major piece of legislation relating to the NHS introduced by the Blair government and covered a wide range of issues. Health consumer groups came together to discuss how they could influence the Bill, and the Patients Forum was the focal point for this activity. It arranged meetings with MPs and peers to discuss aspects of the Bill, and opened a dialogue with ministers and civil servants. One of the civil servants interviewed for the study stated that such activities caught the Department of Health unawares, and that greater efforts were made to engage with the groups and address their concerns thereafter.

Groups were anxious about several aspects of the Bill. These included: the lack of clarity about patient and public involvement; professional self-regulation; the establishment and composition of primary care trusts and the impact of the changes on people needing treatment outside their local area, such as specialist treatment and aftercare. A number of groups lobbied MPs individually as well as through the Patients Forum. As a result, several amendments were proposed in the Lords, although some were later reversed in the Commons due to the government's large majority there. However, the government made concessions on some issues. Amendments to impose a requirement on health bodies to consult and involve patients groups and voluntary organizations were rejected, but the government gave assurances that groups would be involved in consultations about the regulations made under the terms of the Bill. Amendments to enable patients to receive out-of-area treatment for specialist hospital treatment and aftercare were also rejected, although again the government gave assurances that patients' interests would be protected and announced that reports on the commissioning of regionally-based specialized services would be published. Notably, this particular concession was a response to concerns raised by professional groups as well as health consumer groups.

Several of the issues raised during debates, returned to the policy agenda later. For example, an amendment to ensure the representation of older people on the Commission for Health Improvement was rejected, only to be subsequently proposed in the *NHS Plan* for England (Cm 4818, 2000). Concerns about the lack of an explicit requirement to consult with patients groups and voluntary organizations also resurfaced later. Commitments to create a new framework for patient and public involvement were also made in the *NHS Plan* and led to the introduction of a statutory duty to consult and involve patients, carers and the public (see Chapter 2).

When interviewed, health consumer group respondents and civil servants claimed that the Patients Forum and other health consumer groups, including the College of Health and Carers National Association, had significant influence on the debates surrounding the Bill, even though they did not secure major changes to the legislation. The groups ensured that important issues were aired and obtained some concessions. Most important though, it made ministers and civil servants aware of the desirability of prior consultation with health consumer groups and the need to work with them more closely on future legislation.

The Carers and Disabled Children Bill

The second example related to the Carers and Disabled Children Bill of 1999/2000 – enacted in 2000. The Carers National Association had been active in promoting previous legislation such as the Carers' Recognition and Services Act, 1995 (introduced by Malcolm Wicks, now a vice-president of the Carers National Association) and the 1996 Carers Direct Payments Act. Both acts had given carers important rights to have their needs assessed and to obtain support. The Carers National Association wanted further legislation to extend these rights, and in particular, to ensure that carers had an independent right to have their own needs assessed, even if the cared-for person had refused an assessment.

In 1999 the government agreed to strengthen carers' rights in the *National Strategy for Carers* (HM Government, 1999), but when the Queen's Speech was published at the beginning of the 1999/2000 session, it made no commitment to new legislation. The Carers National Association suggested to the Department of Health that their objectives could be achieved by a private member's bill.[3] The government agreed to back this. In the event, Tom Pendry, a Labour MP who came second in the private member's bill ballot, agreed to pilot the measure through the Commons. Discussion with the Department of Health and the Carers National Association followed, and the Bill was drafted and introduced into the Commons. The Carers National Association was broadly content with the Bill, but disagreed with the way some clauses had been drafted. Amendments were tabled to deal with most of these. They included clarification of the term 'carer' to exclude paid or volunteer carers, clarification of 'parental responsibility' to extend the rights of parent carers to others exercising parental roles, and a restriction on local authorities' ability to charge and means test carers.

Throughout the passage of the Bill, the Carers National Association was in close touch with civil servants. On one occasion, ministerial support was needed to bring about an important amendment. This was achieved by the personal intervention of one of the Association's key political contacts, who was able to speak to the minister at a crucial stage. The Carers National Association was in a strong position because the MP who introduced the Bill did not have a background in this field, and needed advice and information, which they supplied. Also the government needed the Association to build support for the measure in parliament:

> So for the civil servants, they needed us and the government needed us, to do the lobbying. We wrote to all MPs. We sent briefings to all MPs. We briefed at the committee stage, we were involved in keeping all the other caring organizations informed about progress and reporting back to them. Dealing with the issues that they raised and trying to ensure they were addressed within the bill and things like that. We were sort of [a] conduit really.

The Carers National Association was particularly close to a handful of MPs who strongly supported the measure and tabled amendments. These included Sylvia Heal, who, as noted earlier, had formerly worked for this organization. When the Bill passed through the House of Lords, the Association could rely on the expertise and support of Baroness Pitkeathley, who had previously been its director.

Other examples of influence

In interview, eight respondents from health consumer groups identified at least one example of how they believed they had influenced parliament. In seven of these cases, they believed that this had also had an impact on government policy. These included legislation, such as the Human Fertilisation and Embryology Act 1990 and subsequent statutory regulations. Other examples included service guidelines, such as those on pregnancy loss and the death of a baby, promoted by the Stillbirth and Neonatal Death Society.[4] Parliamentary pressure could also be used to reiterate a policy commitment. For example, the Stroke Association lobbied to ensure that the condition remained an official priority for government. Concerned that the importance of stroke was being downplayed in official guidance, the Association lobbied parliament. Parliamentary questions were tabled and in December 1999 an adjournment debate was held. The government responded by clarifying its position, namely that stroke remained a priority. In several cases, health consumer groups had worked alongside others to influence parliament. For example, a number of groups, including Age Concern and the UKBCC, were active in calling for an extension of automatic breast screening for women aged 65–69 years and over. MPs were persuaded to table questions and motions, including an early day motion that attracted 138 signatures. This change was also supported by the all-party group on breast cancer and by an earlier inquiry by the Health Committee (Health Committee, 1995). Other voluntary organizations also campaigned on this issue, including charities such as Breakthrough Breast Cancer. Importantly, the extension of screening to older women was also supported by the NHS Breast Cancer Screening Programme and by many professionals advising the government. Subsequently, the Department of Health included a commitment to automatic screening to women aged 65–70 by 2004 in the *Cancer Plan*. It should also be noted in this context that breast cancer campaigns are amongst the highest-profile issues in parliament, as well as in the media. In a survey the breast cancer campaign was recalled by 9 per cent of MPs – second only to the NSPCC's 'full stop' campaign which was recalled by 16 per cent of MPs (Future Foundation, 2001).

Another example was the joint campaign against the draft mental health bill in 2002. There were strong concerns about the civil liberty aspects of the proposals and its likely impact on public perceptions of mental illness. A mass lobby of parliament was held in November 2002, which received considerable media coverage. The level of opposition, from professionals, lawyers, social workers and doctors, as well as health consumer groups, persuaded the government not to include the measure in the 2003 Queen's Speech. The debate over these controversial plans continues at the time of writing.

In summary, the examples of influence mentioned above concerned groups that were active in parliament, but this tells us little about why campaigns succeed or not. The bigger picture is important, notably how the health consumer groups work together; how ministers and civil servants view them and their constituency; and the media profile of the groups and the condition. Moreover, parliamentary support is difficult to measure. The De Montfort study tended to focus on activity rather than latent support. But because certain groups did not use parliament over a particular period of time did not mean that they lacked parliamentary links. They may simply have used their contacts only when they needed to.

Conclusion

Despite cynicism about the ability of parliament to shape policy, it is clear that it cannot be ignored by those seeking to influence health policy. Health consumer groups recognized this and appreciated the need for effective parliamentary organization and lobbying. Parliament was not their primary target, but activity in both the Commons and Lords was seen as complementary to other efforts to influence government and the Department of Health. More specifically, parliament was seen as useful in developing political contacts, raising issues and in demonstrating political support for a particular policy.

The effectiveness of parliament in this respect is contingent on the publicity generated by lobbying activities (Silk and Walters, 1995). Parliament, and the political process generally, does not attract the kind of media coverage it once received (Riddell, 1998). In particular, little publicity is usually generated by debates and parliamentary questions alone. Even so, there is awareness that parliamentary activity, in tandem with efforts to influence the media, can be effective in putting pressure on government. This leads on to a discussion of the crucial role played by the media in the health policy process, the subject of the following chapter.

11 Working with the media

The media is widely acknowledged as an important ally and a dangerous enemy by those seeking to influence the policy process. Certainly, no group wishing to influence public policy can afford to ignore it, even those with insider status possessing effective working relationships with government and parliament. As Newton (2001, p. 167) has observed: 'News and current affairs programmes are saturated with special interests, pressure groups, spokesmen and advocates of every conceivable kind, all trying to gain publicity, make their case with public support and influence government policy.' Others have also noted the central importance of the media to groups (Negrine, 1998) and have acknowledged that sympathetic media coverage is an important asset (Wilson, 1984).

Nonetheless, the media's role in the policy process is more subtle than commonly perceived. The media is comprised of many different organizations that together provide a wide range of products and services: printed publications, broadcasting and new information technologies. Ownership is concentrated, both within and across these different media forms, a trend underlined by the emergence of global media corporations (Keane, 1991). This complexity means that its impact on policy is difficult to unravel.

The role of the media in the health policy process

The media and policy

One of the main difficulties in analysing the media is that it has a dual role. It *reports* and *reflects* on events, issues and policies and it can also be regarded as a *policy advocate* that seeks deliberately to influence policy outcomes. In some cases the media, will operate openly, actively highlighting a particular problem or endorsing a specific policy, but usually advocacy is more indirect. For example, a study of abortion politics in the USA (Terkildsen, Schnell and Ling, 1998) found that the media played a crucial role in advocating policy messages through language and symbolism. Others have also noted how the media can shape policy agendas and construct policy problems and issues, in a particular way (Philo, 1996, 1999). The selection of topics for coverage can lead to the neglect of some issues and over-exposure of others. Connections can be made between issues and events to influence people's understanding in such a way that may affect policy choices. Indeed, the power of the media lies in its ability to reinforce or weaken current ways of understanding (Philo, 1999) and thereby build support, or opposition, for particular policy options. Even so, the media is extensively used by policy-makers (spin-doctors, for example) as well as other policy participants (such as pressure groups). Some suggest that its independent impact as a policy advocate has been exaggerated. Although it has been conceded that the media has affected the style and conduct of politics considerably (Ranney, 1983; Newton, 2001), the same may not be true about its influence over policy content.

The media has three weaknesses as a policy actor. First, it is composed of a diverse group of organizations which lack coherence and rarely pull in the same direction. Indeed, the complex mixture of political interests and commercial priorities means that a particular issue may be covered sympathetically by some parts of the media but ignored or treated with hostility by others (Philo, 1999). Moreover, the ability of individual media organizations to push for a particular policy is constrained by their commercial and competitive environment. This means that issues of great public concern cannot be totally ignored and that the target readership must not be alienated. The large media conglomerates must also balance their media interests with other business interests. For those media organizations that accept advertising and sponsorship, there is the added constraint of not offending the external business interests that provide important sources of revenue.

The media agenda is shaped by proprietors and by the editorial imperative to maintain and extend the audience or readership

(Negrine, 1998). Yet the complexity of interests and the tensions between them, mean that the position of the media (or of any particular media organization) on specific policy issues is not always predictable. Moreover, there is often a vacuum within which individual journalists have considerable room for manoeuvre. As Brindle (1999b) has argued, the production of news is more chaotic than most outsiders realize and journalists have considerable freedom to select issues and report them in the way they choose.

A second restriction on the influence of the media over policy is public opinion. Newton (2001) has argued that people's views are quite entrenched and that it is difficult to get them to change their mind. Although the media may play a role in the formation of a particular view in the first place (Eldridge, Kitzinger and Williams, 1997), this point remains valid. As Philo (1996) has observed, people are not 'blank slates' and are able to resist media messages. Individual experiences can enable people to be critical – although even firsthand experience can be challenged by a strong media message, leading individuals to think that their experience is in some way unusual or uncommon (Philo, 1996, 1999). The scope for media influence is therefore greatest where only a few individuals can draw on personal experience.

Finally, the media operates within a framework of regulation that can limit efforts to influence opinion and policy. Although many aspects of media activity are still predominantly subject to self-regulatory mechanisms, media regulation has become increasingly codified. A range of codes sets standards for the press and broadcasting, and increasingly the new information technology media as well. These govern general standards of reporting, in relation to accuracy and privacy, access to institutions such as hospitals and schools, and can also limit programme content and advertising. Codes are reinforced by complaint procedures, which may be used as to challenge the portrayal of an issue, or an imbalance in reporting.

Media and health

It has been widely acknowledged that health 'stories' trigger the attention of the media (Entwhistle, 1995; Brindle, 1999b; Entwhistle and Sheldon, 1999; Jennings, 1999; Doyle, 2000).

The most effective triggers include events of social, political and human significance; those involving drama, action and/or surprise, and those that have an emotional impact, or raise ethical and moral considerations. Issues affecting a large number of people are considered newsworthy, though rare or unusual cases may also attract media interest. Certain population groups also command attention, particularly issues relating to the health of children and women. Jennings (1999) has observed that significant media attention is given to issues involving pain and loss, particularly where culpability and blame can be attributed (see also Chapter 4). Health issues affecting celebrities or high-profile personalities are attractive to the media, as are stories with an element of scandal or a sexual dimension. Topicality is a key consideration. The media are interested in pursuing issues related to those already in the news and topics of current public debate.

Although media interest can be triggered by at least one of these factors, the level and intensity of interest varies. There can be a variation over time: media coverage of maternity issues and HIV/AIDS, both of which enjoyed a high media profile in the early 1990s, waned later in the decade. At any point in time some medical conditions may be more newsworthy than others. By the end of the 1990s, breast cancer was receiving media coverage far in excess of its relative significance in terms of mortality and morbidity compared with other cancers (Henderson and Kitzinger, 1999). One study found that it received a third of all cancer coverage and was headlined four times more often than other cancers (Saywell, Beattie and Henderson, 2000). However, this was not always so. Breast cancer used to be a taboo subject, and its emergence is largely the result of successful campaigning by health consumer groups and charities, rather than unprompted media interest.

Another consideration when looking at media coverage of health, is what has been termed the 'cuddly charity' effect (Hunt, 1993; Deacon, 1999) or the 'halo effect' (Lloyd, 2001). The media has tended to see charities, and voluntary activity more generally, in a favourable light. Some organizations are treated very favourably indeed, particularly if their client group attracts widespread sympathy, such as sick children (Ingram and Schneider, 1993). Groups campaigning for elderly and disabled people have faced more problems in attracting attention. The greater vulnerability of frail elderly people may gain sympathy, but this is often at odds with the philosophy of campaigners and their desire to promote a more positive image of ageing and disability. Mental health groups face a similar problem. Mental health attracts wide coverage, but tends to focus on certain stereotypes which are regarded as unhelpful. Media reporting of dangerous and psychotic behaviour far outweighs the coverage of chronic mental health problems. In one study Philo (1996), found that two-thirds of such media coverage concerned violence to others; 13 per cent related to self-harm; 18 per cent concerned advice or treatment and 2 per cent related to comic images. Only 1 per cent of media coverage challenged the dominant perspectives of mental illness.

A key problem for most health consumer groups is not difficulty attracting media attention, it is ensuring that coverage is appropriate and sympathetic. Negative or hostile coverage may be worse than nothing, since it may reinforce unhelpful images and stereotypes. Frequently, considerable effort is made to influence media content in order to correct such stereotypes. However, health consumer groups always have to compete for media attention, with the professions, drug companies and other commercial interests, and moreover government which can try to influence media reporting of health issues.

According to Karpf (1988), media coverage of health reflects medical dominance. She argues that this was reflected in the uncritically positive portrayal of medicine, medical technology and doctors for much of the immediate post-war period, in both news and drama programmes. She acknowledges that in the 1960s and 1970s other interpretative frameworks – different perspectives on health stories – emerged. More attention was given to self-help, lifestyles and prevention, the environment and social factors and there was greater criticism of doctors. However, she argued that these alternative frameworks did not seriously challenge medical dominance, which was deeply embedded. The coverage of doctors, medicine, and technology was generally positive, and the profession had effective levers to maintain its social authority, the status of its individual experts, and its collective organizations, particularly the British Medical Association, which is highly skilled in media relations.

The Karpf thesis has been challenged. Entwhistle and Sheldon (1999), while acknowledging the credence given to medical views in the media, argue that there is now greater scope for alternative views to be expressed. They noted occasions where journalists adopted a campaigning stance which put them at odds with the professions. Journalists have also drawn on a wider range of interpretative frameworks, including the health consumer perspective. Bury and Gabe (1994) tested the Karpf thesis against actual cases of British television coverage and concluded that portrayals did not necessarily support medical dominance. In practice, coverage was more critical, portraying medicine in a much less glamorous light, and focusing on conflicts between medicine and other stakeholders such as health service managers. They concluded that the representation of health care reflected, and reinforced, arguments that changes were underway in the social relations of health. Another study by Gabe, Gustafsson and Bury (1991), which drew on an analysis of newspaper coverage of tranquillizer dependence, reinforced these conclusions. Their study found that media coverage was not dominated by medical definitions of health, and indeed could challenge conventional values. They concluded:

Rather than seeing the media as either simply expressing public opinion or as carriers of medical interests in the area of health, we see them more literally as mediators, albeit of complex messages and relationships within specific cultural and ideological settings. (Gabe, Gustafsson and Bury, 1991, p. 350)

Other powerful interests seek to influence the media. The pharmaceutical industry, for example, has a huge public relations and marketing budget, which can be deployed not just to promote particular products but to portray the industry in a positive light. The industry believes that it receives unfavourable coverage – largely due to adverse clinical incidents. It is also seen as exploitative, making profits out of illness. Considerable effort and resources are invested in attempting to correct these negative images. As Chapter 8 suggests, health consumer groups can constitute a useful part of this public relations strategy. By campaigning for the wider availability of new drugs, for example, a health consumer group can both increase the demand for industry's products and help to portray a company in a more favourable light.

Governments also seek to influence media coverage of health. As journalists themselves acknowledge, considerable reliance is placed on official briefings and press releases and these can shape the development of particular stories (Brindle, 1999). Attempts to influence the media are not new, as Karpf (1988) points out. In the inter-war period, the Ministry of Health formally vetted media coverage of health. Attempts to shape media coverage today may be less overt than in the past, but the imperatives are similar. As Entwhistle and Sheldon (1999, p.125) have observed, 'media reports of events in the health service are of key importance to politicians as one of the main currencies of success or failure'. The handling of health issues has been used to judge the overall competence of the government. During the 1990s the Conservative government recognized this and strengthened news management operations at the Department of Health. Matters came to a head in 1994 when a leaked memo from a senior figure in the Conservative government (the so-called Maples Memorandum) stated that: 'The best result for the next 12 months would be zero media coverage of the National Health Service' (Beckett and Brown, 1994).

Under New Labour an even greater emphasis has been placed on 'spin' and news management across all areas of government (Brindle, 1999b; Jones, 2002). The concern to manage media coverage of health matters has increased. Following extensive media pressure in winter 1999/2000, the Labour government launched the *NHS Plan* for England (Cm 4818, 2000) and allocated additional resources. This elevated health even higher in the scale of official priorities and underlined it as one of the key issues on which the government's record would be judged, strengthening the imperative to influence media coverage in this field.

Health consumer groups and the media

Extent of contact

Given its importance, it would be expected that health consumer groups would make considerable efforts to influence the media. Indeed, the De Montfort study showed a high frequency of contact between groups and the media. The questionnaire data indicated that a higher percentage of groups reported contact with the media than with government or parliament. Over a quarter of groups had at least weekly contact with the media, just under half had at least monthly contact, while over three-quarters reported at least quarterly contact. Only 14 per cent of groups claimed to have had no contact with the media in the previous three years.

The questionnaire also indicated that groups saw the media as a key means of influencing policy. Three-quarters stated that links with the media were 'very important' or 'important', slightly more than the proportion judging links with central government as 'very important' or 'important'. Almost two-thirds of groups stated that a lack of media support was 'very important' or 'important'. The significance of the media was further reflected in the large majority of groups (87 per cent) stating that the public profile of their organization was a 'very important' or 'important' consideration.

Media contact varied according to the type of group. Fewer formal alliance organizations reported that they were in contact with the media on a weekly basis (18 per cent) compared with condition-based (24 per cent) and population-based (46 per cent) groups. Nearly 70 per cent of population-based groups stated that they were in contact with the media at least monthly, compared with just under half of formal alliance organizations and condition-based groups. Formal alliance organizations placed links with the media below parliament and central government in terms of their importance as non-financial resources in the policy process. Only 46 per cent of formal alliance organizations believed these links to be 'very important' or 'important', compared with almost all population-based groups and three-quarters of condition-based groups. As Table 11.1. shows, there was also some variation by condition area. Mental health groups were by far the most frequently in contact with the media on a weekly basis, arthritis groups the least frequently. However, there was less variation in the responses by condition area at the 'at least monthly level'. Mental health groups and heart and circulatory disease groups were also more likely than other groups to perceive links with the media as 'very important' or 'important' when influencing policy.

The questionnaire showed that groups were in contact with a wide range of different media. This included broadsheet and

Table 11.1   Health consumer groups' extent of contact with the media and ranking of importance of the media, by condition area

	'At least weekly' contact (%)	'At least monthly' contact (%)	Contact with media 'very important' or 'important' (%)
Arthritis and related conditions	13	40	50
Cancer	18	50	64
Heart/ circulatory disease	17	42	83
Maternity/ childbirth	25	44	67
Mental health	40	50	85

Source: Questionnaire data set 1999.

tabloid newspapers, magazines, television and radio. They were keen to influence coverage in news stories and factual programmes as well as fiction and drama.

Why did groups seek media coverage?

In interviews for the De Montfort study groups identified a range of reasons why they sought media coverage. These reasons could be divided into two categories: raising public awareness about the group or condition and using the media to influence policy-makers. In practice, groups acknowledged that these different rationales were often closely related. They were aware that good publicity in the media could enable them to satisfy a number of objectives. For example, a newspaper feature article on skin cancer may raise public awareness, by describing how to avoid it and how to seek help, as well as enable a group to market services such as help-lines and counselling. This might also generate public and corporate donations to cancer groups and highlight the specific problem of skin cancer, leading to greater support for policy interventions, new initiatives and additional resources for services in this field.

In seeking to raise awareness and improve understanding, an important motive mentioned by several groups was to correct unhelpful stereotypes. The mental health groups in particular continued to challenge the stigma of mental illness. The Mental Health Foundation, for example, stated that it was trying to 'challenge media descriptions of mental health'. Another organization, Mental Health Media, had been established specifically for the purpose of promoting a more positive image of people with mental health problems and learning difficulties. Mental Health Media provided health consumer groups with media skills training and also targeted news, documentary and drama programmes in order to encourage a more positive view of mental illness.

Even so, media coverage could reinforce unhelpful stereotypes. Several groups noted that the media's demand for specific cases could portray a misleading or inaccurate picture of the condition. Interestingly, two cancer groups made similar observations:

> I have major, major concerns...over providing a member...on a platter as it were, for a journalist who's already written the story. I'm not kidding, they will literally phone and say 'can I have a young woman, preferably blonde, not overweight, two children ideally', you know and we're sort of there thinking 'Well, what messages are we conveying there?' (gi36)

> It is something that we [discuss] in the office, you know, somebody else wanting a blonde patient with breast cancer under the age of 25. (gi31)

This finding is reflected in other research. According to Saywell, Beattie and Henderson (2000, p. 59):

> Breast cancer is made newsworthy in most media reporting by focusing on the experiences of young and either maternal or sexual female bodies. This is influenced by perceptions of femininity which focus on the breast as an icon of feminine worth. This is not necessarily the way in which women understand or experience breast cancer.

Arthritis groups, including Arthritis Care, were also concerned about unhelpful stereotypes in the way the condition was portrayed in the media:

> Another tension is that they will often want to try and portray people with arthritis in a very negative light as being people who are suffering and who have this dreadful disease and so on, and yet, our whole philosophy is about trying to be positive and saying you can live with this disease and learn to manage it. It doesn't mean that your life's come to an end. Be positive.

Arthritis Care, along with other groups, made the link between the media's role in shaping public attitudes, and the impact that these could have on policy formation:

> Well, we're very aware that... [an] important aspect of influencing policy is trying to create the right climate of opinion and to do that you've got to influence the media.

Another crucial factor was the way in which the media could draw policy-makers' attention to problems. For example, the Stillbirth and Neonatal Death Society (SANDS) commented that the media was an effective way of demonstrating the anger of parents and the need for an appropriate policy response. Another group, Group Action into Steroid Prescribing, also believed that the media was a vital tool when undertaking campaigns: 'We needed the voice, again, of the media, because they [the government] just take no notice otherwise.' Groups saw government as being very concerned about adverse media coverage. The Blair government was viewed as 'particularly sensitive to adverse media coverage' (gi28) by one mental health group. Its respondent saw health consumer groups' efforts to influence the media as a crucial factor in policy influence. He went on: 'If you're not getting your message across in the media, then you're not getting your message across to government' (gi28). Another perspective on groups' reasons for engaging with the media was provided by an informant with considerable experience of working in health consumer groups and the voluntary sector, and who had served on several government committees. He commented that while the media was generally accessible to health consumer groups, it was often the main recourse for groups lacking other means of influence. In his words, 'If you had little power and few resources, then the media had to be your friend' (si12).

Influencing the media

Attracting media attention

The interview data confirmed that groups faced few barriers when seeking to make contact with the media and that they found that the media were generally attracted by health issues. However, research findings confirmed that the dramatic, emotional or sensational aspects of a story were particularly attractive to journalists. Several groups – including those in mental health – criticized the disproportionate attention on crisis and drama, while noting the media's tendency to exaggerate problems. Others were also concerned about this, the Patients Association referring to the media's thirst for 'horror headlines'. The UK Breast Cancer Coalition (UKBCC) also expressed concern about the media's construction of stories as reinforcing the notion of crisis, which was not necessarily in patients' interest.

The De Montfort study found several examples of journalists taking an interest in health issues as a result of their own experiences and those of close friends and relatives. This confirmed to some extent Jennings' (1999) point that part of the attractiveness of pain and loss experiences to the media lies in their pervasiveness. Groups capitalized on this by contributing material to inquiring journalists, highlighting examples, and pitching directly into the debate. For example, in late 1997 *The Observer* carried a number of articles by reporter Martin Bright describing the plight of his 88-year-old grandmother following her admission to hospital after a stroke. He described how she had spent hours on a trolley, before being admitted to a mixed ward where her diabetes and glaucoma were ignored and where she was left without food and drink. He also showed how she was neglected following admission to a women's geriatric ward, where relatives found her on one occasion lying in her own faeces. *The Observer* received hundreds of letters on the subject, and Help the Aged provided important backup for its coverage.[1] Together they established what became known as the Dignity on the Ward campaign, which was also strongly supported by other consumer and professional groups, including the Patients Association, the Royal College of Nursing and leading geriatricians.

There are further examples of journalists actively campaigning on an issue, such as Marjorie Wallace, who wrote an influential series of articles about schizophrenia for *The Times* in the mid-1980s.[2] Her copy vividly brought to public attention the desperate plight of those suffering from the condition and their families. Her campaign was extremely successful in raising awareness about schizophrenia and the poor quality of services in this field. In 1986 Wallace was named 'Campaigning Journalist of the Year' for her articles at the British Press Awards. In the same year she founded Schizophrenia A National Emergency.

Some groups had more opportunities than others to contribute to the media, because the issues they dealt with were more newsworthy. This is related to the characteristics of issues, discussed earlier in the chapter. The high media profile of breast cancer was acknowledged, along with its success in securing a substantial amount of coverage relative to other cancers and other conditions. In contrast groups in areas such as stroke and arthritis faced an uphill struggle, perceiving that their stories were not particularly attractive to journalists. Arthritis Care, for example commented:

> Yes, its very frustrating, because you know that in their eyes the arthritis often is not seen as such a sexy subject as things that happen to children or cancer-related issues and things like that. So it can be a bit of a struggle at times and you can put a huge amount of work into something and then find that only one journalist turns up and they give you three lines of copy.

The reason given for this was the association of these diseases with elderly people, which according to the groups lacked appeal among journalists. Although some issues received coverage, such as the Dignity on the Ward campaign, because of the sense of scandal and injustice surrounding the case.

Formal alliance organizations, who, as already noted, had less frequent contact with the media than other groups, also had fewer opportunities to get their message across to the media. As the respondent from one group stated:

> A lot of our messages are not ones that interest the media. They are low key, change of language, change of approach, culture and shift of resources. It's not dramatic like some of the health service messages...[We] are less able to do that...[we] are more strategic, more long-term. (gi19)

This was particularly problematic for alliances that covered a range of conditions. Their key messages were broad rather than specific, and therefore lacked a particular focus. It was also more difficult for them to exemplify their points by referring to an individual patient around whom a story could be constructed. It has also been argued that voluntary groups representing ethnic minorities face particular difficulties in attracting media coverage (Deacon, 1999). There was some evidence to support this view from the interview data generated by the De Montfort study. Groups representing patients from minorities perceived that the media was not very interested in them and received few inquiries from journalists.

Media strategy and resources

The better-resourced voluntary organizations tend to be more strategic and well organized in relation to the media (Pharoah and Welchman, 1997; Deacon, 1999). Indeed a distinction has been made between resource-rich groups and resource-poor groups, with the latter finding it difficult to secure sustained media coverage in the face of competition from the former (Miller, 1998). With specific regard to health consumer groups the De Montfort study found that overall income was linked to media contact (see Table 11.2) with the wealthiest groups tending to have more frequent contact with the media.

However, as Miller (1998) and Deacon (1999) acknowledge, even groups with limited resources can have a media presence and can influence debate, particularly if they have an effective political strategy and are seen as a credible organization by journalists. Indeed, health consumer groups with relatively low incomes, and those that did not have specialist public relations staff, were still able in certain circumstances to attract media attention. For example, the National Cancer Alliance said it had 'never, never ever used a professional' and had 'never been systematic' in their

Table 11.2 Percentage of groups having contact with the media 'at least monthly' or 'quarterly', by income group

Income band	'At least monthly' contact (%)	'At least quarterly' contact (%)
£100 000 or less	38	68
£100 001–£1 000 000	52	84
£1 000 001 and over	86	93

Source: Questionnaire data set 1999.

use of the media. Yet they had sent out press releases and had attracted 'a lot of publicity'. In some cases groups had very good access to the media, out of all proportion to their size and resources. The Zito Trust believed it had established very good links with the media, its respondent commented: 'We've never had a dedicated PR function. We've never had to have one. Jayne came to the Zito Trust with a massive amount of media following'. As a consequence the organization, though 'sometimes struggling to survive financially' was 'able to pull in the broadest of media coverage possible'.

Although the resource-poor groups could be proactive, it was those with more resources, such as a publicity budget, or access to specialist public relations skills that were more so. A number of groups employed press or publicity officers, including Help the Aged, National Childbirth Trust, MIND (National Association for Mental Health), Age Concern, and SANDS for example. Others were able to access resources to improve their media relations. In some cases this meant drawing on the skills of members or getting access to training. The UK Federation of Small Mental Health Agencies (UKFSMHA) acting director was a journalist and some members had experience of journalism. Arthritis Care had trained staff in media skills including 'techniques for turning round a negative interview into something positive'.

But several groups acknowledged there was a downside to a proactive strategy. Extensive interest from journalists and from the public could prompt a large number of queries and a failure to respond adequately could damage a group's credibility. As the interviewee from one group commented:

What we do try to do is comment on things that we think we have an expertise in... we don't want to become rent-a-quote. We could end up in a situation in responding to any and every cancer story, I mean obviously there's one in the media every day... We'd rather have a clearly defined area of expertise and I think specialist health journalists recognize that. (gi31)

Groups with specialist public relations staff emphasized their wide range of contacts and used many different types of media. For example, Age Concern used electronic media, local and national newspapers, and specialist press. Groups in this position emphasized the importance of tailoring the message to the specific type of media. As one group put it, a different approach was needed for the populist *GMTV* compared to the more in-depth *The World Tonight*.

Television news and documentaries

Groups were keen to influence the content of factual programmes on television. In most cases groups were involved in an advisory role following an approach from programme makers. For example the Stroke Association mentioned that it had been asked to nominate professional experts to talk about new treatments for a forthcoming documentary. In other cases, groups approached programme makers with ideas, and if successful would then offer information and advice. One case, however, did not fit this conventional pattern, and illustrates how groups can contribute to 'undercover' investigative journalism and have an impact on policy.

During the mid-1990s, a maternity group became involved in 'undercover reporting' about the treatment of pregnant women prisoners. There were allegations that they were shackled in hospital, chained to beds and having to give birth with prison officers being present. The group had been contacted by a woman prisoner, and aware of the prisoner's distress, an officer of the organisation visited her in hospital. A photograph of the prisoner in handcuffs later was passed to Channel 4 News. She was filmed on the postnatal ward (Boseley, 1996). The screening of the film caused a political furore, placing enormous pressure on the authorities to improve conditions for pregnant women prisoners. Combined with pressure from professional groups (such as the Royal College of Midwives) and other health consumer groups, the Prison Service altered its rules. Prisoners taken to hospital to give birth would not be handcuffed. Furthermore, the rule that women should not be shackled during labour would be enforced. Women visiting clinics for antenatal checks were allowed to have restraints removed unless there was an exceptionally high risk of an escape.

Drama

Media coverage of health is not confined to news and documentaries. Indeed, health is frequently the subject of drama programmes, giving health consumer groups much scope for influence. In the UK, a particularly important role is played by 'soap operas' (or 'soaps'), regular dramas that attract large audiences (Henderson, 1999). Writers, striving for realism (within the constraints of audience satisfaction ratings, viewing figures and of course the 'watershed') contact health professionals and health consumer groups for advice. By the same token, groups representing patients contact regular dramas with ideas for storylines and in some cases are engaged as advisors. One of the most successful examples of co-operation between drama producers and a health consumer group was that between *EastEnders* and the National Schizophrenia Fellowship (now Rethink) on the 'Joe Wicks' storyline. This teenage character had schizophrenia, and the charity was heavily involved in the portrayal. The group met the actors and the production team, saw the original storyline and advised on sections of the script. The characterization was widely seen as challenging conventional attitudes towards the condition and received several accolades, including a Mental Health Media award.

Despite attempts to reflect reality, the need to produce effective drama for a large audience necessarily means that storylines are condensed, overplayed or absent (Henderson, 1999). Health consumer groups are often critical about this, and indeed monitor portrayals to evaluate their accuracy and fairness, contacting programme makers when they are dissatisfied. For example, the National Childbirth Trust has criticized programmes for reinforcing negative perceptions of breastfeeding. While most groups accept that drama is primarily about entertainment rather than health education, the fact that drama programmes are seen by large audiences can reinforce inaccurate perceptions and even raise expectations. Specific concerns have been raised about the speed of referral and treatment, as in the case of Peggy Mitchell's breast cancer (*EastEnders*), or the spread or development of the disease as in the case of Alma Halliwell's cervical cancer (*Coronation Street*). Nonetheless, such dramas do seem to have an important impact on public awareness. Following the latter storyline, for example, CancerBACUP experienced an increase in calls to its help-line and the portrayal was held partly responsible for a 21 per cent increase in smear tests in the Greater Manchester area alone (Wright, 2003).

Celebrities

It is a fairly common practice for celebrities to become associated with charities. This has the dual effect of showing celebrities in a favourable light, while generating publicity for charities. However, the De Montfort study found few examples of such links. Celebrities who were identified usually had some connection with the condition and included people from the world of light entertainment such as the late Dame Thora Hird (Stroke Association), Pam Ferris (Carers National Association – now Carers UK), Annette Crosby (National Osteoporosis Society) and Terry Wogan (Arthritis Care).

Celebrity illness can exert a powerful impact on society. It can dramatically raise awareness of a condition, as happened following the death of the actor Rock Hudson from AIDS in the 1980s (Shilts, 1987). It can also challenge existing public beliefs about a disease, as in the case of the Canadian actor Michael J. Fox, who went public with his diagnosis of Parkinson's Disease, demonstrating that the condition was not confined to the elderly (Fox, 2002). Moreover, Fox's story may have encouraged others to acknowledge their condition, build mutual support networks and campaign for better research and care. Similarly the public acknowledgement that former President of the United States of America, the late Ronald Regan, had Alzheimer's Disease was said by one interviewee to have raised the profile of the condition and boosted support for the Alzheimer's Disease Society.

While welcoming publicity, groups were aware that support from celebrities could be double-edged. In particular, they were concerned that celebrity endorsement gave them little control over how the condition and related issues were portrayed. For example, one group noted that when a British comedian announced that he had a serious arthritic condition this actually undermined attempts to inform the public about the condition. Another problem mentioned was that supportive celebrities might not fully understand the issues, and might be unable to give credible responses to inquiries by journalists. In some instances, celebrity messages might mislead or fail to draw out the wider lessons for the public, and for policy. For example, in the case of cancer, it has been argued that celebrity experiences frequently exaggerate the advantages of screening programmes (Hopkins, 2000).

Impact of groups on the media

Many groups believed that they had positively influenced media attitudes. Even those that had experienced difficulty in attracting appropriate media coverage were optimistic about their efforts to influence the media. The respondent from the Stroke Association, for example, believed its press office was successfully challenging negative attitudes about the condition:

> They have helped to change the attitudes of journalists toward stroke. It's no longer a dead end 'shove the mother in the corner and let her die type of thing'. There are things that can be done and so the attitudes are changing and we're pushing at some open doors. There's still problems, there's still attitudes that have to change but the press office is ticking along nicely.

Similarly, some of the mental health groups mentioned success in changing media attitudes, and promoting a more positive view of mental illness. Most groups in this field believed that they worked well with the media and although there remained a tendency to focus on issues such as suicide and homicide by mentally ill people, there was at least a greater willingness to consider other issues and perspectives.

Groups representing elderly people identified examples where they believed they had strongly influenced policy through the media. Age Concern believed that its campaign against the inappropriate use of 'Do Not Resuscitate' orders – which was part of a broader assault on discriminatory practices in the NHS (see Chapter 5 and Gilchrist, 1999) – was a huge success. It was supported by many health care professionals and by other health consumer groups, such as MENCAP. The media picked up the issue and highlighted individual cases where do not resuscitate orders had been allegedly used without consent. The furore led the Department of Health to clarify the requirements for NHS bodies in this area in September 2000. Subsequently, the Royal College of Nursing and the BMA introduced new guidelines on resuscitation which emphasized the need for consultation with patients and relatives.

Likewise, Help the Aged felt that the Dignity on the Ward campaign was effective in getting discrimination against the elderly on the agenda. They believed that it had produced a direct response from government, which set up an inquiry into the care of elderly people in hospital (HAS 2000 Project Team, 1998). Both of the Age Concern and Help the Aged campaigns were also instrumental in promoting policies on minimum standards of care for elderly people and countering age discrimination in the NHS as part of the Older People's national service framework (DoH, 2001b).

A 'some you win, some you lose' philosophy was evident from many of the groups' accounts. Dealing with the media was often described as a struggle, but not without benefits. In general, the groups believed that efforts to influence the media in order to secure coverage for their concerns, and to promote accurate images of the condition, were worthwhile.

Dilemmas of media involvement

Involving users in the media

The media often required actual patients and carers to illustrate and strengthen their particular story. Given the difficulties of identifying individuals and persuading them to appear or allow their experiences to be used, the media needed health consumer groups to act as intermediaries. In one survey of self-help groups, 15 per cent of groups reported the use of patients' stories for articles in the media (Yalphe *et al.*, 2000, p. 178). The De Montfort study also found a willingness among groups at national level to participate in this process. For example, MIND noted that it had 'set up things with users who've had particular experiences and are prepared to provide case histories'. They realized that the media needed access to people with direct experience of conditions, according to Age Concern for example: 'Stories have to have human content if they are going to sell. Without case studies they won't work. If we don't have someone to illustrate the story, the story will die.'

In some cases journalists were clear about the type of person they wished to include. The British Cardiac Patients Association observed 'radio and television will both ring the office, and say we are following up on "x", can you supply us with patients for programmes?' On one occasion they were asked to provide four females between the age of 55 and 60 who had received a valve replacement. Other groups which helped the media to identify cases included: the Patients Association, Action for Sick Children, and the Twins and Multiple Births Association (TAMBA).

Health consumer groups acknowledged that the selection of patients and carers for such purposes posed a dilemma. Some people, particularly the elderly, were reluctant to be publicly identified as having health problems. On the other hand, other individuals actively sought publicity, and there was a tendency for this identified among some parents of sick children. The danger was that the most vociferous case was not always typical. There was also the problem of reinforcing media stereotypes noted earlier with regard to breast cancer. A further problem was confidentiality. When 'supplying' patients for media purposes, groups usually consulted membership databases, but would not give any details to journalists without first securing the willingness of the individual approached to participate. Even so, groups were concerned that people might not fully understand the intrusive nature of the media and some offered advice or training to support those wishing to get involved.

Compromises and the media agenda

The need to secure publicity meant that groups had to play by the media's rules. Groups tailored their message in such a way that media attention was attracted – by emphasizing the triggers mentioned earlier, or by simplifying the message. In some situations, groups had been reluctant to raise issues because of fears of a hostile or indifferent media response.

Groups were well aware that the media was using them to further its own agenda. Some spoke of the need to control the story. According to TAMBA, 'It is a big battle with the media because they have their own agenda'. Groups also accepted that the media had its own motives: 'The media wouldn't do the stories if they didn't think they were going to get something out of it as well' (gi14).

According to a mental health group, the dangers of being manipulated were real:

> Generally speaking, it's more of a partnership type stuff and what you have to avoid is where they're controlling you. Because you're so desperate to get the coverage, you'll just do whatever they say. (gi23)

Another respondent from a mental health group, when asked if he trusted the media, responded with 'not an inch!' (gi21). An interviewee from a generic patients group observed that 'Journalists have an ability to always misquote or misread information that you supply them' (gi27). Several groups referred to their perception that the media's emphasis on drama and sensationalism could misrepresent situations, and coverage could therefore be counterproductive.

Generally, groups accepted that they had to play the media on their terms. As one mental health group stated 'You can sometimes control the way it's going to come out but rarely to a great degree' (gi23). Others believed that in general terms any publicity was helpful. According to an interviewee from an arthritis group: 'I'm just happy to get a mention at all. Even if they've robbed a bank...I would be quite excited because any mention you get is better than no mention' (gi39). Others disagreed. As a respondent from a maternity group stated: 'I am not one of those people who espouses the view that all [coverage] is good news and a slagging off...is better than not being in the press' (gi35).

Conclusion

This chapter has shown that most health consumer groups had regular contact with the media, and that it represented a major point of contact for most groups. Most saw media contact as an important way of influencing the policy process, as well as raising the profile of the organization, and increasing awareness and understanding of the condition. The media was seen as a powerful means of shaping attitudes and perceptions about conditions, and as having the potential to correct unhelpful misrepresentations and stereotypes. They recognized that the media had its own agenda and ways of working that could actually reinforce negative images of the condition. However, they realized that messages had to be tailored to the media's needs and that there were inevitable compromises to be made as a result.

Groups appreciated the many and varied opportunities to influence the media and acknowledged they could provide several things valued by the media: an authoritative source of information and comment, as well as access to actual patients and carers. There were differences between groups, however. Some claimed they had been hampered by a lack of resources and skills. But although the resource-rich groups certainly had more contact, credible but resource-poor groups were not excluded from the media. Some groups faced greater barriers due to existing stereotypes or because the issues they were concerned about were less attractive but they nonetheless made efforts to counteract these negative images, with some success. Several examples were found where groups had used the media not simply to challenge or change attitudes, but to pressure government into action. In most cases, such groups were acting in concert with others, such as other voluntary associations and professional organizations.

Perhaps the key role of the media in terms of policy is the impact it can have on a groups' standing and credibility within policy debates. Health consumer groups are more often than not portrayed sympathetically. As a result they are likely to be taken seriously by the public, and also by the government, who place great emphasis on judgements about a group's credibility. Of course, media coverage can work the other way too, exposing divisions within or between groups (as has happened in the past in the mental health field). It could also undermine a group by revealing its lack of expertise or its unrepresentativeness. On balance, however, the media were seen as allies of health consumer groups rather than enemies, and added weight to their campaigns to influence public opinion and policy-makers.

12

Conclusion: speaking for patients and carers?

What have we discovered about health consumer groups? In particular, what can we say about their activities and role in the health policy process? This concluding chapter reflects on the findings of the De Montfort study in the light of questions raised in Chapter 1. It also identifies areas where further research might be undertaken.

Health consumer groups: diversity and commonality

Diversity

The research showed that health consumer groups are extremely diverse, a common finding in research on voluntary sector organizations. Some focused on a particular condition area, others were concerned with a range of services for a population, and other had a different focus arising from their status as formal alliances.

In terms of their primary activity, some groups put more stress on mutual support, while others focused more sharply on the policy process and this varied according to the type of group. Formal alliance organizations were more likely than other groups to see their primary activity as influencing policy. Variations were also evident between condition areas. Groups in mental health placed more emphasis on the primary importance of influencing policy than groups in other condition areas.

The size of groups in terms of income, membership and staffing was a major variable. Larger groups could be fully active across a range of activities while smaller groups tended to specialize. Size also affected the internal structure of groups. Many larger groups had local branches and formal systems of representation while smaller groups operated more informally. There were also considerable differences in the political skills and expertise of groups, and in the quality of their political contacts and relationships. Finally, although most groups had been formed since the 1980s, a large minority were set up in the decades following the Second World War and a few dated back to an earlier period. The prevailing values at formation continued to have an influence on purpose and structure. Many groups established in recent years were likely to have been formed by people who had lived with a condition, while groups that emerged in earlier periods tended to be established for philanthropic reasons or to extend the social rights of vulnerable people.

Common characteristics

Despite these differences, the research data showed that health consumer groups share many values, a common discourse, perceptions and ways of working. Groups see issues from the perspective of the patient, user or carer. Most groups in the study were membership organizations and where they were not, those living with an illness or condition were integrated into the organization in some way. Thus, central to health consumer groups is a belief in the importance of the knowledge gained from personal experience, in this instance experience related to some form of pain and loss associated with an illness or condition, whether direct or indirect. This drives the commitment to forms of voluntary association where experience can be shared, identity constructed and collective action determined.

Interview data on group formation showed that empathy, self-interest and altruism had all been motivating factors in recent group formation and that the dominant values across the sector included support for services that are publicly provided, provide equality of access, are user-centred, recognize social rights and do not stigmatize those with particular conditions. As a consequence, all health consumer groups, with varying degrees of emphasis depending on size and resources, carry out a similar range of activities that aim to provide support and influence policy.

In terms of working processes, health consumer groups are constituted through informal networks as well as through more more formal structures. These networks provide channels of communication for the transmission of information and knowledge and are a form of social resource used to provide both mutual support and to determine action. Group leaders place a high value on consultative and participative processes to engage members and participants. Written forms of communication and email are widely used to inform their constituency, while conferences, lobbying events and the media are used to reach a wider audience.

The networks of interconnection within groups help to develop expertise based on their collective experience of a particular condition or illness and this can generate political resources. In a number of chapters of the book it has been demonstrated that the expertise of health consumer groups is valued by other stakeholders and government, about which more will be said below.

As health consumer groups are voluntary associations, they face similar concerns and dilemmas, particularly with regard to funding and raising the resources necessary for survival and development. They had a common interest in the health policies pursued by government, in understanding and influencing the policy process and in how to deal with health professionals, the pharmaceutical industry, research charities and the media. Indeed, across all types of group and condition areas, influencing national policy was regarded by a majority of health consumer groups as an important activity.

A contribution to social capital?

Four potential external benefits may be derived from health consumer group activity. First, information on particular conditions is provided for a wider public, not just members. For example, virtually all health consumer groups ran help-lines, produced leaflets and many had websites which were accessible to non-members. Second the specific activities of health consumer groups may generate policy developments and improvements in service provision for people affected by a condition or illness, again not just members. Third, as political actors, their contribution to the policy process may lead policy makers to become more sensitive to the needs and preferences of users and carers generally. Fourth, their expertise in patient and public involvement may facilitate the development of mechanisms through which views of users and carers are incorporated in decision–making processes at all levels of the health care system.

This links with the wider debate on social capital, as noted in Chapter 5. Indeed the research findings support the view that health consumer groups are characterized by trust relationships. Trust is based on a shared experience of dealing with a particular condition and a related commitment to social and political action. This action makes a positive contribution to civil society through the democratic process as well as providing benefits for members and for the wider public in terms of improved services and information. Although there is some evidence that health consumer groups have contributed to social capital in this way, such groups cannot necessarily bridge existing social divisions within society. More research is needed on socio-demographic characteristics of health consumer groups, the relationship between leaders and rank and file members, the links between local and national groups, and on activities and institutions that encourage the bridging of social divisions.

A health consumer movement?

The broad characteristics of new social movements have been described in Chapter 1. New social movements develop from shifts in values and perceptions in the personal world of everyday life and are sustained through new forms of discourse, informal interaction and loose forms of association. Collective action develops through informal channels and may take a variety of forms. We suggest that over the past decade a health consumer movement has emerged. There is evidence of a shared discourse, shared values and perceptions; there are networks of interaction and collaboration.

Evidence to support the existence of a health consumer movement can be found in a particular language and discourse adopted by health consumer groups. For example, the category of 'the mentally ill' has long been replaced by terms such as 'people with mental health problems' or 'survivors' of a mental illness or 'people living with a mental illness'. As a consequence of the cumulative experience and research carried out by cancer groups the term 'the cancer journey' has been used to reflect not only perspective of the person who is faced with a particular diagnosis but the notion that a process is involved and that needs will change over time. Indeed, the process itself will follow a particular pattern which can to some extent be prepared for. The illness journey, and the knowledge of the processes involved, have been developed with varying degrees of explicitness for different conditions. Another term that is now widely used and reflects a shift in thinking is 'the expert patient': that is, someone with a knowledge based on experience which can include both clinical and lay knowledge. The idea of an expert patient suggests a partnership relationship with health professionals.

Shared values and perceptions

The shared perspectives and values of health consumer groups explains the extensive social networks and formal and informal alliances between them. In Chapters 2 and 6, a number of examples are given of the collaboration that has developed over the past decade between health consumer groups. It could be argued that this joint action would not have been possible without a shared set of assumptions and perceptions about what form of collective action should be taken across the sector. Although government has on occasion encouraged alliances and joint-working, it has not been directed from above but has grown out of interconnections between groups.

Collaboration within and across condition areas

In the 1960s and 1970s, a number of groups within the maternity and childbirth field were formed to develop a more woman-centred approach to birth. A sense of their own identity developed in terms of a struggle against medically-dominated and hospital-based forms of delivery. Many mental health groups adopted a similar stance in seeing themselves as speaking for those living with a mental illness, while mental health users themselves and their carers increasingly wished to articulate their own needs and priorities. Members of groups were united by a particular sense of identity and, in their case, a struggle against a medical model and the existing assumptions of service providers. Similar forces shaped the internal organization of arthritis groups in the late 1980s and the 1990s. Larger groups reorganized to represent more directly the views of people with arthritis and a number of new groups formed with a focus on particular illnesses. A shared perception of the needs of carers also drove the formation and amalgamation of carers' groups in the late 1980s.

In all these cases, people living with a particular condition saw their interests as marginal to mainstream concerns and took action either to change the form of existing groups or to form new ones, to forge a common identity and determine a programme of action. This movement has more recently driven the formation of a number of cancer groups and groups for people who have various types of long-term illness.

The identification and transmission of a shared discourse and shared interests has both encouraged and facilitated the extensive collaboration between groups within the same condition area and, more recently, across different groups. As Chapters 2 and 6 show, in the late 1980s, there was collaboration between carers' groups, and in the late 1980s and early 1990s a well-documented collaboration between maternity and childbirth groups. The establishment of both formal and informal alliances during the 1990s is also evidence of the identification of common interests. During the research, and referred to in Chapter 10, a number of mental health groups also developed a common political agenda, in opposition to the second Blair government's plans to change legislation relating to compulsory care. However, collaboration has been greater within some condition areas than others. Where groups had a clear policy objective that was against mainstream views, they were more likely to collaborate either to get an issue on the government agenda or to bring about a change in public perceptions. Cancer groups remain more fragmented than other condition areas. Paradoxically, this may be because they enjoy priority status and have not had to collaborate in order to survive.

Evidence of networking and various forms of alliance, some also involving the wider consumer sector, has been evident from the mid-1990s. While each condition area pursued its interests within a narrower policy arena, they were also part of a wider network of larger population groups such as Age Concern, specialist groups such as the College of Health and general consumer groups such as the National Consumer Council and the Consumers' Association. It is also worth pointing out that a number of those interviewed in the research used the term 'health consumer sector' to refer not only to voluntary groups concerned with aspects of health and illness but also to general and quasi-statutory consumer groups. Membership of the health consumer constituency was defined by values, a commitment to reflecting the perspective of the health care user rather than by formal organizational characteristics.

An aspect of new social movements in health that we did not set out to investigate, but emerged from the data, related to issues of gender, class and ethnicity. The women's movement was one of the early social movements and voluntary activity has also been associated with gender. The influence of the women's movement was strongly reflected in organized action in relation to maternity and childbirth, cancer and carers' issues. But gender may have had a broader impact. Women have secured leadership positions in many health consumer groups. Notably, most of the health consumer group interviewees in the De Montfort study were women (see Chapter 5). Further research is required to examine the activities of women in leadership roles in the voluntary sector more generally.

It has also been argued in the literature that new social movements, as opposed to old social movements that grew out of conflicts between capital and labour, find support from an educated middle class (Gouldner, 1979; Rootes, 1995). A professional background, a previous history of activism, as well as negative experiences related to the diagnosis and treatment of a disease were common characteristics of those who had established groups. There was also evidence among those we interviewed of mobility of those in leadership positions within the voluntary sector and between the voluntary sector and the civil service. Of course, it is only a minority of people that join groups anyway, and people do not mobilize around all conditions in the same way. Indeed, the barriers to participation vary across different condition areas. People may be aware of a group but they may not wish to join, either because they are too ill or because they may not want to associate with people who are at an advanced stage of the illness (Small and Rhodes, 2000). There appears to be under-representation of ethnic minorities, both within groups and across the sector as a whole. Because health consumer groups claim to be inclusive, and wish to be seen as representative, many make considerable efforts to involve ethnic minority groups without obvious success at the national level, although at the local level the picture is more positive.

Strategy and tactics

While the increase in health consumer groups, both in terms of the numbers of recently formed groups and the growth of alliances, coupled with the acknowledgement of their expertise and values, suggests a new social movement, it could not be said to be 'radical' in terms of strategy and tactics. Although the dominance of professional paternalism may be challenged by some groups and new patterns of service espoused by others, health consumer groups have tended to work closely with NHS providers and to respond constructively to overtures from government and professional associations to contribute to policy initiatives. In other words, the movement has been facilitated by state and professional sponsorship. In relation to the latter, most groups in the De Montfort study worked closely with the medical profession. The cancer, heart and circulatory disease groups largely work within the dominant medical paradigm. However, more research needs to be undertaken into these relationships. It is not self-evident that a group formed with support from a health professional, or groups with substantial numbers of professional members or associates, will necessarily be dominated by them. As Epstein (1996) has observed, knowledge, diagnoses and treatment options are all areas for negotiation.

The literature on new social movements suggests that when more conventional political channels of influence are closed, the media may play a crucial role in highlighting issues (Philo, 1996; Jennings, 1999). In the UK, the media has been generally supportive of health consumer groups. Indeed the main targets for critical analysis have been governments or powerful interests such as medicine or the pharmaceutical industry. Yet, as argued in

Chapter 11, not all coverage has supported the views for which a particular group may wish to gain support. Tabloid newspapers in particular may reinforce negative public opinion on some issues, notably in mental health. Most health consumer groups pay close attention to media relations. However, it is evident that most pursue strategies through conventional political channels, through government institutions and parliament, and by building relationships with professional organizations. Even when mobilizing grassroots members to pressure decision-makers, these efforts focused on conventional methods such as contacting MPs, letter writing and petitions. There was hardly any evidence of the type of direct action activities sometimes associated with new social movements.

Further research is needed on the recent history of health consumer groups to support and develop these arguments. The De Montfort research drew on a particular selection of groups, and data were drawn from group leaders rather than rank and file members. In particular, there is a gap in our knowledge on the internal dynamics of groups, of both the relationship between leaders and rank and file members and whether and how collective identities are constructed.

The role of groups in the policy process

Access to the policy process

As noted in Chapter 1, the role health consumer groups in the policy process can be understood in terms of policy networks. In particular, changes in the composition and operation of policy may be associated with policy outcomes. A general observation, that health policy networks are becoming more open (Moran, 1999; Ham, 2000), is supported by the De Montfort study. It is certainly no longer appropriate to describe health policy networks as closed policy communities that exclude patients, users and carers. Indeed, as already noted, health consumer groups are active participants and have made an impact on policy agendas, decisions and the implementation process.

Greater opportunities for health consumer groups to participate in health policy networks have arisen from changes in the political environment. The democratic deficit in the NHS and the lack of accountability to local communities and to service users has been seen as a policy problem, and so has the role of the state as a monopoly provider. The voluntary sector as a health and social care provider has come into greater prominence and attention has been paid to developing relationships between the sector and central government, as discussed in Chapter 2. The Labour government's desire to claim public support for its reform programme and the recognition of the expertise of patients, users and carers has also provided an extended range of opportunities for participation.

Chapter 9 showed that government now consults widely with health consumer groups and representatives of groups are now included on various policy-making fora as a matter of course. However, groups did not simply benefit from a fortuitous change of circumstances. They were proactive in setting new agendas and redefining policy problems and both these strategies enhanced their position within the policy process. First, they are now seen as legitimate representatives of patients, users and carers' interests. Second, there has been a shift in what government has seen as policy problems and priorities, reflected in the setting of national service standards and guidelines for good practice and the 'modernisation' of the NHS with a 'patient-centred' focus.

The extension of political opportunities

These processes require both professional and user expertise to provide a balanced perspective. This acknowledgement of the expertise of health consumer groups and their position in representing a constituency may have political advantages for government in bringing in different voices and interests to counter those of professionals and the drugs industry. Indeed, the De Montfort study found that health consumer groups have been incorporated into institutional structures. Incorporation means that groups have been included within the decision-making process – but they are also bound to some extent by this involvement. This was evident in the Patient Partnership Strategy of the 1990s and in the efforts of the Blair government to increase the proportion of patients, user and carer representatives on official bodies. Meanwhile, as discussed in Chapter 7, some professional associations

began to collaborate with user and carer groups following the 1990
health reforms. Subsequently, the medical establishment has sought
assistance from groups representing patients in achieving radical
changes in systems of self-regulation – a process forced upon
them in the wake of repeated examples of poor medical practice,
rising medical negligence claims and new systems for clinical
governance. As the later chapters of this book show, health
consumer groups are represented on a range of bodies alongside
professionals, and professional associations themselves gain legitimacy by being seen to be working in partnership with groups
representing patients, users and carers.

As discussed in Chapter 1, Baumgartner and Jones (1993)
explain the incorporation of new groups into decision-making
structures in terms of their ability to suggest solutions to new
problems or address old problems in new ways and thus challenge current institutional structures that exclude them. However,
although the existing 'policy monopoly' (in Baumgartner and
Jones' terminology) has been challenged, it has not been broken.
The dominant interests in health care, such as the medical profession
and the drugs industry, remain powerful. Nevertheless, from the
perspective of health consumer groups, they are now engaged as
policy actors alongside these interests.

During the 1990s, health consumer groups built up a network
of influential contacts in Whitehall and parliament. They were
assisted by what Kingdon (1995) calls policy entrepreneurs, people
able to take advantage of the 'windows of opportunity' that occur
in political agenda setting. Where such opportunities are available,
such policy entrepreneurs are able to push forward particular
ways of addressing policy problems. He also argues that policy
entrepreneurs have been particularly successful when they can
claim a particular expertise and speak for a wider constituency,
have good political contacts or negotiating skills and are persistent in
pursuit of a cause. Some individuals associated with the health
consumer world meet these criteria and have been widely
acknowledged as making a particular contribution, such as
Baroness Cumberlege in relation to maternity care, Baroness
Pitkeathley with respect to carers and Baroness Jay, who as health
minister supported the cause of those living with HIV/AIDS
and cancer. However, there are many people who have founded
groups, set up and pushed forward alliances, whose contribution

is acknowledged within the health consumer community but who are less well known outside it.

In short, both high-profile individuals associated with health consumer groups, leaders of groups and activists have seized political opportunities for greater involvement in the policy process and shown persistence in pushing for a greater acknowledgment of the perspectives of patients, users and carers. These two forces of 'pull and push' have led to greater opportunities for participation in the policy process. The extent to which these have been taken, however, depends on the group, and on the specific options available. The priority accorded by government to an issue is important in creating an opportunity and this enhances the ease of access to policy-makers. However, as Chapter 9 showed, expertise, the ability to speak for a constituency and to provide evidence to support arguments were factors that increased the likelihood of influencing the policy outcome. Given the importance of research and evidence, larger and better-resourced groups with a large membership were likely to wield greater influence, although in the current political environment access was relatively open. Indeed, civil servants argued that size of the constituency was less important than being able to draw on experience about a particular condition.

Insider/outsider status: are some more equal than others?

In the pressure group literature, as noted in Chapter 1, considerable emphasis has been placed on the closeness of a group's political contacts with government. Insider status, where groups are regularly consulted on policy is regarded as enhancing influence. However, the De Montfort study found that Whitehall was relatively accessible to groups. However, there did seem to be a clear difference between peripheral and core insiders (Maloney, Jordan and McLaughlin, 1994), with only a few health consumer groups achieving this latter status.

It is perhaps the 'quality of access', rather than simply making contact with government, that is important in gaining influence over policy. As noted in Chapter 9, quality of access was variable, it appears to depend on factors such as informal contacts, expertise and skill in the political process, and knowledge of the 'rules of the game'. The resources of a group are also important because they enable the group to improve access, for example undertaking internal consultations and research, and by employing specialist policy staff.

The status of a group can be enhanced by its activities. It may earn insider status through recognition of its expertise or by playing by Whitehall rules. But the attainment of insider status can be a double-edged sword. It may align a group with unpopular policies or may enable government to manipulate the group more effectively to its own ends. As we saw, some groups did not want to be tainted by such close proximity to government and preferred to be outsiders. In some cases they continued to work with other groups that had a closer relationship with ministers and civil servants, leaving the option for using confrontational tactics open.

Health consumer groups have a difficult dilemma. They may wish to access government in order to exert influence over policy, but, given their limited political resources, they can be manipulated. On the other hand, an outsider strategy leading to abstention from contact with government, rarely pays off – though strong media and parliamentary support can help shape the wider political agenda. Perhaps it is understandable that many groups adopt what Whiteley and Winyard (1987) called an open strategy. They seek an effective working relationship with government while building support in parliament and in the media. In terms of self-reported influence, groups that adopted an open strategy were more effective than those that focused their efforts wholly on government. An open strategy may also be more effective where groups are challenging a well-entrenched policy monopoly, such as medicine, and need to build support in alternative policy arenas (Baumgartner and Jones, 1993).

The evidence so far suggests that the health consumer interest has been incorporated within national level decision-making structures. However, does this necessarily mean that the health consumer interest has overcome the institutional biases that protect dominant interests? (Salter, 2003). More specifically, has an important shift taken place in the balance of power between patients, users and carers on the one hand and professionals, in particular the medical profession, on the other?

As discussed in Chapter 1, Alford's analysis of structural interests placed the community interest in a weak position in the system of health care politics, in particular with regard to the dominant medical profession. Representatives of the repressed community interest faced institutional bias and could only exert influence by mobilizing extraordinary political resources. The De Montfort study, however, found that health consumer groups are actively involved in the policy process, exerted some influence over policy, shared a set of assumptions and were capable of mounting an organized campaign. As noted, there is evidence to suggest that they were regarded by government and by other participants as important policy actors, and were increasingly incorporated within policy-making institutions. Moreover as noted, there was also evidence of strong partnerships between professionals and groups, especially in maternity with the longstanding links between the Royal College of Midwives and maternity groups, and between cancer specialists and the cancer groups. It appears that in these and other fields, groups and professionals have a shared interest in developing guidelines for good practice; in raising awareness and moving issues into mainstream policy agendas and in increasing the flow of resources to condition areas that concern them.

The research showed that although most groups had a firmer foothold in the policy process than a decade ago, there is variation between them. Two important factors affecting incorporation are, first, whether a particular issue was high on the government policy agenda or not and, second, the size and resources of a particular health consumer group. However, participation in the policy process also carries costs. There are costs in terms of time and resources and of opportunities for member activities foregone. Larger groups, with more extensive resources, particularly where a specific and targeted contribution could be made to a current policy issue, found that they were pushing on an open door and their contribution was sought and valued by civil servants and ministers. For example, the cancer and mental health groups were well represented in drawing up policy frameworks. Where issues were not currently on the agenda, such as maternity issues, groups had to employ alternative strategies to obtain access to decision-makers.

In terms of impact, several examples of where groups had an impact on the policy process have been referred to in the later chapters of the book. For example, the Dignity on the Ward campaign clearly influenced the political agenda. Health consumer groups also successfully pressed for the introduction of the *Expert Patients Programme*, and in certain instances both initiated and shaped legislation, as in the case of the Carers and Disabled Children Act 2000. Finally, health consumer groups have also made a contribution to the development of national service frameworks and their implementation.

Despite having gained access to the policy process, when compared to the representation of professional interests health consumer groups still face an institutional bias. The interests of health professionals, and particularly medicine, have been systematically incorporated at various levels in government since the establishment of the NHS. Despite the political will to consult with a wider range of interests and a general suspicion of medical dominance, scientific medicine and its methodologies provide the expertise of first resort and medical interests are powerfully represented in the highest echelons of government. An illustration is the recent creation of the post of national director for patient experience and public involvement, who joins the ranks of a cadre of medical national directors within the Department of Health. From the limited research available to date on policy bodies such as the National Institute for Clinical Excellence and the national service frameworks, clinical scientific paradigms continue to dominate. On the other hand it could be argued that these offer arenas for struggle where new forms of knowledge, or new answers to the issues of the day may eventually gain acceptance.

However, it could be argued that the Alford model is itself flawed. It cannot account for the variation between health consumer groups as representatives of the community interest nor the emergence of political opportunities that favour the health consumer interest. In the context of UK health policy, the later chapters of this book show that some health consumer groups, in relation to selected issues, can call on significant political resources in terms of contacts, networks and influence.

Other dominant interests

It is also pertinent to consider the position of health consumer groups with regard to commercial interests, notably the drugs industry, which has been viewed as a powerful player in the health care system (Hogg, 1999). While health consumer groups were able to co-operate in their relations with government, they were divided in their attitudes to the pharmaceutical industry. Pharmaceutical companies were seen to be concerned with profit and, as corporate entities, too powerful for any relationship to be equal. Many health consumer groups therefore feared that they would be manipulated if they accepted funding and/or did not wish to be associated with a pharmaceutical company. Some accepted funding for specific activities and others sought to codify 'ground rules' for these arrangements, in order to protect themselves against accusations of being manipulated. A number of groups collaborated closely with the industry, though explicit joint working on policy was rare. However, there is certainly room for further research into the precise relationship between the industry and health consumer groups, and the impact they may have on each other.

The representative role of health consumer groups

One fundamental question remains. How justified are health consumer groups' claims to speak for patients, users and carers? As discussed above, groups in the study were shown to be concerned with equality of access to services and the social rights of people within their membership. They drew on the knowledge and expertise of their members in order to represent their interests. How far was this justified in terms of their own systems and structures? It was shown that there were a variety of mechanisms for encouraging participation. What we do not know is how the leadership is seen by grassroots members. Critics of voluntary organizations in general have argued that their formal democratic structures are often poorly developed and even these are vulnerable to elite takeover (Kramer, 1981; Foley and Edwards, 1999). Some of those interviewed in the De Montfort research commented that that the same few people tended to appear as representatives of health consumer groups on official committees. As noted in Chapter 9, the term 'usual suspects' was used pejoratively to refer those who are perceived as an emerging elite. Some groups reported that they had a small active membership, and one commented it was 'punching above' its weight. However, the numbers participating in national level policy fora are relatively small and may reflect the need to build capacity in the sector. Nevertheless, it is incumbent on both government in seeking representatives and health consumer groups in their activities to remain accountable to their constituency. How did health consumer groups measure up in this respect?

Two forms of accountability can be distinguished: formal mechanisms for election to office and annual general meetings, and less formal accountability through consultative and participatory processes. Most health consumer groups had some structure of election and/or systems of reporting to management boards or boards of trustees. Annual general meetings could also have a symbolic function of rallying the membership. However, those interviewed gave much greater importance to downwards accountability to members, clients, local branches or groups through informal networks and interactions through newsletters, conferences and surveys, activities that have been described in Chapter 5. A large majority of group leaders believed that they were responsive to suggestions from the grassroots and saw themselves as facilitators of initiatives coming from below. This may reflect expectations that groups, above all, should be open and transparent rather than depend on formal mechanisms of accountability – a point made by Taylor and Warburton (2003) in their study of local 'third sector' groups. This study also found that government was agnostic about how group representativeness was achieved. The quality of a group's research and expertise was also seen as a key form of legitimacy – both points consistent with our findings.

It is obviously important that all groups are open and accountable to those they claim to represent. Charity law provides some framework of regulation to safeguard donors and to ensure that charities meet standards of financial and managerial probity – though it is acknowledged that there is scope for improvement here. In addition, where groups receive funding for projects they are accountable to the funding bodies.

Does it matter if a group is dominated by a small elite? A group with a small or non-existent membership might be accused of representing 'astroturf', creating the illusion of public support, rather then genuinely representing their constituency (see Chapter 1). It is possible that leaders may misrepresent their membership or that a group may be captured by professional or commercial interests. However, there was little evidence of this from the De Montfort research. At most, a few groups could be said to have been run by a like-minded elite and who adopted a rather paternalistic approach to the membership. Even here there was a strong sense of mission to improve the welfare of these members. There was nothing in our data to suggest that groups were being used as a personal 'hobby horse' or as a means of misrepresenting patients views.

As the role of health consumer groups expands, more formal requirements may be placed upon them to be open, accountable, inclusive and democratic (see Chapter 2). But it is important that these objectives do not undermine the other forms of participation. These are crucial to the social and political resources of the groups and contribute to the political process more generally. If government is serious about producing policies through a form of associative or participatory democracy, as suggested by Hirst (1994), it will have to strengthen the capacity of health consumer groups to make a contribution to policy development, in order to counter the existing institutional biases mentioned above. In particular, health consumer groups must be recognized as full partners in the decision-making process, and must have nominal equality with other participants and in the longer term 'be able to win' on some of their objectives (Schmitter, 2001). Evidence from Chapter 4, on government funding for groups, shows that this was linked and geared to project grants to support the government's agenda. Compared to some other countries such as Holland (Dekkers, 1997), health consumer groups in the UK received only minimal financial support. Groups saw this as a major barrier to participation and the matter needs to be addressed if health consumer groups are to become full partners in the policy process.

Final comments

In conclusion, we would argue that health consumer interests are represented through structures and networks that are beginning to be embedded in the policy process. It is acknowledged that patients, users and carers have valuable perspectives and that policy-makers wish to draw on this. At the same time, research and other methodologies are developing to generalize that experiential knowledge in ways that can challenge clinical knowledge. Meanwhile, new structures of patient and public involvement have been introduced. These represent in one sense a challenge to health consumer groups, as they could displace some of their functions at local and national level. On the other hand, the new structures can be seen as creating further opportunities for involvement in policy processes. What will eventually happen is unclear. However, both statutory bodies and health consumer groups have a key role in enabling patients, users and carers to have a voice, thus promoting a more inclusive and effective model of governance in health care.

Appendix 1: Methodology

The sample

Rather than conduct a survey of all national health consumer groups, the research team decided to focus on five condition areas: arthritis and related conditions; cancer; heart and circulatory disease (focusing upon heart disease and stroke); maternity and childbirth; and mental health. These were chosen in order to cover a range of conditions including life-threatening illness, through chronic conditions and life-changing events. The aim was also to cover a high proportion of morbidity, mortality and health expenditure and include some key government priorities. In drawing up the sample, exclusion criteria were applied as shown below:

Table A1.1 Exclusion criteria by condition area

Arthritis and related conditions	Disability organizations were excluded as these had been covered in other studies.
Cancer	Groups whose primary purpose was to provide palliative care were excluded.
Heart and circulatory disease	Groups dealing overwhelmingly with health promotion issues, such as ASH were excluded.
Maternity and childbirth	This was defined from conception to delivery. Groups dealing with fertility issues abortion and birth control were excluded.
Mental health	Groups dealing primarily with learning disabilities or solely with alcohol and drug addiction were excluded.

A number of umbrella groups and health consumer groups whose interests covered some or all of these condition areas were identified and included in the sample. Inclusion and exclusion criteria were also drawn up to identify other voluntary organizations in the voluntary health sector to be included or excluded, see Table A1.2 overleaf.

All groups serving the whole of the UK were included. However, those serving only Scotland, Northern Ireland, Wales, England/Scotland or England/Northern Ireland were excluded. Groups operating solely at regional or local level were excluded.

Table A1.2   Inclusion and exclusion criteria, questionnaire sample

Inclusion criteria	Exclusion criteria
Groups in the five condition areas	Research charities
Umbrella groups	Professional and occupational associations
Population groups	Organizations representing statutory bodies General consumer organizations Organizations that only provide telephone help-lines Local and/or regional groups General disability groups

Despite having clear inclusion and exclusion criteria, the lack of prior information about many groups meant that decisions about inclusion and exclusion had to be taken after receiving back their questionnaire responses. In some cases, this led to the removal of organizations from the sample (see also below).

Identifying groups

There was no definitive directory that listed all national health consumer groups, so a variety of printed and online sources were used to identify the sample. General sources included the National Council of Voluntary Organizations' *Voluntary Agencies Directory* and the *British Directory of Associations*. Specialist sources were also identified for some of the condition areas. For example, a list of arthritis specialist support groups was provided in *Arthritis News*, Arthritis Care's bi-monthly magazine. The *Midwives Information and Resource Service* had published a directory of support groups in the maternity sector. The membership lists of umbrella groups, the College of Health's database and health related websites often gave contact details of relevant support groups. Of particular importance was the internet site *Patient UK* (http://www.patient.co.uk), which included a directory of support groups. In total 243 health consumer groups were identified that had the potential for inclusion.

Phase 1: the questionnaire

A structured questionnaire with some open questions was drawn up. The questionnaire had four sections. The first section focused on the aims, activities and formation. Section two addressed resources and income. Section three looked at their structure and decision-making processes. The final section addressed involvement in the policy process and asked questions about the type and frequency of involvement; the purpose and frequency of contact with stakeholders and the barriers and facilitators to involvement. Questions were mainly precoded to facilitate data analysis using SPSS[1]. There were some open-ended questions that were later included in the analysis of qualitative data. A coding framework was developed for inputting the data and to allow comparisons to be made between different condition areas and types of groups.

Following a pilot, the questionnaire was sent out in Autumn 1999 to 243 organizations. A number (n=57) were excluded as they were found not to fit the inclusion criteria. The final response rate was 66 per cent (n=123). The response rate by condition area is provided in the table below:

Table A1.3   Questionnaire response rate by condition area

Condition area	Response rate	
	n	(%)
Arthritis and related conditions	18	64
Cancer	19	54
Heart and circulatory disease	13	72
Maternity and childbirth	18	86
Mental health	24	67
Multiple condition groups	31	72
All groups	123	66

Source: Questionnaire data set 1999.

A number of problems were encountered, illustrating the wider problems of researching the voluntary health sector. Contact details were sometimes inaccurate; a few groups no longer existed and groups were so diverse that that some questions were not applicable to all. Despite contacting 85 per cent of groups before sending the questionnaire in order to identify the most appropriate respondent, this information was not always accurate. For example, the receptionist of a maternity/childbirth group identified the librarian as being the member of staff dealing with policy issues – even though it turned out that the organization had a dedicated policy officer. In other cases, the wrong name or job title was provided. There was also a turnover of staff, often between different groups in the same sector. Some groups did not respond due to other priorities such as a fundraising event or a particular campaign. In some large organizations, information was required from several people and took time to complete. In a few very small groups, the key person was in hospital or caring for someone receiving medical treatment and it understandably proved difficult to get a response.

Categorising health consumer groups

A particular feature of the voluntary health sector is its complexity and diversity. Those health consumer groups that remained in the sample could not be described as a homogenous group. They differed in their aims, activities and structures. They included groups that existed to support their members or clients and well as groups that attempted to affect policy through influencing wider audiences, such as the public, professionals, businesses and government. The groups differed in the extent to which they focused on influencing these audiences, and which audiences they chose to serve.

The De Montfort study identified different ways to analyse the groups:

● First the similarities/differences between condition areas i.e. arthritis, cancer, heart/circulatory disease, maternity/childbirth, mental health were considered. Groups whose interests spanned these conditions were called multiple condition groups. The aim was to identify whether different condition areas adopted different structures, strategies or tactics. The working assumption was that the condition area itself could help explain relative success/failure of the groups.

● Second a typology based on the constituency of the groups, that is, who they sought to promote or represent:

  – Condition-based groups: national organizations that sought to promote and or represent the interests of patients, users and carers in relation to specific conditions. Some groups dealt with a specific disease or condition, i.e. cancer or arthritis. Other groups supported patients/users whose experiences related to two or more diseases/conditions, for example, the Kawasaki Syndrome Support Group was found on lists of both arthritis support groups and heart support groups.

  – Population-based groups: national organizations that sought to promote/represent interests of all patients, users and carers, or specific sections of the community (e.g. carers, elderly, children, ethnic people) across any condition.

  – Formal alliance organizations: national organizations whose membership included other autonomous national organizations. Formal alliance organizations were identified within and across condition areas. For example, the Long-term Medical Conditions Alliance brought together groups across numerous condition areas, but the Children's Heart Federation brought together groups within the heart sector. Groups that only brought together local groups were not categorized as formal alliance organizations.

● The third categorization adopted was based on the characteristics of health consumer groups. In their study of the activities of voluntary organizations working in the poverty field, Whiteley and Winyard (1987) identified four key features of the organizations' activities (see Chapter 1). In the analysis of the questionnaire, the research team attempted to identify whether these features were also present in the health consumer groups sector. These features offered clues to the aims, strategies, and procedures of the groups underpinned the deliberations on group influence, as discussed in Chapters 9 to 11.

The assumption was that organizations with different characteristics played different roles and that comparison between these typologies would be possible. Although it should be noted that direct comparisons between a specific 'condition area' and a particular 'type of group' were not valid because of double-counting.

Phase 2: interviews with health consumer groups

Following a small number of exploratory interviews, an interview schedule was developed to explore the internal activities and values of health consumer groups as well as their external relationships, networks and experiences of the policy process in interviews with a stratified sample of health consumer group leaders. These were selected to reflect differences in condition area, constituency, age, size of membership, and characteristics as defined by Whiteley and Winyard. Representatives from 39 health consumer groups were interviewed. Each interview was given a code number, which is used in the text to reference anonymous quotes. The prefix 'gi' denotes an interview with a health consumer group respondent, while 'si' refers to an interview with a stakeholder respondent (government, research charity, drugs industry representative, Member of Parliament, and so on). The interviews lasted between 45 and 90 minutes. In some instances more than one representative of the organization was present, and in the case of four groups more than one interview took place. The majority of the interviews were taped and transcribed. In the remainder, notes were taken and written up. To develop a grounded theory, the data were entered in NVIVO, a qualitative data analysis software package. An initial coding framework was developed to categorize the data according to the internal dynamics of groups and their inter-group and external relations with other health stakeholders. Based on reading and re-reading the data, each researcher developed a framework of themes that drew on theories referred to in Chapter 1. These were agreed by the research team, and a coding framework devised. Each researcher allocated the data using open and axial coding to the various themes. Data were cross-checked for consistency and fit. Each researcher drafted memoranda on specific topics such as the social and political resources of health consumer groups; the role of networks and alliances; the strategies for engagement with stakeholders as well as stakeholders' views of health consumer groups and their contribution to the policy process. Despite the diversity of health consumer groups, the method allowed for generalization and the identification and explanation of negative cases through the use of the constant comparative method (Glaser and Strauss, 1967).

Phase 3: interviews with stakeholders

The aim of the third phase of the research was to assess the ways in which the 'lay interest' was represented in the policy process. It sought stakeholders' views of the advantages and limitations of the 'lay interest' and how they perceived impact on the policy process. 31 interviews were undertaken, lasting from 45 to 90 minutes. In some instances more than one representative of the organization was present. Detailed notes were taken at the interview and written up. Theory-based themes were identified within each category of stakeholder to provide a basis for coding and analysis.

Phase 4: triangulation

Following the production of first drafts of various chapters of the book, six additional interviews were undertaken with people from the political elites in the voluntary health sector and government (including former health ministers) to provide a check on our interpretation of the data.

Advisory group

An advisory group, comprising academics, individuals from health consumer groups and civil servants, provided advice and support to the research project during the course of the study. The group met four times and also provided feedback on research instruments and analysis, when required.

Other activities

Professor Allsop was appointed as a member of the Patients Forum Development Project advisory committee in 1999. In 2001 she was appointed to the advisory panel of the Department of Health-funded scoping study for a national patients' body.

Appendix 2: The Interviews[2]

Individuals from the following organizations were interviewed:

Action for Sick Children
Afiya Trust
Age Concern, England
Arachnoiditis Trust
Arthritis Care
Arthritis Research Campaign
Association for Community Health Councils in England and Wales
Association for Improvements in the Maternity Services
Association of the British Pharmaceutical Industry
British Cardiac Patients Association
British Heart Foundation
British League Against Rheumatism (renamed Arthritis and
    Musculoskeletal Alliance in 2002)
British Medical Association
Cabinet Office
Cancer Black Care
Cancer Research Campaign
CancerBACUP
Cancerlink (merged with Macmillan Cancer Relief in 2001)
Carers National Association (renamed Carers UK in 2001)
Children's Heart Federation
College of Health (closed in 2003)
Consumers' Association
Contact a Family
Department of Health
Family Heart Association (merged with British Hyperlipidaemia
    Association and renamed Heart UK in 2002)
Genetic Interest Group
Group Action into Steroid Prescribing
Help the Aged
HM Treasury
Long-term Medical Conditions Alliance
Macmillan Cancer Relief (merged with Cancerlink in 2001)
Maternity Alliance
Mental After Care Association

Mental Health Foundation
Mental Health Media
MIND (National Association for Mental Health)
National Ankylosing Spondylitis Society
National Association of Patient Participation
National Cancer Alliance
National Childbirth Trust
National Consumer Congress
National Heart Forum
National Schizophrenia Fellowship (renamed Rethink – Severe Mental
    Illness in 2002)
Patients Association
Patients Forum
Richmond Fellowship
Royal College of Midwives
Royal College of Nursing
Royal College of Obstetricians and Gynaecologists
Royal College of Physicians
Royal College of Psychiatrists
Sainsbury Centre for Mental Health
Stillbirth and Neonatal Death Society
Stroke Association
Twins and Multiple Births Association
UK Breast Cancer Coalition (merged with Breakthrough Breast Cancer
    in 2004)
UK Federation of Smaller Mental Health Agencies
Young Minds
Zito Trust

In addition, six MPs and peers were interviewed.

Notes

Introduction

1   ESRC Grant Number R000237888.

Chapter 1

1   The Bristol case involved allegations of poor standards of paediatric heart surgery at the Bristol Royal Infirmary during the 1990s. Parents of children who had died or become disabled following surgery campaigned for an investigation, aided by a member of staff who 'blew the whistle' on his colleagues. Following an inquiry by the GMC, the senior surgeon involved and the chief executive of the Trust (who was also a doctor) were dismissed by the Trust and struck off the medical register. Another surgeon was dismissed and had special conditions imposed on his registration by the GMC. A further inquiry by Professor Sir Ian Kennedy QC led to nearly 200 recommendations on how to create a more patient-centred NHS and avoid such a situation occurring again.
2   Each interview had a specific reference code. Anonymised references in the text use this code to protect confidentiality (see p. 306).

Chapter 2

1   In 2000, the NHSE was reintegrated into the wider Department of Health. The post of Permanent Secretary of the Department of Health and Chief Executive of the NHS were also combined.
2   The Commission for Health Improvement has been given additional functions and powers and is now known as the Healthcare Commission an abbreviation of the Commission for Healthcare Audit and Inspection.
3   Community Health Councils survived in Wales.
4   Clause 20 (c) of the 2002 Act.
5   In 2003 it was announced that the Department of Health was to be restructured again, with a smaller number of directorates. As the

book went to press, the government proposed the abolition of the CPPIH but additional support for patients' forums.

Chapter 3

1 see Arthritis Research Campaign website: http://www.arc.org.uk.
2 In the *National Service Framework for Older People* it is stated that arthritis will be addressed in the next review.
3 In April 2003 the Confidential Enquiry into Stillbirths and Deaths in Infancy merged with the Confidential Enquiry into Maternal Deaths to form the Confidential Enquiry into Maternal and Child Health, which has a wider brief, including children up to age 16.
4 Cutting the perineum to increase the size of the vaginal opening in childbirth.
5 The National Perinatal Epidemiology Unit was set up in 1978 by the Department of Health and is based in Oxford.
6 The alliance agreed on three principles: a woman's need for continuity in care; a woman's right to have choice over the type of care and the place of birth, and a woman's right to control her own body at all stages of pregnancy and childbirth.
7 The Expert Maternity Group was chaired by Baroness Cumberlege. It took evidence from 62 groups, visited 13 centres, used other Department of Health research and commissioned a MORI survey which contacted 1005 women.
8 The Department of Health has also appointed national clinical directors for: Clinical Governance (1999), Older People's Services (2000), Children's Services (2001) and Primary Care (2001).

Chapter 4

1 The interview sample showed similar trends, suggesting that the groups interviewed were broadly representative of the full data set on most criteria (see Table 4.2). However, there was a small over-representation of condition-based groups with higher incomes and greater longevity in the interview sample. This was not intentional (see Appendix 1). However, as established and larger groups they were likely to play a more active role in the policy process and could provide more information on the interaction with government – the purpose of the study.
2 Since the study, at least two new national health consumer groups were formed in the arthritis (National Rheumatoid Arthritis Society) and heart and circulatory disease sector (Blood Pressure Association),

two interview groups merged with other organizations and one ceased to operate.

3   The Feversham Committee (1936–39) on voluntary mental health associations recommended that the Central Association for Mental Welfare (1913), the National Council for Mental Hygiene (1922) and the Child Guidance Council (1927) amalgamate (MIND, 1996).

4   The UK Breast Cancer Coalition was founded by four women with experience of breast cancer. It brings together national, regional and local charities, trade unions and individuals to campaign on breast cancer issues. For the purposes of the De Montfort study it was classified as a formal alliance organization.

5   In the arthritis area, the National Ankylosing Spondylitis Society was said in interview to have been 'kick started by a doctor' at the Royal National Hospital for Rheumatic Diseases in Bath.

6   'Services' refers to services for members or clients. 'Policy' to raising awareness as well as influencing local or national policy.

7   A Charities' Bill was included in the 2003 Queen's Speech. The proposed legislation is likely to provide a new legal definition of charity, based on 'public benefit' and require larger charities to provide more detail on finances and effectiveness (Shifrin, 2003).

8   In 2002, the Department of Health established a Section 64 Review Group to assess the efficiency and effectiveness of the scheme, the Group reported in September 2003, making 31 recommendations, including a two-stage application process and more detailed rejection letters.

9   Charities are unable to reclaim value-added-tax on their non-business activities. It is estimated that charities pay out £400m in irrecoverable value-added-tax each year (Benjamin, 2003).

Chapter 5

1   See also MIND's mission statement – see www.mind.org.uk/About + Mind/Mind + Mission/.

2   The Database of Individual Patient Experience (DIPEx) provides narrative accounts of personal experience of major illness and medical conditions to patients, their friends, family and carers, and the medical profession. More details on the DIPEx charity can be found at www.dipex.org.

3   An automated external defibrillator is a small piece of equipment which can administer an electric shock to a heart to restore normal rhythm following a cardiac arrest. In July 1999, the government announced a national defibrillator programme to install automatic

external defibrillators in public places such as shopping centres and railway stations.

4 This included fundraising, organizing and running events, and committee work.

5 Of the 39 groups we interviewed, 25 were represented by women, 11 by men and 3 by both women and men.

6 Yule (2000) refers to women in local government, but the point also applies to other spheres.

7 Gilligan (1982) has argued that women have a distinctive form of moral reasoning that focuses on the 'ethic of care' whereas men are more closely associated with the 'ethic of justice' that stresses formal rules and abstract rights.

Chapter 6

1 In 1999 the government provided funding for the Patients Forum to develop its role as the primary umbrella group in the health consumer group sector. Government had also worked through the Patients Forum to co-ordinate discussions around new proposals for patient and public involvement in the NHS, developments discussed in Chapter 2. The growth in membership suggests that the development project was succeeding, but could also indicate that health consumer groups are positioning themselves in order to develop closer links with policy-makers.

Chapter 7

1 Three interviews were with doctors representing the Royal Colleges. Their role is to supervise postgraduate specialist education and subsequent specialist practice, so they share some regulatory tasks with the General Medical Council. A fourth interview was with a senior officer from the British Medical Association. Two interviews were undertaken with the Royal College of Nursing, one with the Royal College of Midwives and one with a senior nurse within the Department of Health.

2 The Royal College of General Practitioners was the first Royal College to establish a patient's liaison group in 1983.

3 There are major problems of definition but the 'lay interest' is here defined as non-health professional interests (see Davies, 2001).

Chapter 8

1 The scope of the research was limited to collecting data on the groups in the sample and their relationship with the pharmaceutical industry, not the medical technology industry as a whole except where the interview groups referred to this. Furthermore, due to limitations on time, interview data was limited to the trade association of the industry, the ABPI which has developed a code of practice for relationships with patients (ABPI, 2001) and secondary data from other sources.

2 A maximum price scheme to protect the NHS from significant increases in the price of generic medicines was introduced in August 2000. Prior to this, the NHS has relied on competition in the market to regulate prices. The scheme has been periodically reviewed, with new arrangements due to be implemented in 2004.

3 In early 2004, the ABPI published a briefing paper on industry support and patient groups. The briefing paper (ABPI, 2004) made it clear that the ABPI Code of Practice covering relationships with the general public, by definition covered relationships with patient groups.

Chapter 9

1 According to *The Guardian* (2000), the prime minister's special advisor on health has taken an interest in mental health, and has been instrumental in the introduction of policy initiatives such as *NHS Direct* and walk-in centres.

2 Since the research was undertaken, the Department of Health has reviewed its relationships with user and carer organizations (see p. 46).

3 NICE has encouraged groups to submit such data and has produced guidance and documentation to assist groups.

4 Although highly regarded, in 2003 the College of Health closed due to financial instability (Gould, 2003, p. 4).

5 One stakeholder interviewee commented that the British Cardiac Patients Association's rise had been 'meteoric' (si9).

Chapter 10

1 See, for example, the debate on the second reading of the Carers and Disabled Children's Bill 2000 (Hansard, 2000).

2 By 2003 this had grown to a total of 266 groups: 40 health-related and 30 focused on specific conditions.

3 Every year backbench MPs get the opportunity to introduce their own legislation in the form of a private member's bill. MPs enter a ballot to decide who gets priority for introducing a private member's bill. Often successful MPs are approached by government and interest groups to introduce a particular measure on their behalf. The time for consideration of such measures is limited. Moreover, government can easily veto bills by refusing to give them parliamentary time or ultimately introducing a 'whip' in order to defeat the bill.

4 See: DoH (1995b) *New Guidelines for Professionals on Pregnancy Loss and the Death of a Baby*, 95/508, 2 November (London, DoH).

Chapter 11

1 Dignity on the Ward articles:

Bright, M. (1997) 'She was dying for a cuppa, literally', *The Observer*, 28 September, 26.

Durham, M. and Bright, M. (1997) 'Join our campaign for the old', *The Observer*, 5 October, 2.

Bright, M. (1997) 'Observer Campaign Dignity on the Ward Week Three: Readers respond with a flood of mail relating to their experiences, support grows across Britain', *The Observer*, 12 October, 18.

Bright, M. (1997) 'Dignity on the Ward Charity calls for an abuse inquiry. Help the Aged backs *Observer* funding a damning report on neglect', *The Observer*, 26 October, 18.

Bright, M. (1997) 'Dobson to act after *Observer* campaign', *The Observer*, 2 November, 1.

Bright, M. (1998) 'Dignity on the Ward: My Gran didn't suffer in vain', *The Observer*, 2 November, 6.

2 The series was called 'The forgotten illness':

Wallace, M. (1985) 'Spectrum: Well freedom is a life sentence', *The Times*, 16 December, 10.

Wallace, M. (1985) 'Spectrum: A patients cry – can nobody help', *The Times*, 18 December, 8.

Wallace, M. (1985) 'Counting the cost of a daughter's death: the forgotten illness schizophrenia', *The Times*, 23 December, 3.

Appendixes

1 There may be slight differences in the statistics presented here compared with those presented in earlier publications by members of the research team. These minor differences have occurred as a result of rounding and, in a few cases, following further analysis of the data.
2 The research team agreed not to reveal the name of the individuals interviewed.

References

ABPI (2001) *Code of Practice for the Pharmaceutical Industry together with the Prescription Medicines Code of Practice Authority Constitution and Procedure* (London, Association of the British Pharmaceutical Industry).

ABPI (2002) *Facts and Statistics from the Pharmaceutical Industry* [www] Available from: http://abpi.org.uk/statistics/intro.asp (Accessed 17 October 2002).

ABPI (2004) *Patient Groups, Industry Support and Medicines* (London, Association of the British Pharmaceutical Industry).

Active Community Unit (2000a) *Compact: Getting It Right Together: Funding, A Code of Good Practice* (London, Home Office).

Active Community Unit (2000b) *Compact: Getting It Right Together: Consultation and Policy Appraisal, A Code of Good Practice* (London, Home Office).

Active Community Unit (2001a) *Compact: Getting It Right Together: Black and Minority Ethnic Voluntary and Community Organizations, A Code of Good Practice* (London, Home Office).

Active Community Unit (2001b) *Compact: Getting It Right Together: Volunteering a Good Practice Guide* (London, Home Office).

Administration Committee (1995) (HC 494) *1st Report 1995/96: All-party and Parliamentary Groups* (London, HMSO).

Adonis, A. (1990) *Parliament Today* (Manchester, Manchester University Press).

AIMS and NCT (1997) *A Charter for Ethical Research in Maternity Care* (London, AIMS and NCT).

Alford, R. (1975) *Health Care Politics* (Chicago, IL, University of Chicago Press).

Allen, I., Bourke-Dowling, S. and Williams, S. (1997) *A Leading Role for Midwives? Evaluation of Midwifery Group Practice Development Projects* (London, Policy Studies Institute).

Allsop, J. and Mulcahy, L. (2001) 'Dealing with clinical complaints', in Vincent, C. (ed.), *Clinical Risk Management: Enhancing Patient Safety*, 2nd edition (London, BMA Books).

Allsop, J. and Saks, M. (2002) 'Introduction', in Allsop, J. and Saks, M. (eds) *Regulating the Health Professions* (London, Sage).

Allsop, J. and Taket, A. (2003) 'Evaluating user involvement in primary care', *International Journal of Healthcare Technology and Management*, 5, 34–44.

Allsop, J., Jones, K., Meerabeau, L., Mulcahy, L. and Price, D. (2004) *Regulation of the Health Professions: A Scoping Exercise Carried Out on Behalf of CRHP (February 2004)* (London, CRHP).

Almond, G.A. and Verba, S. (1989) *The Civic Culture: Political Attitudes and Democracy in Five Nations* (Newbury Park, CA, Sage).

Anderson, W., Florin, D., Gillan, S. and Montford, L. (2002) *Every Voice Counts: Primary Care Organisations and Public Involvement* (London, King's Fund).

Anheier, H.K. and Kendall, J. (2002) 'Interpersonal trust and voluntary association: examining three approaches', *British Journal of Sociology*, **53**(3), 343–62.

Anheier, H.K. and Romo, F.P. (1992) *The Philanthropic Tradition*, Paper presented at the 1992 convention of the American Sociological Association, Pittsburgh.

Appleby, J. and Coote, A. (eds) (2002) *Five-year Health Check: A Review of Government Health Policy 1997–2002* (London, King's Fund).

Ashcroft, J. (1999) *Arthritis: Getting It Right* (London, Arthritis Care).

Audit Commission (1997) *First Class Delivery: Improving Maternity Services in England and Wales* (London, Audit Commission).

Audit Commission (2000) *Forget Me Not: Mental Health Services for Older People.* (London, Audit Commission).

Baggott, R. (1995) *Pressure Groups Today* (Manchester, Manchester University Press).

Baldwin, M. (1990) 'The House of Lords', in Rush, M. (ed.), *Parliament and Pressure Politics* (Oxford, Clarendon).

Barber, B. (1984) *Strong Democracy: Participatory Politics for a New Age* (Berkeley, CA, University of California Press).

Barlow, J., Turner, A. and Wright, C. (1998) 'Long term outcomes of an arthritis self-management programme', *British Journal of Rheumatology*, **37**, 1315–19.

Barnes, M. and Bowl, R. (2001) *Mental Health and Empowerment* (London, Palgrave).

Barnes, M., Harrison, S., Mort, M., Shardlow, P. and Wistow, G. (1999) 'The new management of community care: User groups, citizenship and co-production', in Stoker, G. (ed.) *The New Management of British Local Governance* (London, Macmillan).

Bastian, H. (1998) 'Speaking up for ourselves', *International Journal of Technological Assessment in Health Care*, **14**(1), 3–23.

Baumgartner, F. and Jones, B. (1993) *Agendas and Instability in American Politics* (Chicago, IL, University of Chicago Press).

Beckett, M. and Brown, G. (1994) *The National Health 'Secret Service': What the Tories are Hiding about the NHS* (London, Labour Party).

Beech, B. (1991) *Who's Having Your Baby? A Health Rights Handbook for Maternity Care* (London, Bedford Square Press).

Benjamin, A. (2003) 'Charities spurn call to "move on"', *Guardian, Society Pages*, 16 July, 4.

Beresford, P. and Holden, C. (2000) 'We have choices: globalisation and welfare user movements', *Disability & Society*, **15**(7), 973–89.

Billis, D. (1993) 'Sector blurring and nonprofit centres: the case of the UK', *Nonprofit and Voluntary Sector Quarterly*, **22**(3), 241–57.

Billis, D. and Glennerster, H. (1998) 'Human services and the voluntary sector: towards a theory of comparative advantage', *Journal of Social Policy*, 27(1), 79–98.

Blood Pressure Association (2003) *Funders* [www] Available from: http://www.bpassoc.org.uk/about_theBPA/funders.htm (Accessed 7 July 2003).

Borkman, T. (1999) *Understanding Self-help/Mutual Aid: Experiential Learning in the Commons* (New Brunswick, NJ, Rutgers University Press).

Boseley, S. (1996) 'The shame I felt in chains – I just wanted to die', *Guardian*, 11 January, 1.

Boseley, S. (2000) 'On patient power', *Guardian*, G2, 19 September, 9.

Boseley, S. (2002) 'Psychiatrists to join protest over bill: Mental health groups plan to march on Whitehall over planned detentions', *Guardian*, 29 July, 6.

Bourdieu, P. (1991) *Language and Symbolic Power* (Introduction by John B.Thompson) (Cambridge, Polity Press).

Bourdieu, P. and Passeron, J.-C. (1977) *Reproduction: In Education, Society and Culture* (London, Sage).

Bower, H. and Boseley, S. (1999) 'A culture that kills', *Guardian*, 16 March, 15.

Bright, M. (1997) 'She was dying for a cuppa, literally', *Observer*, 28 September, 26.

Bright, M. (1997) '*Observer* Campaign Dignity on the Ward, Week Three: Readers respond with a flood of mail relating to their experiences, support grows across Britain', *Observer*, 12 October, 18.

Bright, M. (1997) 'Dignity on the Ward: Charity calls for an abuse inquiry. Help the Aged backs *Observer*, funding a damning report on neglect', *Observer*, 26 October, 18.

Bright, M. (1997) 'Dobson to act after *Observer* campaign', *Observer*, 1 November, 1.

Bright, M. (1998) 'Dignity on the Ward: my gran didn't suffer in vain', *Observer*, 2 November, 6.

Brindle, D. (1999a) 'Elderly "neglected by NHS"; Ministers told to act on health discrimination', *Guardian*, 8 November, 2.

Brindle, D. (1999b) 'Media coverage of social policy: a journalist's perspective', in Franklin, B. (ed.), *Social Policy, The Media and Media Representation* (London, Routledge).

Bristol Inquiry (2001) *Learning from Bristol: Public Inquiry into Children's Heart Surgery at the Bristol Royal Infirmary 1984–1995*. Chair Professor [now Sir] Ian Kennedy (London, The Stationery Office).

British Heart Foundation (2002) *Statistics Database: CHD Statistics Annual Compendium*, 2002 edition (London, BHF).

Brown, P. (1984) 'Marxism, social psychology, and the sociology of mental health', *International Journal of Health Services*, 14(2), 237–63.

Browne, W.P. (1990) 'Organised interests and their use of niches: a search for pluralism in a policy domain', *Journal of Politics*, 52(2), 477–509.

Bury, M. (1982) 'Chronic illness as a biographical description', *Sociology of Health and Illness*, **4**, 167–82.

Bury, M. and Gabe, J. (1994) 'Television and media coverage: medical dominance or trial by media?' in Gabe, J., Kelleher, D. and Williams, G. (eds), *Challenging Medicine* (London, Routledge).

Busfield, J. (2003) 'Globalization and the pharmaceutical industry revisited', *International Journal of Health Services* **33**(3), 581–605.

Butler, T. (1993) *Changing Mental Health Services* (London, Chapman & Hall).

Buttle, F. and Boldrini, J. (2001) 'Customer relationship management in the pharmaceutical industry: the role of the patient advocacy group', *International Journal of Medical Marketing*, **1**(3), 203–14.

Byrne, P. (1997) *Social Movements in Britain* (London, Routledge).

Cabinet Office (1998) *Service First: The New Charter Programme* (London, Cabinet Office).

Cabinet Office, Performance and Innovation Unit (2002) *Social Capital: A Discussion Paper* (London, Cabinet Office).

Calnan, M., Cant, S. and Gabe, J. (1993) *Going Private: Changing Expectations about Health Care?* (Buckingham, Open University Press).

Campbell, J. and Oliver, M. (1996) *Disability Politics* (London, Routledge).

CancerBACUP (2002) *Funding for Cancer Services: An Independent Audit of Cancer Networks in England* (London, CancerBACUP).

Carlisle, D. (2002) 'For better or for worse?', *Health Service Journal*, 20 June, 40.

Cartwright, L. (1998) 'Community and the public body in breast cancer media activism', *Cultural Studies*, **12**(2), 117–38.

Cawson, A. (ed.) (1985) *Organised Interests and the State: Studies in Meso-corporatism* (London, Sage).

CERT (2002) *Campaign for Effective and Rational Treatment* [www] Available from: http.www.cert-uk.com/pages/about_us.htm (Accessed 24 September 2002).

CESDI (1999) *Confidential Enquiry into Stillbirths and Death in Infancy 6th Annual Report* (London, Confidential Enquiry into Maternal and Child Health).

Chalmers, I., Enkin, M. and Keirse, M. (eds) (1989) *Effective Care in Pregnancy and Childbirth* (Oxford, Oxford University Press).

Chamberlain, G. and Patel, N. (eds) (1994) *The Future of Maternity Services* (London, RCOG Press).

Charities Aid Foundation (2002) *The Charitable Sector in the UK – An Overview* (West Malling, Charities Aid Foundation).

Charity Commission (2001) CC2 – Charities and the Charity Commission (version 10/01) [www] Available from: www.charity-commission.gov.uk (Accessed 30 April 2001).

Charmaz, K. (1983) 'Loss of self: a fundamental form in suffering in the chronically ill', *Sociology of Health and Illness*, **5**, 168–98.

Cigler, A. and Loomis, B. (1995) 'Contemporary interest group politics: more than more of the same', in Cigler, A. and Loomis, B. (eds) *Interest Group Politics* (Washington, DC, Congressional Quarterly Press).

Clarke, K., Gray, D., Keating, N. and Hampton, J. (1994) 'Do women with acute myocardial infarction receive the same treatment as men?' *British Medical Journal*, **309**, 563–6.

Clement-Jones, V. (1985) 'Cancer and beyond: the formation of BACUP' *British Medical Journal*, **291**, 1021–3.

Cm 555 (1989) *Working for Patients* (London, HMSO).

Cm 849 (1989) *Caring for People: Community Care in the Next Decade and Beyond* (London, HMSO).

Cm 1599 (1991) *The Citizen's Charter: Raising the Standard* (London, HMSO).

Cm 1986 (1992) *The Health of the Nation: A Strategy for England* (London, HMSO).

Cm 3807 (1997) *The New NHS: Modern, Dependable* (London, The Stationery Office).

Cm 4100 (1998) *Getting it Right Together: Compact on Relations between Government and the Voluntary and Community Sector in England* (London, HMSO).

Cm 4386 (1999) *Saving Lives: Our Healthier Nation* (London, HMSO).

Cm 4818 (2000) *The NHS Plan: A Plan for Investment, A Plan for Reform* (London, HMSO).

Cm 6079 (2003) *Building on the Best: Choice, Responsiveness and Equity in the NHS* (London, The Stationery Office).

Cmnd 6233 (1975) *Better Services for the Mentally Ill* (London, HMSO).

CNA (2000) *Caring on the Breadline: The Financial Implications of Caring* (London, CNA).

Coburn, D. and Willis, E. (2000) 'The medical profession: knowledge, power and autonomy', in Albrecht, G., Fitzpatrick, R. and Scrimshaw, S. (eds), *The Handbook of Social Studies in Health and Medicine* (London, Sage).

Cohen, J. and Rogers, J. (1995) 'A proposal for reconstructing democratic institutions', in Cohen, J. and Rogers, J. (eds) *Associations and Democracy* (New York, Verso).

Cole, P. (2001) 'Movers and shakers', *Health Service Journal*, 30 August, 23–7.

Colebatch, H.K. (1998) *Policy (Concepts in the Social Sciences Series)* (Buckingham, Open University Press).

Coleman, J.S. (1990) *Foundations of Social Theory* (Cambridge, MA, Harvard University Press).

Coleman, J.S. (1993) 'A rationale choice perspective on economic sociology', in Smelser, N. and Sweberg, R. (eds), *The Handbook of Economic Sociology* (Princeton, NJ, Princeton University Press).

Collier, J. (1989) *The Health Conspiracy* (London, Century).

Commission on the Future of the Voluntary Sector (1996) *Meeting the Challenge of Change. Voluntary Action in the 21st Century. The Report of the Commission on the Future of the Voluntary Sector* (London, NCVO).

Commission for Health Improvement and Audit Commission (2001) *NHS Cancer Care in England and Wales* (London, CHI).

Connolly, M., McKeown, P. and Milligan-Byrne, G. (1994) 'Making the public sector more user friendly? A critical examination of the Citizen's Charter', *Parliamentary Affairs*, 47(1), 23–36.

Consumers' Association (2001a) *Response to High-level Working Group on Innovation and Provision of Medicines Consultation* [www] Available from: http://pharmacos.eudra.org/F3/g10/p7.htm (Accessed 15 May 2003).

Consumers' Association (2001b) *National Institute for Clinical Excellence: A Patient-centred Inquiry* (London, Which?).

Cooper, L., Coote, A., Davies, A. and Jackson, C. (1995) *Voices Off: Tackling the Democratic Deficit in Health* (London, Institute for Public Policy Research).

Cope, R. (1989) 'The compulsory detention of Afro-Caribbeans under the Mental Health Act', *New Community*, 15(3), 343–56.

Coulter, A. (2002) *The Autonomous Patient: Ending Paternalism in Medical Care* (London, The Stationery Office).

Coulthard, M., Walker, A. and Morgan, A. (2002) *People's Perceptions of their Neighbourhood and Community Involvement: Results from the Social Capital Module of the General Household Survey 2000* (London, The Stationery Office).

Covington, G. (2001) From article 'Joining the army' on PMLive.com (www.PMLive.com) (Accessed 15 May 2003).

Crossley, N. (1999) 'Fish, field habitus and madness: the first wave of mental health users movements in Great Britain', *British Journal of Sociology*, 50(4), 647–70.

Dahrendorf, R. (1993) 'Die Zunkunftder Bugergesell schaft', in Guggenberg, B. and Hansen, K. (eds), *Die Mitter Westdeutscher Verlag* (Opladen, Leske & Budrich).

Davies, C. (2001) *Lay Involvement in Professional Regulation: A Study of Public Appointment-holders in the Health Field* (School of Health and Social Welfare, The Open University).

Davies, C. and Beach, A. (2000) *Interpreting Self-regulation: A History of the United Kingdom Central Council for Nursing, Midwifery and Health Visiting* (London, Routledge).

Day, P. and Klein, R. (1997) *Steering not Rowing? The Transformation of the Department of Health: A Case Study* (Bristol, The Policy Press).

Deacon, D. (1999) 'The construction of voluntary sector news', in Franklin, B. (ed.), *Social Policy, the Media and Media Representation* (London, Routledge).

Deakin, N. and Wright, A. (eds) (1990) *Consuming Public Services* (London, Routledge).

Declerq , E. (1998) 'Changing childbirth' in the United Kingdom: lessons for US health policy', *Journal of Health Politics, Policy and Law*, 23(5), 833–59.

Dekker, P. and Broek, A. van den (1998) 'Civil society in comparative perspective: involvement in voluntary associations in North America and Europe', *Voluntas*, 9(1), 11–38.

Dekkers, A.F.M. (1997) 'The experience of the Netherlands: the Dutch Federation of Patient and Consumer Organizations', in Kranich, C.

and Bochen, J. (eds), *Patientenrechte und Patientenunterstützung in Europa* (Baden-Baden, Nomos) (English translation from the author).

Different Strokes (2003) *Introduction* [www] Available from: http://www.differentstrokes.co.uk/intro/htm (Accessed 20 June 2003).

Dillon, J. and Gould, M. (2000) 'Drug firm set up 'patient' groups', *The Independent*, 9 April, 8.

DoH (1991) *The Patient's Charter: Raising the Standard* (London, HMSO).

DoH (1995a) *A Policy Framework for Commissioning Cancer Services: A Report by the Expert Advisory Group on Cancer to the Chief Medical Officers of England and Wales: Guidance for Purchasers and Providers of Cancer Services* (London, DoH).

DoH (1995b) *New Guidelines for Professionals on Pregnancy Loss and the Death of a Baby*, 95/508, 2 November (London, DoH).

DoH (1998a) *Modernising Mental Health Services: Safe, Sound and Supportive* (London, DoH).

DoH (1998b) *Modernising Health and Social Services: National Priorities Guidance for 1999/2000–2001/02* (London, DoH).

DoH (1998c) *Section 64 General Scheme of Grants Application Form and General Notes of Guidance 1999/2000* (London, DoH).

DoH (1999a) *Patient and Public Involvement in the New NHS* (London, DoH).

DoH (1999b) *Clinical Governance: Quality in the New NHS* (London, DoH).

DoH (1999c) *Report of the Expert Committee: Review of the Mental Health Act 1983* (Chair Genevra Richardson) (London, DoH).

DoH (1999d) *National Service Framework for Mental Health: Modern Standards and Service Models* (London, DoH).

DoH (2000a) *The NHS Cancer Plan: A Plan for Investment, A Plan for Reform* (London, DoH).

DoH (2000b) *The Nursing Contribution to Cancer Care: A Strategy Programme of Action in Support of the National Cancer Programme* (London, DoH).

DoH (2000c) *National Service Framework for Coronary Heart Disease* (London, DoH).

DoH (2000d) *National Survey of Patients: Cancer, National Overview 1999/2000* (London, DoH).

DoH (2001a) *The Expert Patient: A New Approach to Disease Management for the 21st Century* (London, DoH).

DoH (2001b) *National Service Framework for Older People* (London, DoH).

DoH (2001c) *Making It Happen: A Guide to Delivering Mental Health Promotion* (Leeds, DoH).

DoH (2002a) *Compact: A Dynamic Mechanism for an Evolving Relationship with the Voluntary and Community Sector* (London, DoH).

DoH (2002b) *Hospital Episode Statistics 2000/01* (London, DoH).

DoH (2002c) *NHS Maternity Statistics England 1998–99 to 2000–01* (London, DoH).

DoH (2002d) *National Suicide Prevention Strategy for England* (London, DoH).

DoH, Welsh Office, Scottish Department of Health Department of Health and Social Services Northern Ireland (1998) *Why Mothers Die. Report on Confidential Enquiries into Maternal Deaths in the UK 1994–1996* (London, The Stationery Office).

Donnison, J. (1988) *Midwives and Medical Men: A History of the Struggle for the Control of Childbirth*, 2nd edition (London, Historical Publications).

Dowding, K. (1995) 'Model or metaphor? A critical review of the policy approach network', *Political Studies*, **43**(1), 136–58.

Doyal, L. (ed.) (1998) *Women and Health Services* (Buckinghamshire, Open University Press).

Doyle, H. (2000) 'Health scares, media hype and policy making', in Hann, A. (ed.), *Analysing Health Policy* (Aldershot, Ashgate).

Dryzek, J. (1987) *Rational Ecology Environmental and Political Economy* (Oxford, Blackwell).

Dubs, A. (1989) *Lobbying: An Insiders Guide* (London, Pluto).

Dunning, M., Needham, G. and Weston, S. (1997) *But Will it Work, Doctor? Report of the Second Conference* (London, King's Fund).

Durham, M. and Bright, M. (1997) 'Join our campaign for the old', *The Observer*, 5 October, 2.

Eaton, L. (2002) 'In search of true asylum', *Health Service Journal*, 20 June, 38–9.

Edwards, C. (2000) 'Accessing the user's perspective', *Health and Social Care in the Community*, **8**(6), 417–24.

Eldridge, J., Kitzinger, J. and Williams, K. (1997) *The Mass Media and Power in Modern Britain* (Oxford, Oxford University Press).

Elston, M. (1991) 'The politics of professional power: medicine in a changing health service', in Gabe, J., Calnan, M. and Bury, M. (eds), *The Sociology of the Health Service* (London, Routledge).

English Nursing Board (2000) *Report of the Board's Midwifery Practice Audit 1999–2000* (London, ENB).

Entwhistle, V. (1995) 'Reporting research in medical journals and newspapers', *British Medical Journal*, **310**, 920–3.

Entwhistle, V. and Sheldon, T. (1999) 'The picture of health media coverage of the health service', in Franklin, B. (ed.), *Social Policy, the Media and Media Representation* (London, Routledge).

Epstein, S. (1996) *Impure Science: Aids, Activism, and the Politics of Knowledge* (Berkley and Los Angeles, CA, University of California Press).

Evers, A. (1995) 'Part of the welfare mix: the third sector as an intermediate area between market economy, state and community', *Voluntas*, **6**(2), 159–82.

Expert Maternity Group (1993) *Changing Childbirth. Part 1: Report of the Expert Maternity Group* (London, HMSO).

Fazackerley, A. and Parker, S. (2001) 'SANE and MIND – a relationship on the mend', *The Guardian*, [www] Available from: http://society.

guardian.co.uk/news/story/0,7838,437604,00.html (Accessed 8 April 2003).

Fogarty, M. (1990) 'Efficiency and democracy in large voluntary organisations', *Policy Studies*, 11(3), 42–8.

Foley, M. and Edwards, B. (1999) 'Is it time to disinvest in social capital?', *Journal of Public Policy*, 19(2), 199–231.

Food Commission (2002) 'Health charities boost food company profits', *Food Magazine*, 57, Apr/Jun, 12–13.

Fox, M.J. (2002) *Lucky Man: A Memoir* (London, Ebury).

Future Foundation (2001) Press Release 17 January (London, Future Foundation).

Gabe, J., Gustafsson, U. and Bury, M. (1991) 'Mediating illness – newspaper coverage of tranquilliser dependence', *Sociology of Health and Illness*, 13, 332–53.

Gander, P. (2000) From article 'Oops! Sorry' on PMLive.com (www.PMLive.com) (Accessed 15 May 2003).

Garcia, J., Redshaw, M., Fitzsimmons, B. and Keene, J. (1998) *First Class Delivery: A National Survey of Women's Views of Maternity Care* (London, Audit Commission/NPEU).

Genetic Interest Group (1999) *Working Together: Annual Report 1998/9* (London, GIG).

Giddens, A. (1990) *The Consequences of Modernity* (Cambridge, Polity Press).

Giddens, A. (1991) *Modernity and Self-Identity* (Cambridge, Polity Press).

Gilchrist, C. (1999) *Turning Your Back on Us: Older People and the NHS* (London, Age Concern, England).

Gilligan, C. (1982) *In a Different Voice: Psychological Theory and Women's Development* (Cambridge, MA, Harvard).

Glaser, B.G. and Strauss, A.L. (1967) *The Discovery of Grounded Theory; Strategies for Qualitative Research* (New York: Aldine de Gruyter).

Gould, M. (2003) 'Unfinished business: cash strapped college closes after 20 years of innovative work', *The Guardian*, Society Pages, 29 October, 4.

Gouldner, D.W. (1979) *The Future of Intellectuals and the Rise of the New Class* (New York, Oxford University Press).

Grant, W. (1995) *Pressure Groups, Politics and Democracy in Britain* (Hemel Hemstead, Harvester).

Grant, W. (2000) *Pressure Groups and British Politics* (Basingstoke, Palgrave Macmillan).

Gray, V. and Lowery, D. (1998) 'To lobby alone or in a flock', *American Politics Quarterly*, 26(1), 5–35.

Greener, I. (2003) 'Performance in the NHS: The insistence of measurement and confusion of content', *Public Performance and Management Review*, 26, 237–50.

Guardian (2000a) 'The 15 most powerful people in health', 14 November, [www] Available from: www.societyguardian.co.uk (Accessed 21 November 2000).

Guardian (2000b) 'Removing the barriers to better care in arthritis', *The Guardian*, 15 November, 7.

Guardian (2001) 'Britain's mean business: wanted: a revolution in corporate giving', *The Guardian*, 6 November, 19.

Gulland, A. (2002) 'Hospitals struggle to cope with stroke care says Royal College', *British Medical Journal*, **325**, 179.

Habermas, J. (1984) *The Theory of Communicative Action*, Volume 1: *Reason and the Ratonalization of Society* (Boston, MA, Beacon Press).

Habermas, J. (1991) *The Theory of Communicative Action*, Volume 1: *Reason and the Ratonalization of Society* (Oxford, Polity).

Ham, C. (2000) *The Politics of NHS Reform 1988–97: Metaphor or Reality?* (London, King' Fund).

Ham, C. and Alberti, K. (2002) 'The medical profession, the public and the government', *British Medical Journal*, **321**, 838–42.

Hanf, K. and Scharpf, F.W (eds) (1978) *Interorganisational Policy Making* (London, Sage).

Hansard (1995a) *House of Commons Official Report: Carers (Recognition and Services) Bill*, **258**, 21 April 1995, Col. 425.

Hansard (1995b) *House of Commons Official Report: Carers (Recognition and Services) Bill*, **258**, 21 April 1995, Col. 461.

Hansard (1999) *House of Commons Official Report: Arthritis*, **341**, 13 December 1999, Cols 124–30.

Hansard (2000) *House of Commons Official Report: Carers and Disabled Children Bill*, **343**, 4 February 2000, Cols 1335–9.

Harrison, S. (1999) 'Clinical autonomy and health policy: past and future', in Exworthy, M. and Halford, S. (eds), *Professionals and the New Managerialism in the Public Sector* (Buckingham, Open University Press).

Harrison, S., Hunter, D.J., Marnoch, G. and Pollit, C. (1992) *Just Managing: Power and Culture: the National Health Service* (London, Macmillan).

Health Advisory Service (1998) *Not Because They Are Old: Independent Inquiry into the Care of Older People in Acute Wards in General Hospitals* (London, HAS).

Health Committee (1992) (HC 29-I) *2nd Report 1991/2: Maternity Services* (London, HMSO).

Health Committee (1995) (HC 324) *3rd Report 1994/5: Breast Cancer Services* (London, HMSO).

Health Committee (1999) (HC 549-I) *6th Report 1999/2000: Procedures Related to Adverse Clinical Incidents and Outcomes in Medical Care* (London, The Stationery Office).

Health Committee (2000) (HC 373) *4th Report 1999/2000: Provision of NHS Mental Health Services* (London, The Stationery Office).

Health Committee (2001a) (HC 301) *3rd Report 2000/01: Head Injury: Rehabilitation* (London, The Stationery Office).

Health Committee (2001b) (HC 308) *4th Report 2000/01: The Provision of Information by the Government Relating to the Safety of Breast Implants* (London, The Stationery Office).

Health Committee (2002) (HC 515-I) *2nd Report 2002/03: National Institute for Clinical Excellence* (London, The Stationery Office).

Health Committee (2003a) (HC 464-I) *4th Report 2002/03: Provision of Maternity Services* (London, The Stationery Office).

Health Committee (2003b) (HC 696) *8th Report 2002/03: Inequalities in Access to Maternity Services* (London, The Stationery Office).

Health Committee (2003c) (HC 796-I) *9th Report 2002/03: Choice in Maternity Services* (London, The Stationery Office).

Heart (2002) 'Provision of services: Fifth report on the provision of services for patients with heart disease', *Heart*, **88** (supplement III), iii1–iii59.

Heinz, J.P. (1993) *The Hollow Core: Private Interests in National Policy Making* (Cambridge, MA, Harvard University Press).

Henderson, L (1999) 'Producing serious soaps', in Philo, G. (ed.), *Message Received: Glasgow Media Group Research 1993–1998* (London, Longman).

Henderson, L. and Kitzinger, J. (1999) 'The human drama of genes: media representations of inherited breast cancer', *Sociology of Health and Illness*, **21**, 560–78.

Henderson, S. and Peterson, A. (eds) (2002) *Consuming Health: The Commodification of Health Care* (London, Routledge).

Herxheimer, A. (2003) 'DIPEx: Fresh insights for medical practice', *Journal of the Royal Society of Medicine*, **96**(5), 209–10.

High Level Group on Innovation and Provision of Medicines (2002) *High Level Group on Innovation and Provision of Medicines: Recommendations for Action. G10 Medicines-Report* (Brussels, European Commission).

Hirschmann, A.O. (1970) *Exit, Voice and Loyalty: Responses to Decline in Firms, Organizations, and States* (Cambridge, MA, Harvard University Press).

Hirst, P. (1994) *Associative Democracy* (Cambridge, Polity Press).

Hirst, P. (2002) 'Renewing democracy through associations', *Political Quarterly*, **73**(4), 409–21.

HM Government (1999) *Caring About Carers: A National Strategy for Carers* (London, The Stationery Office).

HM Treasury, The Public Inquiry Unit (2002) *The Role of the Voluntary and Community Sector in Service Delivery: A Cross-Cutting Review* (London, HM Treasury).

Hogg, C. (1999) *Patients, Power and Politics: From patients to citizens* (London, Sage).

Hogg, C. (2002) *National Service Frameworks: Involving Patients and the Public* (London, Patients Forum).

Hogg, C. and Graham, L. (2001) *Patient and Public Involvement in the NHS: What is Needed at National Level?* (London, Patients Forum).

Hogg, C. and Williamson, C. (2001) 'Whose interests do lay people represent? Towards an understanding of the role of lay people as members of committees', *Health Expectations*, **4**(1), 2–9.

Hojnacki, M. (1997) 'Interest groups' decisions to join alliances or work alone', *American Journal of Political Science*, **41**, 61–87.

Hojnacki, M. (1998) 'Organised interests advocacy behavior in alliances', *Political Research Quarterly*, **51**(2), 437–59.

Home Office (1990) *Efficiency Scrutiny of Government Funding of the Voluntary Sector* (London, Home Office).

Hopkins, J. (2000) 'Celebrity illnesses raise awareness but can give the wrong message', *British Medical Journal*, **321**, 1099.

Hugman, R. (1994) 'Consuming health and welfare', in Keet, R., Whitely, N. and Abercrombie, N. (eds), *The Authority of the Consumer* (London, Routledge).

Hunt, M. (1993) 'Uncuddly charities out in the cold', *Third Sector*, 16 December, 8–9.

Illman, J. (2000) *The Expert Patient* (London, ABPI).

Independent (1997) 'Shopping: NCT resolves row over Sainsbury deal', *The Independent*, 8 December, 9.

Ingram, H. and Schneider, A. (1993) 'The social construction of target populations: implications for politics and policy', *American Political Science Review*, **87**, 334–47.

Intercollegiate Stroke Working Party, Royal College of Physicians (2002) *National Sentinel Audit of Stroke* (London, Royal College of Physicians).

Irvine, D. (2003) *The Doctor's Tale: Professionalism and Public Trust* (Oxford, Radcliffe Medical Press).

Jenkins-Smith, H. and Sabatier, P. (1993) *Policy Change and Learning: An Advocacy Coalition Approach* (Boulder, CO, Westview).

Jennings, M.K. (1999) 'Political responses to pain and loss: Presidential Address 1998 American Political Science Association', *American Political Science Review*, **93**(1), 1–15.

Jensen, T. and Froestad, J. (1988) 'Interest organizations – a complex answer to political poverty', *Tidsskrift for rettssosiologi*, **5**(2), 88–117.

Johnson, M. and Jowell, R. (2001) 'How robust is British civil society?' in Parks, A., Curtice, J., Thomson, K., Jarvis, L and Bromley, C. (eds), *British Social Attitudes, 18th Report: Public Policy, Social Ties* (London, Sage), 175–97.

Johnson, T. (1995) 'Governmentality and the institutionalization of expertise', in Johnson, T., Larkin, G. and Saks, M. (eds) *Health Professions and the State in Europe* (London, Routledge).

Jones, J.B. (1990) 'Party committees and all-party groups', in Rush, M. (ed.), *Parliament and Pressure Politics* (Oxford, Clarendon).

Jones, N. (2002) *The Control Freaks: How New Labour Gets its Own Way* (London, Politico's).

Jones, R. (2000) 'Manifesto for the third millennium', *The Patient's Network*, **5**(3), 23–4.

Jordan, A.G. (1981) 'Iron triangles, woolly corporatism and elastic nets: new images of the policy process', *Journal of Public Policy*, **1**(1), 95–123.

Jordan, A.G. and Richardson, J. (1987) *Government and Pressure Groups in Britain* (Oxford, Clarendon Press).

Judd, D. (2003) 'How the internet changed my life', *Daily Express*, 6 March, 41.

Judge, D. (1992) 'Parliament and interest representation', in Rush, M. (ed.), *Parliament and Pressure Politics* (Oxford, Clarendon).

Karpf, A. (1988) *Doctors in the Media: The Reporting of Health and Medicine* (London, Routledge).

Kay, A. (2001) 'Pharmaceutical policy in the UK', *Public Money and Management*, 21(4), 51–4.

Keane, J. (1991) *The Media and Democracy* (Cambridge, Polity).

Kendall, J. (2000) 'The mainstreaming of the third sector into public policy: voluntary organisations in England in the late 1990s whys and wherefores', *Policy and Politics*, 28(4), 541–62.

Kendall, J. and Knapp, M.R.J. (1999) 'Evaluation and the voluntary (nonprofit) sector: emerging issues' in Lewis, D. (ed.), *International Perspectives in Voluntary Action: Reshaping the Third Sector* (London, Earthscan).

Kendall, J. and Knapp, M. (2000) 'Measuring the performance of voluntary organizations', *Public Management*, 2(1), 106–32.

Kendall, L. (2001) *The Future Patient* (London, IPPR).

Kent, A. (1999) 'Cancer doctors told to become lobbyists', *British Medical Journal*, 319, 874.

Kingdon, J. (1995) *Agendas, Alternatives and Public Policy* (Boston, MA, Little Brown).

Kirkness, B. (1996) *Putting Patients First: The Emerging Role of Patients in the Provision of Health Care* (London, ABPI).

Kitzinger, S. (1987) *Freedom and Choice in Childbirth: Making Pregnancy Decisions and Birth Plans* (Harmondsworth, Penguin).

Klein, R. (1995) *The New Politics of the NHS*, 3rd edition (London, Longman).

Klein, R. (2001) *The New Politics of the NHS*, 4th edition (London, Prentice Hall).

Klein, R. and Lewis, J. (1976) *The Politics of Consumer Representation* (London, Centre for Studies in Social Policy).

Kooiman, J. (ed.) (1993) *Modern Governance: New Government–Society Interactions* (London, Sage).

Kramer, R. (1981) *Voluntary Agencies in the Welfare State* (Berkeley, CA, University of California Press).

Lam, A. (2000) 'Tacit knowledge, organizational learning and societal institutions: an integrated framework', *Organization Studies*, 21(3), 487–513.

Lamb, B. (1997) *The Good Campaigns Guide* (London, NCVO).

Lawton, V. (1999) 'Pharmaceutical from regulations to competition', *Public Money and Management*, 19(4), 4–6.

Lawton-Smith, S. (1999) *Members of Parliament and Mental Health Issues* (London, Mental After Care Association).

Le Grand, J., Mays, N. and Mulligan, J. (1998) *Learning from the NHS Internal Market: A Review of the Evidence* (London, King's Fund).

Lear, J., Lawrence, I., Pohl, J. and Burden, A. (1994) 'Myocardial infarction and thrombolysis: a comparison of Indian and European populations in a coronary care unit', *Journal of the Royal College of Physicians of London*, **28**(2), 143–7.

Levy, L. (1981) 'The National Schizophrenia Fellowship: A British self-help group', *Social Psychiatry*, **16**, 129–35.

Lewin, E. and Olesen, V. (1985) *Women, Health and Healing: Towards a New Perspective* (London, Tavistock).

Lewis, C. (2002) 'Cinderella not yet at the ball', *Health Service Journal*, 20 June, 35–6.

Lewis, J. (1999) 'The voluntary sector and the state in twentieth-century Britain', in Fawcett, H. and Lowe, R. (eds), *Welfare Policy in Britain: The Road from 1945* (Basingstoke, Macmillan).

Lewthwaite, J. and Haffenden, S. (1997) *Patients Influencing Purchasers: A Report of an Action Research Project sponsored by the Long-term Medical Conditions Alliance* (Birmingham, NHS Confederation).

Liu, J., Maniadakis, N., Gray, A. and Rayner, M. (2002) 'The economic burden of CHD in the UK', *Heart*, **88**, 597–603.

Lloyd, J. (2001) The third sector and the fourth estate. The Fourth Hinton Lecture. NCVO Annual General Meeting. [www] Available from: http://www.ncvo-vol.org.uk (Accessed 16 January 2003).

LMCA (1999a) *The Long-term Medical Conditions Alliance: The First Ten Years* (London, LMCA).

LMCA (1999b) *Improving People's Lives: The Agenda for People with Long-term Medical Conditions* (London, LMCA).

LMCA (2000a) *The Long-term Medical Conditions Alliance Annual Review 1999* (London, LMCA).

LMCA (2000b) *Working with the Pharmaceutical Industry Guidelines for Voluntary Health Organisations on Developing a Policy* [www] Available from: http://www.lmca.demon.co.uk/docs/pharmgds.htm (Accessed 15 May 2003).

LMCA (2001a) *Making People's Voices Heard: Enabling People with Long-term Medical Conditions to Contribute to Policy* (London, LMCA).

LMCA (2001b) 'Diary: Party conference meetings', *Connect*, **12**, Autumn, 3.

Long, S. (1999) 'The tyranny of the customer and the cost of consumerism: an analysis using systems and psychoanalytic approach to groups and society', *Human Relations*, **52**(6), 723–43.

Lowi, T. (1969) *The End of Liberalism* (New York, Norton).

Lowndes, V. (2004) 'Getting on or getting by? Women, social capital and political participation', *British Journal of Politics and International Relations*, **6**(1), 47–66.

Luhmann, N. (1979) *Trust and Power* (Chichester, John Wiley).

Lukes, S. (1974) *Power: A Radical View* (London, Macmillan).

Lusignan, S. de (2003) 'The National Health Service on the internet', *Journal of the Royal Society of Medicine*, **96**(10), 490–2.

MacGillivray, A. (2002) *The Glue Factory: Social Capital, Business Innovation and Trust* (London, New Economics Foundation for the Association of Chartered Certified Accountants).

Macpherson, C.B. (1973) *Democratic Theory: Essays in Retrieval* (Oxford, Clarendon).

Maloney, W.A., Jordan, A.G. and McLaughlin, A.M. (1994) 'Interest groups and the policy process: the insider/outsider model revisited', *Journal of Public Policy*, **14**(1), 17–38.

Mansbridge, J. (1992) 'A deliberative theory of interest representation', in Petracca, M. (ed.), *The Politics of Interests: Interest Groups Transformed* (Boulder, CO, Westview).

Marsh, D. and Rhodes, R. (1992) *Policy Networks in British Government* (Oxford, Clarendon).

Martin, G. (2001) 'Social movements welfare and social policy: a critical analysis', *Critical Social Policy*, **21**(3), 361–83.

Maternity Care Working Party (2002) *Modernising Maternity Care – A Commissioning Tool-kit for Primary Care Trusts in England* (London, NCT, RCM, RCOG).

McConnell, G. (1966) *Private Power and American Democracy* (New York, Alfred A. Knopf).

McCurry, P. (2001) 'Just rewards', *The Guardian*, G2, 25 April, 9.

McCurry, P. (2003) 'Cross currents', *The Guardian*, 3 September [www] Available from: www.society.guardian.co.uk/publicmanager/story/0,13002,1034224,00.html (Accessed 10 September 2003).

McNeill, J. (1999) 'Cancerlink: helping people help themselves', *European Journal of Cancer Care*, **8**(1), 12–15.

Medewar, C. (2002) 'Promotion of prescription drugs: trade tactics?', *Consumer Policy Review*, Jan/Feb, 18–30.

Melucci, A. (1995) 'The process of collective identity', in Johnston, H. and Klandermans, B. (eds.), *Social Movements and Culture* (London, University of Minnesota, UCL Press).

Mental Health Foundation (1999) *The Big Picture: Promoting Children's and Young People's Mental Health* (London, MHF).

Michael, A. (1997) *Building the Future Together. Labour's Policies for Partnership between Government and the Voluntary Sector* (London, Labour Party).

Milewa, T., Valentine, J. and Calnan, M. (1998) 'Managerialism and active citizenship in Britain's reformed health service: power and community in an era of decentralisations', *Social Science and Medicine*, **47**(4), 507–17.

Miller, D. (1998) 'Public relations and journalism promotional strategies and media power', in Briggs, A. and Cobley, P. (eds), *The Media: An Introduction* (London, Addison, Wesley and Longman).

MIND (1996) *Fifty Years of Caring: Story of MIND 1946–1996* (London, MIND).

MIND (2002) *Mental Health Statistics Factsheet 5: The Financial Aspects of Mental Health Problems* (London, MIND).

MIND (2003) *Report and Financial Statement for the Year Ended 31 March 2003* (London, MIND).

Moran, M. (1999) *Governing the Health Care State: A Comparative Study of the United Kingdom, United State and Germany* (Manchester, Manchester University Press).

Moran, M. (2002) 'The health professionals in international perspective', in Allsop, J. and Saks, M. (eds), *Regulating the Health Professions* (London, Sage).

Morison, J. (2000) 'The government–voluntary sector compacts: governance, governmentality and civil society', *Journal of Law and Society*, 27, 98–132.

Moynihan, R., Heath, I. and Henry, D. (2002) 'Selling sickness: the pharmaceutical industry and disease mongering', *British Medical Journal*, 324, 886–91.

Murphy, P. (2001) 'Top companies leave charities in cold', *The Guardian*, 5 November, 1.

National Consumer Council (1999) *Models of Self-regulation: An Overview of Models in Business and the Professions* (London, NCC).

National Heart Forum (1998) *Social Inequalities in Heart Disease: Opportunities for Action* (London, NHF).

National Schizophrenia Fellowship (1999a) *Picking Up the Pieces* (London, NSF).

National Schizophrenia Fellowship (1999b) *National Schizophrenia Fellowship: The Voice for Change: Annual Review 1998/9* (London, NSF).

National Schizophrenia Fellowship (2000) *A Question of Choice* (London, NSF).

Nazroo, J.Y. (1997) *The Health of Britain's Ethnic Minorities: Findings from a National Survey* (London, Policy Studies Institute).

NCEPOD (2001) *2001 Report of the National Confidential Enquiry into Perioperative Deaths: Changing the Way We Operate* (London, NCEPOD).

NCVO and Centre for Civil Society (2001) *Next Steps in Voluntary Action: An Analysis of Five Years of Developments in the Voluntary Sector in England, Northern Ireland, Scotland and Wales* (London, NCVO).

Negrine, R (1998) *Politics and the Mass Media in Britain*, 2nd edition (London, Routledge).

Newton, K. (2001) 'The transformation of governance', in Axford, B. and Higgins, R. (eds), *New Media and Politics* (London, Sage).

NHS Management Executive (1992) *Local Voices: The Views of Local People in Purchasing for Health* (London, NHSME).

NHSE (1994) *Priorities and Planning Guidance for the National Health Service 1995/96* (London, NHSE).

NHSE (1995) *Priorities and Planning Guidance for the National Health Service 1996/97* (London, NHSE).

NHSE (1996) *Patient Partnership: Building a Collaborative Strategy* (Leeds, DoH).

NHSE/IHSM/NHS Confederation (1998) *In the Public Interest: Developing a Strategy for Patient Partnership in the NHS* (Leeds, NHSE).

NICE (2000) *Combined Annual Report and Accounts* [www] Available from: http://www.nice.org.uk/article.asp?a=4967 (Accessed on 11 April 2003).

North, N. (1995) 'Alford revisited; the professional monopolisers, corporate rationalisers, community and markets', *Policy and Politics*, 23(2), 115–25.

Norton, P. (1993) *Does Parliament Matter?* (London, Harvester Wheatsheaf).

NRAS (2002) *National Rheumatoid Arthritis Society* [www] Available from: http://www.rheumatoid.org (Accessed 9 July 2003).

Oakley, A. (1986) *The Captured Womb* (Oxford, Blackwell).

OED (1991) *The Oxford English Minidictionary*, 3rd edition (Oxford University Press).

Office of Public Services Reform (2002) *Reforming our Public Services: Principles into Practice* (London, Office of Public Services Reform).

Olson, M. (1965) *The Logic of Collective Action* (Harvard, MA, Harvard University Press).

ONS (2000a) *Living in Britain: Results from the 1998 General Household Survey* (London, The Stationery Office).

ONS (2000b) *Psychiatric Morbidity among Adults Living in Private Households, 2000: Summary Report* (London, ONS).

Osborne, D. and Gabler, T. (1992) *Reinventing Government* (Reading, MA, Addison-Wesley).

Osborne, S. and McLaughlin, K. (2002) 'Trends and issues in the implementation of local voluntary sector compacts in England', *Public Money and Management*, 5, 55–63.

Parker, S. (2002) 'Health charities benefit from worries over NHS', *The Guardian*, 11 October [www] Available from: http://society.guardian.co.uk/Print/0,3858,4521717,00.html (Accessed 13 May 2003).

Passey, A., Hems, L. and Jas, P. (2000) *The UK Voluntary Sector Almanac* (London, NCVO).

Patel, A. and Knapp, M. (1998) 'Costs of mental illness in England', *PSSRU Mental Health Research Review*, 5, 4–10.

Pateman, C. (1970) *Participation and Democratic Theory* (Cambridge, Cambridge University Press).

Paton, C. (1993) 'Devolution and centralism in the National Health Service', *Social Policy and Administration*, 27(2), 83–106.

Peck, E. and Parker, E. (1998) 'Mental health in the NHS: policy and practice 1979–98', *Journal of Mental Health*, 7(3), 241–59.

Pharoah, C. and Welchman, R. (1997) *Keeping Posted: A Survey of Current Approaches to Public Communications in the Voluntary Sector* (London, Charities Aid Foundation).

Phillips, A. (2001) 'The campaigning group born at a bus stop', *The Guardian*, 11 July [www] Available from: http:society.guardian.co.uk/campaigning/story/0,8150,519989,00.html (Accessed 16 January 2003).

Philo, G. (ed.) (1996) *Media and Mental Distress* (London, Longman).

Philo, G. (1999) 'Media and mental illness', in Philo, G. (ed.), *Message Received: Glasgow Media Group Research 1993–1998* (London, Longman).

Plowden, W. (2001) 'England – five years after Deakin', in NCVO and Centre for Civil Society, *Next Steps in Voluntary Action: An Analysis of Five Years of Developments in the Voluntary Sector in England, Northern Ireland, Scotland and Wales* (London, NCVO).

Potter, J. (1988) 'Consumerism in the public sector: how well does the coat fit?', *Public Administration*, 66, 149–64.

Powell, J.A. (2003) 'The doctor, the patient and the world wide web – how the internet is changing healthcare', *Journal of the Royal Society of Medicine*, 90, 74–6.

Prior, L. (2003) 'Belief, knowledge and expertise: the emergence of the lay expert in medical sociology', *Sociology of Health and Illness*, 25 (Silver Anniversary Issue), 41–57.

Putnam, R. (1993) *Making Democracy Work* (Princeton, NJ, Princeton University Press).

Putnam, R. (1995) 'Bowling alone: America's declining social capital', *Journal of Democracy*, 6(1), 65–78.

Putnam, R. (2000) *Bowling Alone: America's Declining Social Capital* (New York, Simon & Schuster).

Quennell, P. (2001) 'Getting their say, or getting their way? Has participation strengthened the patient "voice" in the National Institute for Clinical Excellence?', *Journal of Management in Medicine*, 15(3), 201–19.

Rangnekar, D. and Duckenfield, M. (2002) *Drug development and patient groups and drug development: The Emerging Influence of Patient Groups* (draft), Report for the Patient Groups and Drug Development Seminar, University College London, 16 September 2002. Policy Innovation Group (London, University College London).

Ranney, A. (1983) *Channels of Power: The Impact of Television on American Politics* (New York, Basic Books).

Rayner, M. and Peterson, S. (2000) *European Cardiovascular Disease Statistics 2000 edition* (Oxford, British Heart Foundation Health Promotion Research Group).

RCOG, Royal College of Midwives and National Childbirth Trust (1999) *The Rising Caesarean Rate: A Public Health Issue Conference Report* (London, Profile).

RCOG, Royal College of Midwives and National Childbirth Trust (2000) *The Rising Caesarean Rate – Causes and Effects for Public Health*, Conference Report (London, RCM, RCOG, NCT).

Rethink (2003) *Corporate Partnership* [www] Available from http://www.rethink.org/fundraising/corporate_partnership.html (Accessed May 19 2003).

Revenson, T.A. and Cassell, J.B. (1991) 'An exploration of leadership in a medical mutual help organisation', *American Journal of Psychology*, 19(5), 683–97.

Rhodes, R. (1997) *Understanding Governance* (Buckingham, Open University Press).

Richardson, J. (2000) 'Government, interest groups and policy change', *Political Studies*, **48**, 1006–25.

Richardson, J. and Jordan, A.G. (1979) *Governing Under Pressure* (Oxford, Martin Robertson).

Riddell, P. (1998) *Parliament Under Pressure* (London, Victor Gollancz).

Riker, W. (1962) *The Theory of Political Coalitions* (Harvard, MA, Yale University Press).

Rogers, A. and Pilgrim, D. (1991) 'Pulling down churches: accounting for the British mental health users movement', *Sociology of Health and Illness*, **13**(2), 129–48.

Rogers, A. and Pilgrim, D. (2001) *Mental Health Policy in Britain*, 2nd edition (Basingstoke, Palgrave).

Rootes, C. (1995) 'The new class: the higher education and the new politics', in Maheu, L. (ed.), *Social Movements and Social Classes* (London, Sage).

Rorsman, B., Grasbeck, A., Hagnell, O., Lanke, J., Ohman, R., Ojesjo, L. and Otterbeck, L. (1990) 'A prospective study of first incidence depression', *British Journal of Psychiatry*, **156**, 336–42.

Rowden, R. (2002) From article 'Power to the patient' on PMLive.com (www.PMLive.com) (Accessed 15 May 2003).

Rush, M. (1990) *Parliament and Pressure Politics* (Oxford, Clarendon).

Sabatier, P.A. (1999) 'The need for better theories', in Sabatier, P.A. (ed.), *Theories of the Policy Process* (Boulder, CO, Westview).

Salisbury, R.H. (1987) 'Who works with whom? Interest groups alliances and opposition', *American Political Science Review*, **81**(4), 1217–34.

Salter, B. (1996) 'Medicine and the state: redefining the concordat', *Public Policy and Administration*, **10**(3), 60–87.

Salter, B. (1999) *Medical Regulation and Public Trust: An International Review* (London, King's Fund).

Salter, B. (2003) 'Patients and doctors: reformulating the UK health policy community', *Social Science and Medicine*, **57**(5), 927–36.

Sashidaran, S. and Francis, E. (1993) 'Epidemiology, ethnicity and schizophrenia', in Ahmad, W. (ed.) (1993) *Race and Health in Contemporary Britain* (Buckinghamshire, Open University Press).

Savage, W. (1986) *A Savage Inquiry: Who Controls Childbirth?* (London, Virago).

Saward, M. (1990) 'Co-option and power: who gets what from formal incorporation', *Political Studies*, **38**, 588–602.

Saywell, C., Beattie, L. and Henderson, L. (2000) 'Sexualised illness: the newsworthy body in media representations of breast cancer', in Potts, L. (ed.), *Ideologies of Breast Cancer: Feminist Perspective* (Basingstoke, Palgrave).

Schmitter, P. (1979) 'Still the century of corporatism', in Schmitter, P. and Lehmbruch, G. (eds.), *Trends Towards Corporatist Intermediation* (Beverly Hills, CA, Sage).

Schmitter, P. (2001) 'Participatory governance in a multi-level context', in Grote, J.R. and Gbikpi, B. (eds), *Participatory Governance, Political and Societal Implications* (Opladen, Leske & Budrich).

Science and Technology Committee (2000) (HC 332-I) *6th Report 1999/2000: Cancer Research: A Fresh Look* (London, The Stationery Office).

Science and Technology Committee (2002) (HC 444) *1st Report 2001/2002: Cancer Research: A Follow-up* (London, The Stationery Office).

Shackley, P. and Ryan, M. (1994) 'What is the role of the consumer in health care?', *Journal of Social Policy*, 23(4), 517–41.

Shell, D. (1993) *The House of Lords* (London, Harvester Wheatsheaf).

Shifrin, T. (2003) 'Draft bill signals major overhaul of charity law', *The Guardian* [www] Available from http://society.guardian.co.uk/futureofpublicservices/story/0,8150,1093646,00.html (Accessed 4 February 2004).

Shilts, R. (1987) *And the Band Played On: Politics, People and the AIDS Epidemic* (London, Penguin).

Siddall, R. (2002). 'Heart services set for tougher targets', *Health Service Journal*, 7 March, 8–9.

Silk, S. and Waters, R. (1995) *How Parliament Works*, 3rd edition (London, Longman).

Silver, E. (1999) 'Equity in access to health care and medicines', *The Patients Network*, 4(10), 3–5.

Singleton, N., Meltzer, H. and Gatward, R. (1997) *Psychiatric Morbidity among Prisoners in England and Wales* (London, The Stationery Office).

Small, N. and Rhodes, P. (2000) *Too Ill to Talk? User Involvement and Palliative Care* (London, Routledge).

Smith, M.J. (1993) *Pressure, Power and Policy* (Harlow, Prentice Hall).

Social Exclusion Unit (1998) *Rough Sleeping: Report by the Social Exclusion Unit* (London, Social Exclusion Unit).

Social Services Committee (1983) (HC 209) *1st Report 1983/84: Griffith's Management Inquiry* (London, HMSO).

Stacey, M. (1976) 'The health service consumer: a sociological misconception', in Stacey, M. (ed.), *The Sociology of the National Health Service, Sociological Review Monograph 22* (Keele, University of Keele).

TAB (2002a) *Patient and Public Involvement in Health: Interim Report on the Work of the Transition Advisory Board to the Department of Health* (London, TAB).

TAB (2002b) *Patient and Public Involvement in Health: Key Messages for the Commission for Patient and Public Involvement in Health and the Department of Health. The Final Report of the Transition Advisory Board on Patient and Public Involvement in Health* (London, TAB).

Taylor, M. (1999) 'Between public and private: accountability in voluntary organisations', *Policy and Politics*, 24(1), 57–72.

Taylor, M. and Warburton, D. (2003) 'Legitimacy and the role of UK third sector organisations in the policy process' *Voluntas*, 14(3), 321–37.

Terkildsen, N., Schnell, F.I. and Ling, C. (1998) 'Interest groups, the media and policy debate formation: an analysis of message, structure, rhetoric and source cues', *Political Communication*, 15, 45–61.

Tew, M. (1998) *Safer Childbirth? A Critical History of Maternity Care*, 3rd edition (London, Free Association Books).

Thomas, J. and Paranjothy, S. (2001) *The National Sentinel Caesarean Section Audit Report, Royal College of Obstetricians and Gynaecologists Clinical Effectiveness Support Unit* (London, RCOG).

Thorne, S., Ternulf-Nyhlin, K. and Patterson, B. (2000) 'Attitudes toward patient expertise in chronic illness', *International Journal of Nursing Studies*, 37, 303–11.

Trojan, A. (1989) 'Benefits of self-help groups', *Social Science and Medicine*, 29, 225–32.

Tyler, S. (2002) 'Comparing the campaigning profile of maternity user groups in Europe – can we learn anything useful?', *Health Expectations*, 5(2), 136–47.

UKCC (2000) *Strategy for Public Involvement* (London, UKCC).

UKFSMHA (2000) 'Victim of our own success', *Small Voices*, Spring, 6.

Van der Zeijden, A. (2003) 'Corrections – the International Alliance of Patients' Organisations', *British Medical Journal*, 4 August, [www] Available from: http://bmj.bmjjournals.com/cgi/eletters/326/7400/1208 (Accessed 16 June 2004).

Vincent, J. (2002) *Relations between Central Government and Voluntary Organisations which Provide Health Services in Scotland and England*. PhD thesis, South Bank University, London.

Waine, B. (1992) 'The voluntary sector: the Thatcher years', in Manning, N. and Page, R. (eds), *Social Policy Review 4* (London, Social Policy Association).

Waldegrave, W., Secrett, C., Bazalgette, P., Gaines, A., Parminter, K. (1996) *Pressure Group Politics in Modern Britain*, Occasional Paper (London, Social Market Foundation).

Wallace, H. and Mulcahy, L. (1999) *Cause for Complaints: An Evaluation of the Effectiveness of the NHS Complaints Procedure* (London, The Public Law Project).

Wallace, M. (1985) 'Spectrum: Well freedom is a life sentence', *The Times*, December 16, 10.

Wallace, M. (1985) 'Spectrum: A patients cry – can nobody help', *The Times*, December 18, 8.

Wallace, M. (1985) 'Counting the cost of a daughter's death: the forgotten illness, schizophrenia', *The Times*, December 23, 3.

Walshe, K. (2003) *Regulating Healthcare: A Prescription for Improvement?* (Maidenhead, Open University).

Wanless, D. (2002) *Securing our Future Health: Taking a Long-term View* (London, HM Treasury).

Ware, A. (1989) *Between Profit and State: Intermediate Organisations in Britain and the US* (Cambridge, Polity Press).

Watts, E.J. (1997) 'Cancer self-help groups are underused', *British Medical Journal*, **315**, 812.

Weeks, J., Aggleton, P., Mckevitt, C., Parkinson, K. and Taylor-Laybourn, A. (1996) Community and contracts: tensions and dilemmas in the voluntary sector response to HIV and AIDS, *Policy Studies*, **17**(2), 107–23.

Which? (2002) *Patients Groups* [www] Available from: http://sub.which.net/health/reports/aug2002he4/printreport.html (Accessed 15 May 2003).

Which? (2003) 'Who's injecting the cash?', *Which* (April), 24–5.

Whincup, P., Emberson, J., Lennon, L., Walker, M., Papacosta, O. and Thomson, A. (2002) 'Low prevalence of lipid-lowering drug use in older men with established coronary heart disease', *Heart*, **88**, 25–9.

White, D. (2000) 'Consumer and community participation: a reassessment of process, impact and value', in Albrecht, G., Fitzpatrick, R., Scrimshaw, S. (eds), *The Handbook of Social Studies in Health and Medicine* (London, Sage).

Whitehead, S. (2000) From Article 'Power to the patient' on PMLive (www.PMlive.com) (Accessed 15 May 2003).

Whiteley, P.F. and Winyard, S.J. (1987) *Pressure for the Poor: The Poverty Lobby and Policy-Making* (London, Methuen).

WHO (2001) *World Health Report 2001* (Geneva, WHO).

Williams, G. (1984) 'The genesis of chronic illness', *Sociology of Health and Illness*, **6**, 175–200.

Williams, G. (1989) 'Hope for the humblest? The role of self-help in chronic illness: The case of ankylosing spondylitis', *Sociology of Health and Illness*, **2**, 135–59.

Williamson, C. (1992) *Whose Standards? Consumer and Professional Standards in Health Care* (Buckingham, Open University Press).

Williamson, C. (1998) 'The rise of doctor–patient working groups', *British Medical Journal*, **317**, 1374–7.

Williamson, C. (2000) 'Consumer and professional standards: working towards consensus', *Quality in Health Care*, **9**, 190–4.

Wilson, B., Thornton, J., Hewison, J., Lilford, R., Watt, I., Braunholtz, D. and Robinson, M. (2002) 'The Leeds University Maternity Audit Project', *International Journal of Quality in Health Care*, **14**(3), 175–81.

Wilson, D. (1984) *Pressure: the A-Z of Campaigning in Britain* (London, Heinemann).

Wilson, J. (1996) 'Citizen Major? The rationale and impact of the Citizen's Charter', *Public Policy and Administration*, **11**(1), 45–62.

Wilson, J. (1998) *Working with the Pharmaceutical Industry. Guidelines for Voluntary Health Organizations on Developing a Policy* (London, LMCA).

Wilson, J. (1999) 'Acknowledging the expertise of patients and their organisations', *British Medical Journal*, **319**, 771–4.

Wilson, P. (2001) 'A policy analysis of the expert patient in the United Kingdom: self-care as an expression of pastoral power?', *Health and Social Care in the Community*, **9**(3), 134–42.

Wolfe, C., Rudd, A. and Beech, R. (eds) (1996) *Stroke Services and Research: An Overview with Recommendations for Future Research* (London, Stroke Association).

Wood, B. (2000) *Patient Power? The Politics of Patients' Associations in Britain and America* (Buckingham, Open University Press).

Woolf, A. and Akesson, K. (2001) 'Understanding the burden of musculoskeletal conditions', *British Medical Journal*, **322**, 179–80.

Wright, O. (2003) 'Television death led to 14,000 smear tests', *The Times*, 28 February, 5.

Yalphe, J., Rigge, M., Herxheimer, A., McPherson, A., Miller, R., Shepperd, S. and Ziebland, S. (2000) 'The use of patients' stories by self-help groups: a survey of voluntary organisations in the UK on the register of the College of Health', *Health Expectations*, **3**(3), 176–81.

Youngson, R.M. (1998) *Coping with Rheumatism and Arthritis* (London, Sheldon Press).

Yule, J. (2000) 'Women councillors and committee recruitment', *Local Government Studies*, **26**(3), 31–54.

Index

Active Community Unit, Home
    Office 44–6
Age Concern, England 20, 28, 117,
    175, 212, 234, 250, 252, 257,
    273, 274, 277–9, 289
AIDS/HIV groups 10, 37, 119,
    163, 189
Alford, R. *see* structural interests
alliances 28–31, 33, 47, 80, 81, 135,
    133, 142, 285; benefits 138,
    143, 146–52, 161, 216, 221–2,
    244; costs of collaboration
    150, 155–7, 161; drugs
    industry 193–7; influence in
    policy process 230, 231, 233,
    253–5, 257; informal
    alliances 136, 139–40, 145;
    internal dynamics and
    membership 142, 143, 152–5,
    156–7; joint-working 90, 136,
    138–9, 145, 150, 152, 243–4, 287;
    media 271–2; parliamentary
    alliances 243–4, 251, 257–8;
    policy activity 93, 143, 144,
    149, 216, 221–2, 230, 231,
    253–5; theories 133–4
    (*see also* formal alliance
    organizations)
all-party groups *see* parliament
Alzheimer's Disease Society 28, 39,
    41, 118, 175, 276
Arthritis and Musculoskeletal
    Alliance *see* British League
    Against Rheumatism
arthritis and related conditions: access
    to treatment 51–2, 192, 193;
    drugs industry 193, 194, 195,
    202–3; government 222, 223,
    229; groups 81, 86–7, 92, 93,
    94, 97, 100, 125, 127, 139, 149,
    150, 158, 159, 165, 288; health
    professions 53, 164, 166, 167,
    183; incidence and impact 50;
    joint working 53, 76, 136, 137,
    141, 143, 147, 148–9, 243;
    media 267, 269, 271, 273, 280;

medical research charities 52,
    157, 158; parliament 240, 241,
    242, 245, 251; policies and
    politics 51–3, 159; priority
    status 52, 75, 222, 228, 229
Arthritis Care 30, 39, 51, 83,
    121, 123, 137, 148, 157,
    159, 194, 195, 240, 242,
    269, 271
Arthritis Research Campaign 52,
    157, 158
Association of Community
    Health Councils in England
    and Wales 29, 33, 34, 40
    (*see also* Community Health
    Councils)
Association for Improvements in the
    Maternity Services 68, 85, 138,
    139, 150, 173, 248
Association of the British
    Pharmaceutical Industry *see*
    pharmaceutical industry
Australia *see* Consumers' Health
    Forum, Australia

barriers to participation:
    co-option 13, 14, 181, 191,
    290, 295, 299; consultation
    process 223–5; drugs
    industry 197–8, 203;
    government 34, 35, 47, 126,
    208–9, 212, 223–5, 232, 233,
    234; health professionals 179–81
    (*see also* medical dominance);
    illness 126–7, 217, 289–90;
    priority status 228–9; resources
    35, 98, 102–3, 222, 224,
    225, 294, 295, 296 (*see also*
    resources)
black and minority ethnic groups 27,
    131, 147, 180–1, 217; Afiya
    Trust 84, 92; Cancer Black
    Care 86, 147, 157 (*see also*
    membership, ethnicity)
branches *see* health consumer groups,
    branches